D1710794

HANDBOOK
OF VETERINARY NEUROLOGIC DIAGNOSIS

JOHN E. OLIVER, JR., D.V.M., M.S., Ph. D.

Professor and Head
Department of Small Animal Medicine
College of Veterinary Medicine
University of Georgia
Athens, Georgia

Diplomate,
American College of Veterinary Internal Medicine,
Neurology

MICHAEL D. LORENZ, D.V.M.

Professor and Chief of Staff, Medicine
Department of Small Animal Medicine
College of Veterinary Medicine
University of Georgia
Athens, Georgia

Diplomate,
American College of Veterinary Internal Medicine,
Internal Medicine

W.B. SAUNDERS COMPANY
Philadelphia / London / Toronto / Mexico City / Rio de Janeiro / Sydney / Tokyo

W. B. SAUNDERS COMPANY
Harcourt Brace Jovanovich, Inc.

The Curtis Center
Independence Square West
Philadelphia, PA 19106

Library of Congress Cataloging in Publication Data

Oliver, John E. (John Eoff), 1933–
    Handbook of veterinary neurologic diagnosis.

1. Veterinary neurology—Handbook, manuals, etc.
2. Nervous system—Diseases—Diagnosis—Handbooks,
manuals, etc. I. Lorenz, Michael D. II. Title.
III. Title: Veterinary neurologic diagnosis. [DNLM:
1. Nervous system diseases—Veterinary—Handbooks.
2. Neurologic examination—Veterinary—Handbooks. SF 895
048h]
SF895.044 1983   636.089′680475   82-60567
ISBN 0-7216-6967-0 (pbk.)

Handbook of Veterinary Neurologic Diagnosis   ISBN   0-7216-6967-0

Last digit is the print number: 9   8

DEDICATION

To our families, who gave us the time
To our teachers, who showed us the way
To our colleagues, who kept us honest
And, most of all, to our students, who made it worthwhile

PREFACE

Neurology has been one of the most difficult areas of clinical medicine for students and veterinarians to understand. Traditionally, when neurology was taught, neuroanatomy, neurophysiology, and neuropathology were emphasized. The complexity of the subject overwhelmed the student to the point that nothing made sense.

For the past 8 years we have been assembling a different approach to the teaching of neurology. The approach is based on the following assumptions: neurologic diagnosis is logical, the organization of the nervous system is not as complex as its many parts, the clinical veterinarian does not have to function at the level of the neuroscientist to solve clinical problems, and the basic concepts can be imparted to others. The performance of our students has convinced us that our assumptions are correct. We hope the readers of this book will agree.

John E. Oliver, Jr.
Michael D. Lorenz

CONTENTS

1

CHAPTER

INTRODUCTION

OBJECTIVES AND ORGANIZATION OF THE BOOK

This book is designed to guide the reader through the mechanics and the logic of making a diagnosis when presented with a neurologic problem. A minimal knowledge of anatomy, physiology, and pathology is assumed, but we believe that a detailed understanding of neuroanatomy, neurophysiology, and neuropathology is not needed in order to make a diagnosis adequate for the management of most clinical cases. Using the techniques described in Chapter 3 and the step-by-step logic presented in Chapter 4, the veterinarian should be able to make an anatomic diagnosis without knowing names of tracts or nuclei. The dog is used as the model in this book. Species differences are indicated when appropriate.

The book is organized in two sections. Section I presents the fundamentals necessary for neurologic diagnosis. The objectives of the medical history and some suggestions on history taking pertinent to neurologic problems are presented in Chapter 2. Chapter 3 describes the method of performing a neurologic examination. The anatomic and physiologic bases for each part of the examination are included, but it should be remembered that a diagnosis can be made without a comprehensive understanding of anatomy and physiology. A "cookbook" approach to the localization of lesions in the nervous system is presented in Chapter 4. Using the algorithms and tables provided, the veterinarian can make an anatomic diagnosis. Chapter 5 provides a system for the diagnosis of lesions affecting the autonomic nervous system, especially micturition. Guidelines for the use of ancillary tests, such as radiography, are presented in Chapter 6. The last chapter of Section II provides a foundation for the treatment of diseases of the nervous system.

Section II reviews the most common problems presented in clinical neurology. Starting with "Paresis of One Limb" (Chapter 8) and finishing with "Systemic or Multifocal Signs" (Chapter 17), the section first reviews the anatomic diagnosis and then presents a plan for establishing an etiologic diagnosis. A brief review of major diseases is provided, including suggested diagnostic tests and management of the patient.

This book is not a comprehensive review of neurology. It is intended to provide the tools and the logic necessary to make a neurologic diagnosis. For more information on the anatomy and physiology of the nervous sytem, the books by Jenkins, deLahunta, and Swenson are recommended.[1-3] *Comparative Neuropathology* by Innes and Saunders is the only comprehensive treatise on the neuropathology of animals.[4] Standard veterinary pathology texts are more readily available.[5,6] Brief descriptions of pathologic lesions seen in diseases of the central nervous system (CNS) also are presented in books by Hoerlein and McGrath.[7,8] Palmer reviews the fundamental pathologic changes of nervous tissue.[9] The primary reference for diseases of the nervous system and their treatment is *Canine Neurology* by B. F. Hoerlein.[7] It is the only comprehensive source for diagnostic and therapeutic techniques. References in these chapters are limited to textbooks, review articles, or primary reports that are likely to be available to the veterinarian.

PATHOLOGIC REACTIONS OF THE NERVOUS SYSTEM

Distribution of Pathologic Lesions

FOCAL LESIONS

Many clinical syndromes are characterized by a single, focal lesion of the nervous system. Common examples include tumors, abscesses, hemorrhages, infarctions, spinal or cranial fractures, and herniated intervertebral disks. The first step in neurologic diagnosis is localization of the lesion. The first assumption is that the clinical signs will be explained by a single lesion. Only when the results of the examination demonstrate signs that can be caused only by multifocal or diffuse disease is this assumption discarded.

MULTIFOCAL LESIONS

Some disease processes affect several sites in the nervous system simultaneously. Inflammatory diseases are the most frequent cause of multifocal signs, although metastatic neoplasms or degenerative diseases also may have multifocal signs.

DIFFUSE LESIONS

Infectious diseases that are disseminated by the vascular system frequently have a diffuse distribution. Differentiation of diffuse and multifocal problems may be difficult clinically. A disease affecting most parts of the nervous system may be more severe in certain regions and may present a picture of focal or multifocal disease in the early stages. For example, the distemper virus may cause a brain stem syndrome in the early stages and only later in its course produce signs of cerebral or spinal cord disease.

Morphology of Pathologic Lesions

MASS LESIONS

Many pathologic changes alter cellular function directly and also affect surrounding elements by compression. Examples include tumors, abscesses, herniated intervertebral disks, spinal fractures and luxations, and hematomas. Mass lesions are of clinical importance because surgical removal of the compression is often the treatment of choice.

NONMASS LESIONS

Pathologic changes that do not compress surrounding structures are characteristic of degenerative, metabolic, inflammatory (except abscesses), and toxic diseases. Most of these diseases require medical treatment or are not treatable.

Cellular Pathology

A brief review of histopathologic changes of the CNS will be presented. Pathology texts should be consulted for a more comprehensive discussion.[4-6,10]

LESIONS OF NEURONS

Neurons are the primary functional units of the nervous system. Mature neurons do not proliferate. As a result, diseases often cause a depletion of the neuronal pool.

Neuronal Necrosis. Most pathologic processes ultimately lead to neuronal necrosis. Depending on the cause and the stage of the disease, histopathologic findings may include one or more of the following:

Nerve cell loss, or depopulation, may be recognized when the number of neurons in an area is reduced. It is estimated that at least 30 per cent of the cells must be lost in most areas in order to be recognized.[10] The loss of some cells, for example, Purkinje cells of the cerebellum, may be easier to recognize. *Neuronophagia* is the process of phagocytosis of the neuron and is characterized by a group of macrophages surrounding a degenerating neuron. *Ischemic nerve cell change* results from anoxia of the neuron and is recognized as a shrunken, eosinophilic cell with loss of the Nissl bodies and a pyknotic nucleus.

Chromatolysis. Chromatoloysis of neurons is seen most commonly following injury to the axon. The neuron is swollen. Nissl substance is present at the periphery of the cell, and the nucleus is located eccentrically. Chromatolysis reflects the process of increased activity of the cell for regeneration of the axon. Chromatolytic neurons may recover or subsequently may necrose, depending on the pathologic process.

Abnormal Intraneuronal Material. *Lipofuscin pigment* accumulates in neurons with aging and apparently has no special pathologic significance.

Inclusion bodies, both intranuclear and intracytoplasmic, are most commonly associated with viral diseases. Rabies virus inclusions are intracytoplasmic, whereas distemper virus may be intracytoplasmic or intranuclear.[11] The Lafora body is a mucopolysaccharide intracytoplasmic inclusion body found in human beings and beagle dogs with a form of epilepsy. It also has been found in older dogs with no neurologic deficits. Its significance is not known.

Storage diseases are characterized by intraneuronal accumulations of metabolic products (usually lipids) caused by a deficiency of an enzyme. Neurons are distended with the material and ultimately undergo necrosis. See Chapter 17 for a description of the storage diseases.

LESIONS OF AXONS

Wallerian Degeneration. Severance of an axon or destruction of its neuronal cell body results in degeneration of the axon distally because of the loss of axoplasmic flow from the cell body (Fig. 1–1). The myelin sheath and the motor end plate also disintegrate. The degeneration also occurs proximally for a few milli-

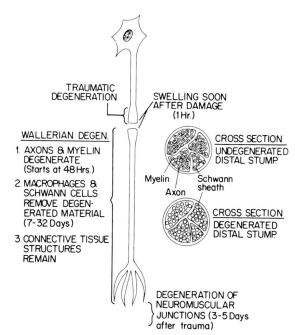

TRAUMATIC DEGENERATION

SWELLING SOON AFTER DAMAGE (1 Hr.)

WALLERIAN DEGEN.

1. AXONS & MYELIN DEGENERATE (Starts at 48 Hrs.)

2. MACROPHAGES & SCHWANN CELLS REMOVE DEGEN- ERATED MATERIAL (7-32 Days)

3. CONNECTIVE TISSUE STRUCTURES REMAIN

CROSS SECTION UNDEGENERATED DISTAL STUMP.

Myelin
Axon
Schwann sheath

CROSS SECTION DEGENERATED DISTAL STUMP.

DEGENERATION OF NEUROMUSCULAR JUNCTIONS (3-5 Days after trauma)

Figure 1–1. Process of nerve degeneration (Wallerian). (From Hoerlein, B. F.: Canine Neurology: Diagnosis and Treatment, 3rd ed. Philadelphia, W. B. Saunders Co., 1978. Used by permission.)

meters, and the cell body becomes chromatolytic. The axon sends out a number of processes, called axonal buds. If the axonal buds can find the nerve sheath, regeneration may occur. The rate of growth is approximately 1 to 3 mm per day, or 1 inch per month. If the axons are blocked by scar tissue, they may continue to grow, forming a swelling called a neuroma.

LESIONS OF SCHWANN CELLS

Peripheral Demyelination. Schwann cells form the myelin covering of peripheral nerves. These cells may be affected selectively in some disease processes, especially polyradiculoneuritis (coon-hound paralysis). Although axon lesions also occur, the predominant finding is a loss of individual Schwann cells, producing segmental demyelination (see Fig. 1–1).

LESIONS OF OLIGODENDROGLIA

Oligodendroglia form the myelin sheaths of axons in the central nervous system. Pathologic changes in oligodendroglia are seen primarily as alterations in myelin.

Central Demyelination. Demyelination is recognized by the loss of staining properties of the myelin sheath. Destruction of myelin

occurs in many pathologic processes, including canine distemper. Leukodystrophies are caused by enzymatic deficiences and are of genetic origin. Globoid cell leukodystrophy is the best example of a leukodystrophy in animals.

Other Lesions of Oligodendroglia. Satellitosis, the clustering of oligodendroglia around neurons, probably has no pathologic significance. Inclusions and storage materials also may be found in oligodendroglia.

LESIONS OF ASTROCYTES

Astrocytes form the bulk of the supporting structure of the central nervous system. They are intimately related to the walls of capillaries and to nonsynaptic portions of neurons. The extracellular space of gray matter is very small; hence, it is assumed that astrocytes are of major importance in the metabolic processes of the neuron. Astrocytes are also highly reactive to disease.

Gliosis. Many disease processes will cause hypertrophy and hyperplasia of astrocytes. Hypertrophy of the cell bodies is called protoplasmic gliosis.

Other Lesions of Astrocytes. Astrocytes may have viral inclusions (canine distemper) or storage material or may undergo necrosis.

LESIONS OF MICROGLIA

Microglia generally are considered to be fixed tissue phagocytes of mesodermal origin. They react to injury to the nervous system by proliferation and assume the role of phagocytes. Recently, it has been proposed that microglia are reserve cells of astroglia. All of the macrophages and other cells seen in inflammation are derived from circulating leukocytes according to this theory.[12]

Neuronophagia. Microglia are at least a part of the population of phagocytes surrounding necrotic neurons. After the neuron is gone, the clumps of cells are called microglial nodules.

Tissue Pathology

NERVOUS TISSUE

Edema. Edema of nervous tissue may occur as a result of a variety of factors. Trauma, hypoxia, hypercarbia, ischemia, venous stasis, toxins, heat, and cold are just a few of the causes. Edema of white matter is primarily extracellular and may lead to demyelination. Edema of gray matter is primarily intracellular and may lead to glial and neuronal death. The brain and the spinal cord are enclosed in rigid compartments; therefore, any swelling of the nervous tissue causes pressure changes as well. Swelling of the cerebrum may cause herniation of the cortex under the tentorium cerebelli, which results in compression of the midbrain. Herniation of the cerebellum through the foramen magnum compresses the medulla oblongata and leads to death of the animal. (See Chapter 14 for a more complete discussion.)

Histologically, edema causes pallor of the white matter, a loose appearance of the gray matter, swollen glial cells, and dilatation of perivascular and pericellular spaces.

Necrosis. Destruction of neural tissue may be caused by a variety of disease processes. The normal architecture is lost and is often associated with edema. Malacia is an area of necrosis of most cellular elements. Gliosis and macrophages are present, especially around the periphery of the lesion. Laminar necrosis (death of nerve cells in some layers of the cerebral cortex) frequently is found following hypoxia.

Hemorrhage. Intraparenchymal hemorrhage is seen most commonly following traumatic injury. Diseases affecting the blood vessels also may cause hemorrhage.

Inflammation. Infiltrates of cells around the vessels are the most characteristic lesions in CNS inflammation. These perivascular cuffs are usually mononuclear (lymphocytes, plasma cells, histiocytes) in viral diseases and polymorphonuclear in bacterial diseases, although mononuclear cells may be seen in chronic bacterial diseases. Perivascular cuffing, however, is not necessarily indicative of an infectious etiology.

Demyelination. Demyelination is defined as a loss of the normal staining properties of the myelin sheath. The distribution of demyelination may be significant in establishing an etiologic diagnosis.

Neoplasia. Primary nerve cell tumors, medulloblastomas, and ganglioneuromas are rare. Gliomas, including astrocytomas, glioblastomas, and oligodendrogliomas, are more common in brachycephalic dogs. Ependymomas and choroid plexus papillomas are relatively uncommon and have no breed predilection. Tumors of supporting structures, such as neurofibromas and meningiomas, are seen more frequently. Metastatic tumors and bone tumors involving the skull or the spinal column may be identified because of the signs of nervous system dysfunction. Neoplasms may produce local destruction of neural elements and may affect surrounding structures by compression or by interference with the vascular system (see Chapter 17).

Ventricular Dilatation. Enlargement of the ventricular system may be caused by atrophy of the cerebrum or may be secondary to obstruction of cerebrospinal fluid circulation (hydrocephalus, see Chapter 14) (Fig. 1–2). Atrophy is characterized by widening of the sulci and the fissures of the cortex with narrowing of the gyri. A mild degree of atrophy is seen in older animals.

MENINGES

There are three layers of connective tissue coverings of the nervous system (see Fig. 1–2). The pia mater is in intimate contact with the nervous tissue and follows the convolutions into the sulci and the fissures. The arachnoid mater is a thin, delicate membrane with small filamentous attachments to the pia mater. The space between the pia mater and the arachnoid mater contains cerebrospinal fluid (CSF). The pia and the arachnoid collectively are called the leptomeninges. The dura mater is a thick, tough layer of connective tissue. The space between the dura mater and the arachnoid mater, the subdural space, is normally only a potential space.

Inflammation. Inflammatory changes in the meninges are typical of inflammation in any connective tissue. Cellular infiltrates may be mononuclear or polymorphonuclear, depending on the etiologic agent. The leptomeninges usually are involved in any inflammatory process affecting the brain or the spinal cord. Infiltrates in the leptomeninges will be reflected in changes in the CSF, which can be sampled as an aid to diagnosis.

Meningeal inflammation may lead to adhesions and fibrosis, interfering with circulation and absorption of CSF with subsequent development of hydrocephalus.

Hemorrhage. Hemorrhage may be extradural, subdural, or subarachnoid. Extradural hemorrhage in the cranial vault usually is caused by skull fractures that lacerate the middle meningeal artery. Hematoma formation is rapid. Subdural hemorrhage usually is caused by laceration of some of the veins that cross from the bony calvarium to the surface of the brain. Hematoma formation may be slow. Subarachnoid hemorrhage may be either ar-

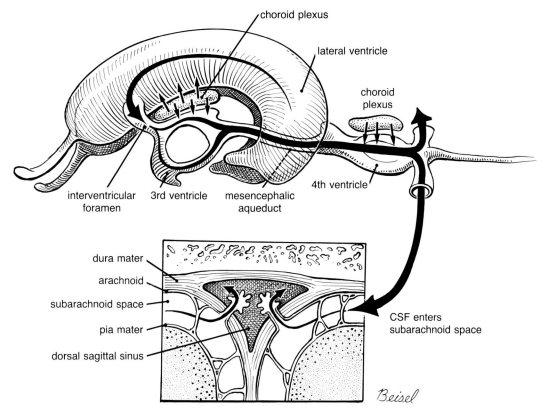

Figure 1–2. Cerebrospinal fluid (CSF) circulates from the lateral ventricles through the interventricular foramina to the third ventricle. It continues through the mesencephalic aqueduct to the fourth ventricle and through the lateral apertures to the subarachnoid space. Absorption occurs primarily through the arachnoid villi in the venous sinuses. The inset illustrates the relationship of the meninges to the brain and the venous sinuses.

terial or venous in origin. It differs from extradural or subdural hemorrhage in that it rarely forms a mass. The blood tends to flow in the CSF pathway. Blood in the CSF acts as a foreign protein, eliciting an inflammatory response, an aseptic meningitis.

Neoplasia. Meningiomas are generally benign tumors that are seen most frequently in cats and in mesaticephalic or dolichocephalic dogs.

CLASSIFICATION OF DISEASES OF THE NERVOUS SYSTEM

The most logical way to approach a diagnosis is to establish relative probabilities for broad categories of disease and then to progress to narrower groups until the process has been identified in a manner that is as finite as possible. The specificity of the diagnosis may depend on a variety of factors, including available knowledge, economics, safety of the patient, available diagnostic tools, and so on.

For example, a metabolic storage disease such as gangliosidosis may be diagnosed definitively only by histologic examination of nervous tissue. Biopsy of the brain can be performed but is not often allowed or recommended. The history of a chronic progressive diffuse encephalopathy in a young animal may be sufficient evidence for a decision.

A convenient scheme for the classification of diseases into broad categories is presented in Table 1–1. The acronym *DAMNIT* was first suggested by Dr. Carl Osborne (personal communication) and is useful for a quick review

Table 1–1. ETIOLOGIC CLASSIFICATION OF DISEASES

D	Degenerative, Demyelinating
A	Allergic, Anomalous
M	Metabolic
N	Neoplastic, Nutritional
I	Inflammatory, Infectious
T	Traumatic, Toxic

of the major categories of disease. This scheme, with minor modifications, will be used throughout this book. Some of the identifying characteristics of each of these categories will be discussed in the next chapter.

REFERENCES

1. Jenkins, T. W.: Functional Mammalian Neuroanatomy, 2nd ed. Philadelphia, Lea & Febiger, 1978.
2. deLahunta, A.: Veterinary Neuroanatomy and Clinical Neurology. Philadelphia, W. B. Saunders Co., 1977.
3. Swenson, M. J.: Duke's Physiology of Domestic Animals, 9th ed. Ithaca, Cornell University Press, 1977.
4. Innes, J. R. M., and Saunders, L. Z.: Comparative Neuropathology. New York, Academic Press, 1962.
5. Jubb, K. V. F., and Kennedy, P. C.: Pathology in Domestic Animals. New York, Academic Press, 1970.
6. Smith, H. A., Jones, T. C., and Hunt, R. D.: Veterinary Pathology. Philadelphia, Lea & Febiger, 1972.
7. Hoerlein, B. F.: Canine Neurology, 3rd ed. Philadelphia, W. B. Saunders, Co., 1978.
8. McGrath, J. T.: Neurologic Examination of the Dog with Clinicopathologic Observations, 2nd ed. Philadelphia, Lea & Febiger, 1960.
9. Palmer, A. C.: Introduction to Animal Neurology, 2nd ed. Oxford, Blackwell Scientific Pub., 1976.
10. Escourolle, R., and Poirier, J.: Manual of Basic Neuropathology, 2nd ed. Philadelphia, W. B. Saunders Co., 1978.
11. Braund, K. G.: Encephalitis and meningitis. Vet. Clin. North Am. 10:31–56, 1980.
12. Kitamura, T.: Dynamic aspects of glial reactions in altered brains. Pathol. Res. Pract. 168:301–343, 1980.

I
SECTION

FUNDAMENTALS

INTRODUCTION

The objectives for the management of a patient with a problem that possibly is related to the nervous system are (1) to determine that the problem is caused by a lesion in the nervous system, (2) to localize the lesion in the nervous system, (3) to estimate the extent of the lesion in the nervous system, (4) to determine the cause or the pathologic process, or both, and (5) to estimate the prognosis with no treatment or with various alternative methods of treatment.

Physical and neurologic examinations establish the presence, the location, and the severity of a nervous system abnormality. This information is vital for formulating a prognosis.

The clinical history yields information that suggests the kind of disease process. The course of the disease also may be an important factor for formulating a prognosis.

TAKING THE HISTORY

Traditionally, the history has been taken by the veterinarian. Paraprofessional personnel were not expected to obtain information other than the signalment (species, breed, age, sex, and so forth). The development of the concept of a *defined data base* in conjunction with a problem-oriented medical record system has provided the impetus for changes.[1] If one establishes a minimum base of necessary information about every patient, or about every patient with a certain problem, then one can obtain that information in a number of ways.

Owner's History

A basic history can be obtained by use of a well-designed questionnaire. The receptionist gives the questionnaire to the client, who completes it in the reception area. A paraprofessional (veterinary technician, nurse) can assist the client in answering difficult questions. The general medical history is available for review by the veterinarian, who notes significant items that may need further clarification (Fig. 2–1). Problem-specific owner histories can be used to supplement the general history.

Role of the Veterinarian

The most important parts of the history should be reviewed with the client by the veterinarian. Misinterpretation of terminol-

2

CHAPTER

NEUROLOGIC HISTORY

Etiology and Prognosis

ogy, of a course of events, or of clinical signs occurs frequently. The veterinarian may need to rephrase questions several times before receiving a meaningful answer.

The manner in which a question is phrased is important. Questions that are felt to imply negligence or ignorance on the part of the client may lead to defensive answers. Questions that suggest a correct answer may lead the client to interpret events incorrectly. All questions should be asked so that the answer "I don't know" is an acceptable alternative; otherwise, the client may hypothesize rather than relate facts.[2]

Neurologic History

SIGNALMENT

The species, breed, age, and sex of the patient provide important clues to the diagnosis. Although there are very few diagnoses that can be positively ruled in or out on the basis of the signalment, many diseases are more or less likely to occur among certain groups of animals.

The incidence of some diseases varies greatly among species and breeds. Many infectious diseases are species-specific, such as canine distemper, feline infectious peritonitis, and scrapie of sheep. Known inherited diseases must be considered, especially in cases involving young animals. Table 2–1 lists many of the diseases with a species or breed predilection. Infectious diseases are listed in Chapter 17.

Figure 2–1. Owner's history.

OWNER'S HISTORY

Directions: To aid the veterinarian in reaching an accurate diagnosis, it is essential for you to provide complete background information about your pet. Please fill out the following questionnaire. Circle "yes" or "no" as appropriate. Answer each question to the best of your ability. If you do not understand a question or have doubts about your answer, leave the question blank or put a question mark(?). The veterinarian will go over the questionnaire with you.

I. Reason for visit (check one)
_____A. Vaccination
_____B. Regular checkup
_____C. Medical or surgical problem

II. Has your pet received the following immunizations?   *Approximate Date*
yes   no A. Serum (puppy shots)   _____
yes   no B. Dog distemper hepatitis vaccination   _____
yes   no C. Rabies vaccination   _____
yes   no D. Cat enteritis (distemper) vaccination   _____
         E. Other (specify) _____

III. Previous illnesses or injuries
        A. Illnesses
yes   no 1. Has your pet ever been sick before the present illness? If yes, list dates and abnormalities
            observed. _____
            _____
            _____
            _____

yes   no 2. Does your pet have allergic reactions to drugs or any allergies? Provide details (name of drug,
            nature of allergy) if possible. _____
            _____

        B. Surgery
        1. Has your pet been spayed or castrated?   _____
        2. Has your pet been declawed?   _____
        3. List dates and other kinds of surgery. _____
            _____
            _____

IV. Environment
        A. Where did you obtain your pet? (check one)
_____1. Raised from own bitch.
_____2. From a breeder.
_____3. From a pet store.
_____4. From a friend.
_____5. The animal was a stray.
_____6. From the Humane Society.
        B. How old is your pet?   _____
        C. How long have you owned your pet?   _____
yes   no D. Does your pet live in your house?
        E. Where do you live? (check one)
_____   Urban area
_____   Rural area
_____   Suburban area
_____   Apartment
        F. How frequently does your pet go outside? (times per day)   _____
yes   no G. Does your pet roam from your property?
        H. What other pets do you have in your home?_____
            _____

Illustration continued on opposite page

I. With what other animals does your pet come in contact? _____
_____

yes no J. Has your pet traveled out of state? _____
When/Where? _____
_____

V. Diet

A. What do you feed your pet? (check one)
_____1. Table leftovers
_____2. Canned food
    a. What brand? _____
_____3. Commercial dry food
    a. What brand? _____
_____4. Semidry food
    a. What brand? _____
yes no B. Does your pet have access to other sources of food?
C. How many times per day is your pet fed? _____
D. How many of the following is your pet being fed?
    1. Packets _____
    2. Cans _____
    3. Cups _____
yes no E. Are you feeding your pet any supplements?
    1. How often? _____
    2. What type? _____
yes no F. Do you give your pet treats?
    1. How often? _____
yes no G. Does your pet have constant access to water?
    1. Source of water _____
yes no   2. Have you noticed a change in the amount your pet drinks?
    _____ a. Increase Amount: _____
    _____ b. Decrease Amount: _____
yes no H. Has your pet gained or lost weight recently?
    1. Would you describe your pet's appetite as:
        _____ 1. Normal?
        _____ 2. Ravenous?
        _____ 3. Selective?
        _____ 4. Absent?

VI. Urination

yes no A. Do you see your pet urinate?
If yes, have you observed any of the following?
    1. Change in frequency of urination
    _____ a. Increased
    _____ b. Decreased
    _____ c. Urinating at night
yes no   2. Straining to urinate
yes no   3. Change in volume of urine
    _____ a. Increased
    _____ b. Decreased
yes no B. Do you see the urine from your pet?
If yes, have you observed any of the following?
yes no   1. Change in color
yes no   2. Presence of blood
yes no   3. Change in odor

VII. Defecation (bowel movements)

yes no A. Do you observe your pet's bowel movements?
B. How many times per day does your pet defecate? _____
yes no C. Have you noticed any change in your pet's stool?
yes no   1. Straining
yes no   2. Blood in the stool
yes no   3. Change in the consistency of stool
    _____ a. Fluid

Illustration continued on following page

_____ b. Soft
_____ c. Hard
yes no 4. Change in odor
yes no 5. Presence of mucus
yes no 6. Change in amount
_____ a. Increase
_____ b. Decrease

VIII. Have you noted any discharges from: (if yes, please describe)
yes no A. Nose?   _____
yes no B. Mouth?   _____
yes no C. Vagina?   _____
yes no D. Anus?   _____
yes no E. Mammary glands?   _____
yes no F. Eyes?   _____
yes no G. Ears?   _____
yes no H. Other sites?   _____

IX. Signs:
yes no A. Has your pet been exhibiting any abnormal behaviors?
            If yes, please describe. _____
            _____

      B. How would you describe your pet?
            _____ 1. Very active
            _____ 2. Active
            _____ 3. Moderately active
            _____ 4. Depressed
      C. How would you describe your pet's endurance?
            _____ 1. Good
            _____ 2. Moderate
            _____ 3. Poor
yes no D. Is your pet exhibiting abnormal signs not already covered?
            If yes, please describe. _____
            _____

      1. How long has your pet been showing these signs? (hours, days,
         weeks, months, years)   _____
      2. Have the signs been constant or intermittent?
      3. Have they gotten worse or stayed the same?   _____
yes no 4. Have you had your pet treated by a veterinarian?
yes no 5. Has any medication been given or procedures performed for these signs?
yes no 6. Was there an improvement with the medication or procedure?
      E. Has your pet shown any of the following signs?
yes no 1. Sneezing
yes no 2. Coughing
            a. Please describe the frequency.   _____
            b. Is the coughing productive?   _____
yes no 3. Vomiting
            a. What is the relationship to meals?   _____
            b. Describe its color.   _____

Figure 2–1 _Continued_

Young animals are more likely to have congenital and inherited disorders and infectious diseases. Older animals are likely to have degenerative and neoplastic diseases.

Although these criteria are not absolute, the probability is much greater that an 8-year-old brachycephalic dog will have a neoplasm of the central nervous system (CNS) rather than a congenital anomaly. In the preliminary (and sometimes in the final) assessment, a diagnosis is an ordering of probabilities.

SIGN-TIME GRAPH

Construction of a sign-time graph is useful for evaluating the course of a disease (Fig. 2–2). The sign-time graph plots the severity of clinical signs (on the vertical axis) against time (on the horizontal axis). A complete history will

Table 2–1. DISEASES WITH A SPECIES OR BREED PREDISPOSITION

Disease	Breed	Disease	Breed
Neural Tube Anomalies		Neuronal abiotrophy†·‡	Swedish Lapland dog
Myelodysplasia (spina bifida, meningocele, myelomeningocele, myeloschisis)*·‡	Manx cat, English bulldog, Boston terrier, Rhodesian ridgeback	Stockard's paralysis†·‡	Great Dane–bloodhound crossbreed, Great Dane–Saint Bernard crossbreed
Hemivertebra, incomplete segmentation*·‡	Brachycephalic dogs	Neurofilament accumulation†·‡	Domestic cat, collie
Spinal dysraphism*·‡	Weimaraner	Wallerian degeneration—brain and spinal cord†·‡	Jack Russell terrier
Vertebral and Disk Abnormalities		Cerebellar cortical atrophy†·‡	Gordon setter
Atlantoaxial luxation*·§	Toy breeds	Cerebellar degenerations†·‡	Airedale, Finnish harrier, Bern running dog, beagle, Samoyed, cattle
Cervical malformation—malarticulation*·§	Great Dane, Doberman pinscher		
Lumbosacral malformation—malarticulation*·§	German shepherd	Cerebellum, Purkinje cell diseases†·‡	Aberdeen Angus, Holstein, Charolais cattle
Spondylosis*·§	Large breeds	Hereditary ataxia, spinocerebellar tracts†·‡	Smooth-haired fox terrier
Intervertebral disk disease*·§	Chondrodystrophic dogs (dachshund, Pekingese, beagle)	Hereditary ataxia†·‡	Jack Russell terrier
		Neuronal dystrophy†·‡	Domestic cat
Neuronal Storage Diseases		Quadriplegia and amblyopia†·‡	Irish setters
Gangliosidosis GM₁†·‡	Korat, Siamese, and domestic cats, beagle, Friesian cattle	Giant axonal neuropathy†,§	German shepherd
		Demyelinating Diseases	
Gangliosidosis GM₂ (Tay-Sachs disease)†·‡	German short-haired pointer	Globoid cell leukodystrophy†·‡	Cairn and West Highland white terriers, domestic cat, beagle, poodle, blue tick hound, mixed-breed dogs, polled Dorset sheep
Gangliosidosis GM₂ (Sandhoff's disease)†·‡	Domestic cat		
Gangliosidosis GM₂, juvenile Type 3†·‡	Yorkshire swine		
Sphingomyelin lipidosis (Niemann-Pick disease)†·‡	Siamese and domestic cats, poodle		
Glycogenosis (Pompe's disease)†·‡	Domestic cat, Lapland dog, sheep, Brahman cattle	Metachromatic leukodystrophy†	Domestic cat
		Dysmyelination†·§	Chow chow
Glycoproteinosis (Lafora's disease)†·‡	Beagle, basset hound, poodle	Demyelination†·§	Miniature poodle
		Miscellaneous Neural Abnormalities	
Ceroid lipofuscinosis†·‡	English setter, Siamese cat, dachshund, Chihuahua, spaniel, cattle, South Hampshire sheep, border collie, Welsh corgi	Degenerative myelopathy or radiculomyelopathy*·§	German shepherd
		Myelopathy (myelinolytic)†·§	Afghan hound
		Lissencephaly†	Lhasa apso
		Hydrocephalus*·§	Toy breeds
		Cerebellar hypoplasia*	Cats (panleukopenia)
Glucocerebroside storage disease (Gaucher's disease)†·‡	Sidney silky dog	Deafness, congenital*·‡	White-coated, blue-eyed cats, Dalmatian, bull terrier
Mucopolysaccharidosis VI†·‡	Siamese and domestic cats	Hypoplasia of retina and optic nerve*·‡	Blue Merle collie
Lipidosis†·‡	Cocker spaniel	Epilepsy*·‡	Beagle, German shepherd, poodle, fox terrier, keeshond
Mannosidosis†·‡	Domestic cat, Angus cattle		
		Hereditary neuraxial edema†·‡	Polled Hereford cattle
Neuronal Degenerative Diseases		***Other***	
Spinal muscular atrophy (amyotrophic lateral sclerosis)†·‡	Brittany spaniel	Scottie cramp*·‡	Scottish terrier
		Occipital dysplasia†	Toy breeds
Neuroaxonal dystrophy†·‡	Domestic cat	Brain neoplasms	
Cerebellar and extrapyramidal neuronal abiotrophy†·‡	Kerry blue terrier	Gliomas†	Boxer, Boston terrier
Cerebellum, brain stem, and spinal cord diseases†·‡	Collie	Meningioma†	Dolichocephalic dogs, cats
		Pituitary adenomas†	Boxer, Boston terrier

*Seen fairly often.
†Seen infrequently or rarely.
‡Known to be an inherited trait in some breeds.
§Suspected to be an inherited trait in some breeds.

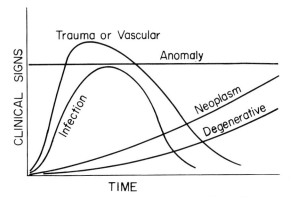

Figure 2–2. Sign-time graph of neurologic diseases. Metabolic, nutritional, and toxic diseases are variable, depending on the cause.

allow the clinician to construct a graph that has no major gaps.[3]

The sign-time graph is not usually drawn and entered on the case record. Rather, it is a useful tool for the clinician to construct mentally.

The time of the onset of some problems may be very exact (e.g., an automobile accident), or it may be very difficult to determine (e.g., neoplastic disease). The first time the client recognized a problem must be taken as the starting point. Sometimes, seemingly unrelated episodes may be the earliest signs and will be recognized only as the complete history is unfolded. For example, an animal with degenerative spinal cord disease may have been observed to stumble or may have had difficulty with stairs some time before clear manifestations of paresis were evident.

The course of the disease as revealed by the sign-time graph provides important information about the cause of the disease (Fig. 2–3). Slowly progressive diseases with an unrelenting course are immediately distinguished from acute diseases. The first step in making an etiologic diagnosis is classifying the problem as acute or chronic and progressive or nonprogressive. With this information, the problem logically falls into a group of diseases (Figs. 2–2 and 2–3 and Table 2–2). The neurologic examination can further narrow the choice of diseases by indicating whether the problem is focal or diffuse (Fig. 2–3). After a general etiologic or pathologic diagnosis is considered, the diagnostic plan can be established so that one can rule in or out each of the probable causes (see specific problems in Chapters 8 to 17).

NEUROLOGIC SIGNS

Signs that are likely to be associated with an abnormality in the nervous system are listed in Table 2–3.

Seizures always indicate a problem in the brain, although the problem may be secondary to a metabolic or toxic condition. Differentiation between seizures and syncope may be difficult and may require wording the questions carefully and interpreting the answers even more carefully.

Table 2–2. CHECK LIST FOR DIFFERENTIAL DIAGNOSIS

Category of Disease		Examples
D	Degenerative	Primary degeneration
		Storage diseases
		Demyelinating diseases
		Neuronopathies
		Intervertebral disk disease
		Spondylosis
		Spondylopathies
		Vascular diseases
A	Anomalous	Congenital defects
M	Metabolic	Nervous system disorders secondary to an abnormality of other organ systems (e.g., hypoglycemia, uremia)
N	Neoplastic	All tumors
	Nutritional	All nutritional problems
I	Inflammatory	Infectious diseases
T	Traumatic	Physical injury
	Toxic	Exposure to all toxic agents (may include tetanus and botulism)

Table 2–3. SIGNS OF ABNORMALITY IN THE NERVOUS SYSTEM

Signs Usually Indicative of Nervous System Abnormality
Seizures, convulsions, fits
Altered mental status
  Stupor, coma
  Behavioral changes
Paresis, paralysis
Proprioceptive deficits
Ataxia
Head tilt
Circling
Tremors and other abnormal movements
Dysmetria
Nystagmus
Hypesthesia, analgesia

Signs That May Indicate Nervous System Abnormality
Syncope, fainting
Weakness
Lameness
Pain, hyperesthesia
Blindness
Hearing deficits
Anosmia
Visceral dysfunction, micturition

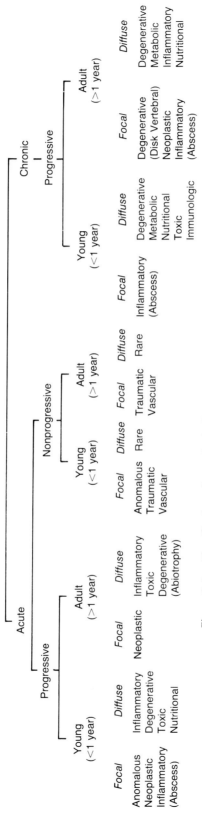

Figure 2–3. Classification of neurologic diseases (in approximate order of frequency).

Stupor and coma are manifestations of abnormal cerebral or brain stem function. Behavioral changes may be caused by primary brain abnormalities or may be secondary to environmental factors.

Paresis and paralysis, signs of primary motor dysfunction, are caused by a neurologic abnormality. Lameness of musculoskeletal origin is differentiated from these signs by the neurologic examination.

Sensory deficits, such as loss of proprioception or hypesthesia (decreased sensation), are always a result of an abnormality in the nervous system.

Pain may be related to neural lesions. The client's observations may be helpful in localizing the animal's pain. A careful physical and neurologic examination is essential in order to verify the signs.

Visual deficits may be caused by an abnormality of the eye or of the nervous system. An ocular and neurologic examination is necessary in order to make a diagnosis. Historical information may be deceptive in the case of visual abnormalities. Animals in their normal surroundings may function normally even though they may be completely blind.

Deficits in hearing are not usually recognized unless they are bilateral. Brain lesions causing bilateral hearing loss are rare.

Loss of the sense of smell (anosmia) is rarely recognized, except in working dogs. Inappetence occasionally may be associated with anosmia.

PROGNOSIS

Providing the owner with a reasonably accurate prognosis is an essential part of clinical neurology. The prognosis is influenced by many variables. The major variables are the location, the extent, and the etiology of the lesion.

The clinical course of the problem provides significant insight into the prognosis. A disease that has a slow progressive course has a much poorer prognosis than one that has passed its peak of severity and is improving (Fig. 2–2). Degenerative and neoplastic diseases, as demonstrated on the sign-time graph, are examples of progressive diseases.

Clinical signs are also valuable clues to prognosis. Spinal cord compression produces signs that vary with increasing compression, as outlined in Figure 2–4. The signs are not related to the location of the tracts in the spinal cord but do correlate with the size of the fibers. When compressed, larger fibers stop functioning earlier than small fibers. Functional recovery is possible until pain sensation is lost. An animal with no response to a painful stimulus has a very low probability of recovery. Animals that do recover frequently have severe motor deficits.

Duration of the lesion is also a significant factor in prognosis. Nervous tissue tolerates injury for only a short time. Spinal cord compression has been studied more thoroughly than have most injuries to the CNS. It has been demonstrated that a spinal cord with compression severe enough to abolish voluntary motor function, but not severe enough to abolish the response to a painful stimulus, has a reasonably good prognosis for recovery if decompression is accomplished within 5 to 7 days. The longer the duration, however, the slower the recovery. If decompression is delayed over 7 days, the probability for recovery is not significantly different regardless of whether decompression is indeed accomplished. Compression abolishing pain sensation has a very poor prognosis after only 2 to 4 hours.

The prognoses in the many disorders affect-

Fiber Size	Function	Signs with Increasing Compression	Prognosis
	Proprioception	Proprioceptive Deficits	Good
	Voluntary Motor	Paresis, Paralysis	Fair
	Superficial Pain	Loss of Cutaneous Sensation	Fair
	Deep Pain	Loss of Deep Pain	Poor

Figure 2–4. Progression of signs in spinal cord compression.

ing the nervous system are discussed throughout the text.

CASE HISTORIES

The following case histories are presented for two purposes. First, they provide examples of the kinds of histories obtained in cases involving neurologic problems and demonstrate the process used in evaluating this information. Second, they can be used to gauge one's understanding of the material in this chapter. After reading the history, but before reading the assessment, draw a sign-time graph and list the most probable categories of disease. Later chapters will include the complete findings in the cases and a final diagnosis. In this chapter, make only a sign-time graph and establish a list of rule-outs.

Case History 2A

Signalment. Canine, West Highland white terrier, female, 6 years old.
History. There are no significant previous medical problems, and vaccinations are current. The dog was found down in the fenced-in back yard 4 days ago. She was unable to walk, although some apparently voluntary movements were noticed in the left thoracic and pelvic limbs. The owners do not believe that conditions have changed since they first found the dog. They do not think the dog is in any pain. Appetite and eliminations are normal, and the dog seems alert and responsive.

Case History 2B

Signalment. Canine, German shepherd, female, 7 years old.
History. The dog has hip dysplasia, which was first diagnosed at 1 year of age. There are no other medical problems, and vaccinations are current. The owners had noticed the dog having difficulty with the pelvic limbs approximately 6 months ago. At first, she just stumbled a bit on the steps or slipped on the kitchen floor. The problem has progressed slowly, and now she can no longer go up steps. They have noticed that she has some swaying of the rear quarters when she walks. Occasionally, she will stumble and fall, even on good footing. They are not aware of any pain. Appetite and eliminations are normal.

Case History 2C

Signalment. Feline, domestic short hair, female, 3 months old.
History. The kitten always has seemed more clumsy than the others in the litter. There were four kittens: One was born dead, and the other two seem normal. This kitten had some difficulty in nursing but has grown well and is alert and active. She has a peculiar

prancing gait and trembles at times. The owners do not think the condition is getting worse. If anything, the kitten is able to get around somewhat better than when she first started walking.

Case History 2D

Signalment. Feline, Siamese, male, 2 years old.
History. The right eye has seemed irritated for the past two months. Uveitis was diagnosed by another veterinarian, but treatment gave only temporary relief. The cat now seems to be lame in the right forelimb. The owners report a trembling of the head when the cat eats. In the last two days, the cat has seemed depressed and has refused to eat. There were no other problems in the past, and vaccinations are current.

Case History 2E

Signalment. Canine, Yorkshire terrier, male, 8 months old.
History. The dog has been vaccinated in your clinic. Although he has had a reasonably good appetite, he has always been thin and small. Recently, the dog has had episodes of abnormal behavior. He paces continuously and resents being held. At times, he stops and just stands and stares straight ahead. If someone tries to pick him up at these times, he appears startled. The episodes usually last for 2 to 3 hours, but on occasion he has seemed abnormal for an entire day. The owners cannot recall any days in the past 3 weeks when the dog did not have an "attack."

Construct a sign-time graph and a list of rule-outs (general categories of diseases) before reviewing the assessments.

ASSESSMENT 2A

This dog's problem is tetraparesis with an acute onset and no progression. There are two primary groups of diseases that fit: trauma and vascular lesions. Inflammatory (infectious) diseases may have an acute onset, but they are usually progressive. Intervertebral disks usually have a slower onset, unless they are associated with trauma.
   Rule-outs:
1. vascular lesion,
2. trauma, and
3. inflammation (low probability).
   Asking additional questions regarding possible sources of trauma proved unrewarding. The neurologic examination of this dog will be discussed at the end of Chapter 3.

ASSESSMENT 2B

The dog's problems are pelvic limb paresis and ataxia with a chronic onset and a progressive course. A number of diseases can be chronic and progressive (see Fig. 2–3). It will be important to establish whether the disease is focal or diffuse when the neurologic examination is performed. With the information we have, we would include degenerative diseases, neoplasia, and inflammation as the primary rule-outs. Metabolic and nutritional diseases are more likely to affect the whole animal.

Rule-outs:
1. degenerative diseases,
2. neoplasia, and
3. inflammation.

ASSESSMENT 2C

The history suggests that the problem is ataxia and tremors of the entire body with the onset at birth and no progression. The onset suggests an anomaly or a birth injury. Either of these problems could be nonprogressive. Most of the other diseases affecting neonates, such as degenerative or inflammatory diseases, are progressive.

Rule-outs:
1. anomaly and
2. trauma.

ASSESSMENT 2D

The cat has ocular disease, trembling of the head, lameness of the right thoracic limb, and depression. The disease is chronic and progressive. Chronic progressive diseases include degenerative, metabolic, neoplastic, inflammatory, and nutritional diseases. If the neurologic examination substantiates that the signs are multifocal in origin, as the history suggests, then metabolic and nutritional diseases would be much lower on the list.

Rule-outs:
1. inflammatory disease,

2. neoplastic disease, and
3. degenerative disease.

ASSESSMENT 2E

The problem is primarily an abnormality in mental status. The neurologic examination is needed in order to determine if there are other abnormalities. The onset is chronic and the course progressive, but the entire syndrome is episodic. Episodic disorders other than seizures are usually metabolic in origin. Toxicities can wax and wane with exposure, but this phenomenon is rare. Structural disorders such as degeneration, neoplasia, and inflammation may have signs that wax and wane, but they rarely have periods of normal activity.

Rule-outs:
1. metabolic disorder and
2. toxic disorder.

Further questioning regarding the timing of the episodes with feeding revealed that the dog was fed morning and evening. The usual diet was canned dog food. The episodes usually occurred 2 to 4 hours after feeding. This situation is typical of hepatic encephalopathy (see Chapter 14).

REFERENCES

1. Weed, L. L.: Medical Records, Medical Education and Patient Care. Chicago, Year Book Medical Publishers, Inc., 1971.
2. Osborne, C. A., and Low, D. G.: The medical history redefined: Idealism vs. realism. Proc. AAHA 207–213, 1976.
3. Oliver, J. E., Jr.: Neurologic examinations: Taking the history. VM/SAC 67:433–434, 1972.

INTRODUCTION

In the neurologic examination, one systematically evaluates the functional integrity of the various components of the nervous system. The examination can be conveniently divided into the following parts: observation; palpation; examination of postural reactions, spinal reflexes, and cranial nerve responses; and sensory evaluation. In every complete physical examination, each of these categories would be investigated in order for problems related to the nervous system to be ruled out. An abbreviated neurologic examination might include the items marked with an asterisk in Table 3–1. Positive findings in any of these tests indicate the need for a complete neurologic examination. The history may provide the first evidence of neurologic disease and often indicates the etiology and the prognosis of the problem (see Chapter 2). Neurologic responses of neonatal dogs are outlined in Table 3–2.

THE NEUROLOGIC EXAMINATION

Observation

During every physical examination, the veterinarian should observe the animal's *mental status, posture,* and *movement.* The animal

3

CHAPTER

NEUROLOGIC EXAMINATION

should be allowed to move around the examination room or an open area while the history is being taken.[1-3]

MENTAL STATUS

Technique. One can obtain a general impression of the animal's behavior by observing its response to environmental stimuli or to people. Natural variations, such as the aggressive cuiosity of puppies, the indifference of older hounds, and the withdrawal of cats, must be recognized as normal behavior. Overt aggression and fear-biting usually can be recognized.

Table 3–1. NEUROLOGIC EXAMINATION

I. Observation*
Mental status
Posture
Movement
III. Postural Reactions
Proprioceptive positioning*
Wheelbarrowing
Hopping*
Extensor postural thrust
Hemistanding and hemiwalking
Placing (tactile)
Placing (visual)
Tonic neck
V. Cranial Nerves
Olfactory
Optic*
Oculomotor*
Trochlear
Trigeminal*
Abducent*
Facial*
Vestibulocochlear*
Glossopharyngeal
Vagus
Accessory
Hypoglossal*
	II. Palpation*
	Integument
	Muscles
	Skeleton
	IV. Spinal Reflexes
	Myotatic
	  Pelvic limb
	    Quadriceps femoris muscle*
	    Cranial tibial muscle
	    Gastrocnemius muscle
	  Thoracic limb
	    Extensor carpi radialis muscle
	    Triceps brachii muscle
	    Biceps brachii muscle
	Flexor*
	Extensor thrust
	Perineal*
	Crossed extensor
	Extensor toe
	VI. Sensation
	Touch
	Hyperesthesia*
	Superficial pain*
	Deep pain†

*Included in a screening examination.
†If superficial pain is absent.

Table 3–2. NEUROLOGIC EVALUATION OF THE NEONATAL DOG*

Motor Responses	Strong	Weak, Variable	Absent or Adult-like
		Age in Days	
Crossed extensor reflex	1–16	16–18	18+ (absent)
Magnus reflex	1–17	17–21	21+ (absent)
Neck extension posture	Flexion 1–4	Hyperextension 4–21	Normotonia 21+
Forelimb placing	4+	2–4	0–2 (absent)
Hind limb placing	8+	6–8	0–6 (absent)
Fore limb supporting	10+	6–19	0–6 (absent)
Hind limb supporting	15+	11–15	0–11 (absent)
Standing on all fours	21+	18–21	1–18 (absent)
Body righting (cutaneous)	1+	0–1	—
Sensory Responses	**Strong**	**Weak, Variable** (*Age in Days*)	**Absent or Adult-like**
Rooting reflex	0–14	14–25	25+ (absent)
Nociceptive withdrawal reflex	0–19	19–23	23+ (adult-like)
Panniculus reflex	0–19	19–25	25+ (adult-like)
Reflex urination	0–22	22–25	25+ (absent)
Visual and Auditory Responses	**Strong**	**Weak, Variable** (*Age in Days*)	**Absent or Adult-like**
Blinking response to light	16+	4–16	0–4 (absent)
Visual orientation	25+	20–25	0–20 (absent)
Auditory startle reflex	24+	15–24	0–15 (absent)
Sound orientation	25+	18–25	0–18

*Modified from Fox, M. W.: The clinical behavior of the neonatal dog. JAVMA 143:1331–1335, 1963.

Anatomy and Physiology. Consciousness is a function of the cerebral cortex and the brain stem. Sensory stimuli from the body, such as touch, temperature, and pain, and from outside the body, such as light, sound, and odors, provide input to the reticular formation. Consciousness is maintained by diffuse projections of the reticular formation to the cerebral cortex (Fig. 3–1). This arousal system is termed the *reticular activating system*.[4] A common cause of decreased levels of consciousness is a disruption of the pathways between the reticular formation and the cerebral cortex.

Assessment. An animal's mental status may be recorded as *alert, depressed, stuporous,* or *comatose,* depending on its level of consciousness (see Chapter 14). Behavioral changes may include *aggression, fear, withdrawal,* and *disorientation.*

Depression describes an animal that is conscious but inactive, is relatively unresponsive to the environment, and tends to sleep when

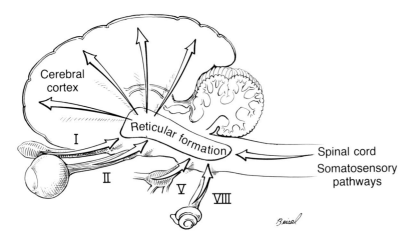

Figure 3–1. The ascending reticular activating system in the brain stem receives sensory information from the spinal cord and the cranial nerves. It projects diffusely to the cerebral cortex, thus maintaining consciousness.

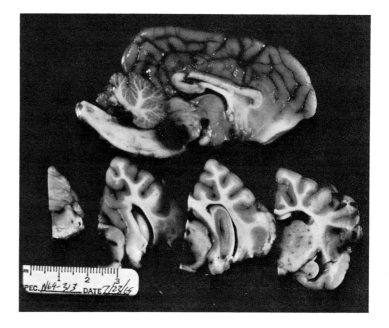

Figure 3–2. The brain of a boxer dog that was hit by a car. Hemorrhage in the brain stem extends from the caudal aspect of the mesencephalon into the rostral pons. This dog was comatose and exhibited decerebrate rigidity. (From Oliver, J. E., Jr.: Neurologic examination. VM/SAC 67:654–659, 1972. Used by permission.)

undisturbed. Depression may be caused by systemic problems, such as fever, anemia, or metabolic disorders. When associated with primary brain problems, depression usually indicates diffuse cerebral cortex disease.

Stupor is exemplified by an animal that tends to sleep when undisturbed. Innocuous stimuli such as touch or noise may not cause arousal, but a painful stimulus will cause the animal to awaken. Stupor usually is associated with partial disconnection of the reticular formation and the cerebral cortex, as in diffuse cerebral edema with compression of the brain stem.

Coma is a state of deep unconsciousness. The animal cannot be aroused even with painful stimuli, although simple reflexes may be intact. For example, pinching the foot will produce a flexor reflex but will not cause arousal. Coma indicates complete disconnection of the reticular formation and the cerebral cortex. The most common cause in small animals is acute head injury with hemorrhage in the pons and the midbrain (Fig. 3–2).[5]

Behavior disorders are often functional, that is, related to environment and training. Primary brain disease, however, also can cause alterations in behavior. The limbic system is a complex organization of nuclei and pathways in the more primitive portions of the brain that relates to behavior (Fig. 3–3). Abnormality in any part of the limbic system may cause abnormal behavior. This type of abnormal behavior is not generally useful for localizing brain lesions (see Chapter 16).

POSTURE

Technique. Abnormalities in posture may be noticed while the history is being recorded and the animal is free to move about. Further observations may require moving the animal to different positions so that its ability to regain normal posture can be evaluated.

Assessment

HEAD. The most frequent abnormality in the posture of the head is a tilt or a twist to one side (Fig. 3–4). Intermittent head tilt, especially if associated with rubbing of the ear, may be associated with otitis externa or ear mites. A continuous head tilt with resistance to straightening of the head by the examiner is almost always associated with an abnormality in the vestibular system (see Chapter 11). Signs may range from tilting of the head or twisting of the head and neck to twisting and rolling of the head, neck, and body.

TRUNK. Abnormal posture of the trunk may be associated with congenital or acquired lesions of the vertebrae or abnormal muscle tone from brain or spinal cord lesions. Deviations in spinal contour consist of (1) *scoliosis*—lateral deviation, (2) *lordosis*—ventral deviation (swayback), and (3) *kyphosis*—dorsal deviation (humpback).

LIMBS. Abnormal posture of the limbs includes improper positioning and increased or decreased extensor tone. A *wide-based stance* is common with all forms of ataxia (see Chapter 11). It also may be seen in cases of generalized

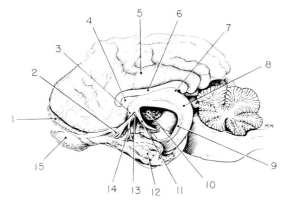

Figure 3–3. Lateral view of the brain showing rhinencephalic structures. *1.* Right olfactory bulb. *2.* Rostral part of rostral commissure. *3.* Precommissural fornix. *4.* Telencephalic septum. *5.* Medial surface of right cerebral hemisphere. *6.* Corpus callosum. *7.* Dorsal commissure of fornix. *8.* Alveus of hippocampus. *9.* Fimbria of hippocampus. *10.* Interthalamic adhesion. *11.* Column of fornix. *12.* Piriform lobe (from dorsal side). *13.* Rostral commissure. *14.* Caudal part of rostral commissure. *15.* Left olfactory bulb. (From Evans, H. E., and Christensen, G. C.: Miller's Anatomy of the Dog, 2nd ed. Philadelphia, W. B. Saunders Co., 1979. Used by permission.)

weakness. Proprioceptive deficits or lower motor neuron (LMN) or upper motor neuron (UMN) lesions may cause the animal to stand with a foot knuckled over (see Chapter 4). Uneven distribution of weight on the limbs may provide a clue to weakness.

Decreased tone in the muscles of the limb often is associated with LMN lesions and will cause abnormal posture. The limbs will be positioned passively, often with the toes knuckled.

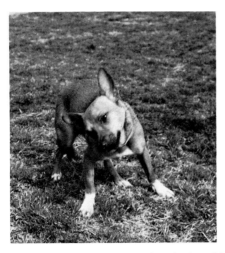

Figure 3–4. A dog with a head tilt and a broad-based stance, which are typical of vestibular disease.

Decerebrate rigidity is characterized by extension of all four limbs and the trunk. It is caused by a lesion in the rostral brain stem (midbrain or pons). Opisthotonos may be associated with decerebrate rigidity if the anterior lobes of the cerebellum are damaged. Opisthotonos is dorsiflexion of the head and the neck.

Increased tone in the extensor muscles is a sign of UMN disease (see Chapter 4). Partial lesions may be manifested as an exaggerated straightness in the stifle and hock joints. Decerebrate rigidity is an extreme form of increased extensor tone. Increased tone in the forelimbs with flaccid paralysis of the hind limbs is called the Schiff-Sherrington phenomenon and is associated with spinal cord lesions between T2 and L4.

MOVEMENT

The animal should be observed for abnormal movements while resting and at gait.

Gait

Technique. The gait should be observed with the animal on a surface offering adequate traction (carpet, synthetic turf, grass). Gaits vary among species and breeds, and one must be knowledgeable of these differences. Some

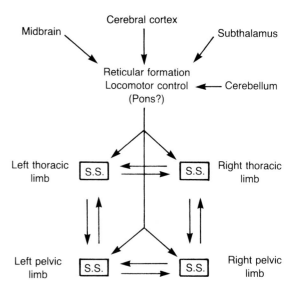

S.S. = Spinal stepping circuit in spinal cord

Figure 3–5. Schematic diagram of automatic control of locomotion. Spinal stepping reflexes are controlled by the brain stem centers for locomotion. Voluntary control is imposed from the cerebral cortex. The cerebellum and other areas coordinate the movements.

breeds of dogs have been selectively developed for characteristic gaits. Because of this breeding, neurologic diseases may have been genetically selected. The gait should be observed from the side and while the animal is moving toward and away from the examiner. The animal should be turned in wide and tight circles and should be backed up. The examiner may exaggerate minimal abnormalities in gait by blindfolding the animal.

Anatomy and Physiology. The neural organization of gait and posture is complex, involving all levels of the nervous system. Limbs are maintained in extension for supporting weight by spinal cord reflexes. Stepping movements also are programmed at the spinal level (Fig. 3–5). Organization of the stepping movement for locomotion occurs at the brain stem level in the reticular formation. Cerebellar regulation of this system makes locomotion smooth and coordinated. Vestibular input maintains balance. Cerebral cortical input to the system is necessary for voluntary control and fine coordination, especially of learned movements (Fig. 3–6).[6–8]

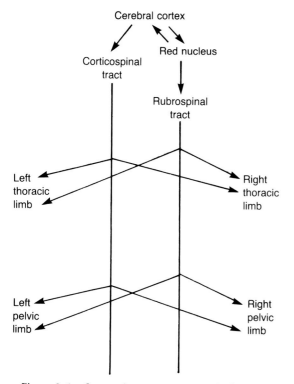

Figure 3–6. System for voluntary control of the limbs. The cerebral cortex controls fine, coordinated movements of the limbs through the corticospinal and corticorubrospinal pathways in addition to its input to the locomotor centers of the brain stem (see Fig. 3–5).

An animal with a cerebral cortex lesion will be able to walk but will not have the precision of movement of a healthy animal. Postural reactions will be grossly abnormal. Rostral brain stem lesions (of the midbrain and the pons) cause decerebrate rigidity, because the voluntary motor pathways that inhibit extensor muscle activity are lost. The substrate for locomotion is still present and may be seen in animals with chronic lesions, but it is usually masked by the increased extensor tone. Lesions in the pons or the medulla will abolish integrated locomotion. Acute lesions of the cerebellum produce rigidity, whereas chronic lesions produce an uncoordinated gait.

Assessment. Abnormalities of gait may include *proprioceptive deficits, paresis, circling, ataxia,* and *dysmetria.*

Proprioception, or position sense, is the ability to recognize the location of the limbs in relation to the rest of the body. A deficit appears as a misplacement or a knuckling of the foot that may not occur with every step. The proprioceptive pathways in the spinal cord are in the dorsal and dorsolateral columns and project to both the cerebellum (unconscious) and the cerebral cortex (conscious) (see the section on sensation in this chapter).

Paresis is a deficit of voluntary movements. Affected limbs will have inadequate or absent voluntary motion, which may be described as *monoparesis*—paresis of one limb; *paraparesis*—paresis of both pelvic limbs; *tetraparesis* or *quadriparesis*—paresis of all four limbs; or *hemiparesis*—paresis of the thoracic and the pelvic limb of the same side.

The suffix *-plegia,* (e.g., paraplegia) may be used to denote complete loss of voluntary movements and is used by some authors to indicate both motor and sensory loss. In this text, paresis indicates partial deficit of motor function, whereas paralysis (-plegia) indicates a complete loss of voluntary movements.

Paresis is caused by disruption of the voluntary motor pathways, which extend from the cerebral cortex through the brain stem to the lateral columns of the spinal cord. They continue to synapse on the LMN in each spinal cord segment that innervates the muscles. Paresis may be of the UMN or the LMN type (see Chapter 4 and Chapters 8 through 10).

A neurologic disease may cause an animal to *circle.* Circling may vary from a tendency to drift in wide circles to forced spinning in a tight circle. Circling is not generally localizing, except that tight circles usually are caused by caudal brain stem lesions. The direction of the circling is usually toward the side of the lesion, but there are exceptions, especially in lesions rostral to the midbrain. Twisting or head tilt associated with circling usually indicates involvement of the vestibular system (see Chapters 4 and 11).

Ataxia is lack of coordination without spasticity, paresis, or involuntary movements, although each of these conditions may be seen in association with ataxia. Truncal ataxia is characterized by poorly controlled swaying of the body. The movement of the limbs is uncoordinated. The feet may be crossed or placed too far apart. Ataxia may be caused by lesions of the cerebellum, the vestibular system, or the proprioceptive pathways (see Chapter 11).

Dysmetria is characterized by movements that are too long (hypermetria) or too short (hypometria). "Goose-stepping" is the most common sign of dysmetria. The stride may be abruptly stopped, forcing the animal to lurch from side to side. Dysmetria of the head and the neck may be most apparent when the animal tries to drink or eat and overshoots or undershoots the target. Dysmetria usually is caused by cerebellar or cerebellar pathway lesions and may be associated with ataxia and intention tremors (see Chapter 11).

Abnormal Movement

Technique. Abnormal movements may occur while the animal is at rest or when it is moving and may be intermittent or continuous. The most frequently recognized movement disorders are *tremors* and *myoclonus.*

Assessment. A *tremor* is produced by alternating contractions of opposing groups of muscles. The oscillatory movements are small and rapid. Tremors from neurologic causes must be differentiated from those induced by fatigue, fear, chilling, drug reactions, or primary muscle disease.

An *intention tremor* is one that is more pronounced when movements are initiated. It is an important sign of cerebellar disease. A *continuous tremor* usually is associated with an abnormality of the motor system.

Myoclonus is a coarse jerking of muscle groups. Myoclonus associated with canine distemper encephalomyelitis is usually a rhythmic jerking of one muscle group, such as the flexors of the elbow or the temporal muscle. The myoclonus of distemper has been called chorea; however, chorea describes irregular, purposeless movements that are brief and that often vary from one part of the body to the other.[9] Two forms of myoclonus may be

seen in the dog. In the acute encephalitis stage, the lesion is probably related to destruction of areas in the basal nuclei.[10] The more common chronic form is related to the interneurons or the LMN at the segmental level.[11] Other movement disorders, such as *cataplexy* and *athetosis,* are much less common or have not been reported in clinical patients. Cataplexy is a sudden, complete loss of muscle tone that causes the animal to fall limp. It usually is seen in association with narcolepsy (see Chapter 15).

Palpation

Technique. After the mental status, posture, and gait of the animal have been assessed the physical examination is initiated. Careful inspection and palpation of the musculoskeletal systems and of the integument may be performed at one time or on a regional basis in conjunction with other parts of the examination. Comparison of one side with the other for symmetry is best accomplished as one step in the examination.[12]

Assessment

INTEGUMENT. Although the skin is not often involved in neurologic disease, careful inspection may reveal clues to the diagnosis. Scars may indicate previous trauma. Worn nails may be associated with paresis or with proprioceptive deficits. Coat and eye color may be related to a hereditary abnormality. For example, blue eyes and a white coat is associated with deafness in cats. Myelomeningocele may be palpated as it attaches to the skin in the lumbosacral region. The temperature of the extremities may be significantly lowered with arterial occlusion.

SKELETON. Careful palpation of the skeletal system may reveal *masses, deviation of normal contour, abnormal motion,* or *crepitation.* Tumors involving the skull or the spinal column may be palpable as a mass. The dorsal spinous processes of the vertebrae should be palpated in order to detect irregularity of contour. Deviations may indicate a luxation, a fracture, or a congenital anomaly. Depressed or elevated skull fractures often can be palpated, especially in animals with minimal temporal muscle mass. Open fontanelles and suture lines in the skull may indicate hydrocephalus. Abnormal motion or crepitation may be detected in fractures and luxations. When spinal luxations or fractures are suspected, manipulation should not be attempted, because additional displacement may cause serious spinal cord

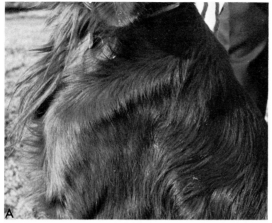

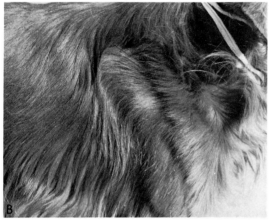

Figure 3–7. Left (*A*) and right (*B*) shoulders of an Irish setter dog with a neurofibrosarcoma involving the right C6 nerve root. Atrophy of the supraspinatus and infraspinatus muscles is prominent on the right side. (From Oliver, J. E., Jr.: Neurologic examination. VM/SAC 67:1327–1328, 1972. Used by permission.)

damage. Peripheral nerve injuries may be associated with fractures of the long bones.

MUSCLES. Muscles are evaluated for *size*, *tone*, and *strength*. All of the muscles should be systematically palpated, starting with the head, extending down the neck and the trunk, and continuing down each limb.

Changes in the *size* of muscles may be apparent from observation as well as from palpation. Loss of muscle mass (atrophy) is the most frequent finding (Fig. 3–7). Atrophy may indicate LMN disease or disuse. Criteria for differentiating the two are presented in Chapter 4. Detection of localized muscle atrophy, which usually accompanies disease of the LMN, is an important localizing sign.

The *tonus* of muscles is maintained through the spinal stretch (myotatic) reflex. Alterations in tone, either increased or decreased, can be detected by palpation and passive manipula-

tion of the limb. Increased tone of the extensor muscles, a common finding in UMN disease, is manifested as an increased resistance to passive flexion of the limb (see Chapter 4 for an interpretation).

The *strength* of muscles is difficult to evaluate, even in the most cooperative patients. The extensor muscles can be evaluated during postural reactions, such as hopping, in which the animal must support all of its weight on one limb (see the section on hopping in this chapter). The flexor muscles can be evaluated by comparing the relative strength of pull during a flexor reflex (see the section on the flexor reflex in this chapter). Loss of muscle strength is usually an LMN sign.

Postural Reactions

The complex responses that maintain an animal's normal, upright position are known as postural reactions. If an animal's weight is shifted from one side to the other, from front to rear, or from rear to front, the increased load on the supporting limb or limbs requires increased tone in the extensor muscles in order to keep the limb from collapsing. Part of the alteration in tone is accomplished through spinal reflexes, but in order for the changes to be smooth and coordinated, the sensory and motor systems of the brain must be involved.

Abnormalities of complex reactions, such as the hopping reaction, do not provide precise localizing information, because lesions in any one of several areas of the nervous system may affect the reaction. The assessment of the postural reactions, however, is an important part of the neurologic examination. Minimal deficits in the function of a key component, such as the cerebral cortex, may cause significant alterations in the postural reactions that are not detected when one observes the gait.

The following postural reactions are listed in a sequence found to be convenient for performing an examination. In an initial screening examination, the reactions marked with an asterisk in Table 3–1 should be tested. If they are normal, it is unlikely that abnormalities will be found in the other reactions.

PROPRIOCEPTIVE POSITIONING REACTION

Technique. Proprioception is the ability of the animal to recognize the location of its limbs without visual information. Although proprioception is a sensory function, the tests described in this section require motor reac-

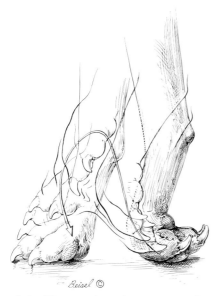

Figure 3–8. The proprioceptive response. Conscious proprioceptive function is tested by placing the dorsal surface of the animal's foot on the floor. The animal immediately should replace it to the normal position. (From Ettinger, S. J.: Textbook of Veterinary Internal Medicine, 2nd ed. Philadelphia, W. B. Saunders Co., 1982. Used by permission.)

tions, so it has been included as a postural reaction.[13]

The simplest method of evaluation is flexing the paw so that the dorsal surface is on the floor (Fig. 3–8). The animal should immediately return the paw to a normal position. Most animals will not allow weight bearing to occur in the abnormal position. Another method is placing the foot on a sheet of cardboard and slowly sliding the cardboard laterally.[14] As the limb reaches an abnormal position, the animal should replace it for normal weight bearing. The first test is the most sensitive for proprioception in the distal extremity, whereas the second test is more likely to detect abnormalities in the proximal portion of the limb. In either method, the examiner should test each foot separately.

Anatomy and Physiology. Proprioceptive information is carried in the dorsal columns and the spinomedullothalamic tract in the dorsolateral fasciculus of the spinal cord, through the brain stem to the sensorimotor cortex (Fig. 3–9). The motor response is initiated by the cerebral cortex and is transmitted to the LMN in the spinal cord (See the section on sensation in this chapter).

Assessment. Because the dorsal columns are very sensitive to compression, abnormali-

ties in proprioceptive positioning may occur before motor dysfunction can be detected (see Chapter 4). The response will be abnormal if there is significant paresis, but other postural reactions, such as hopping, are also affected.

WHEELBARROWING REACTION

Technique. The animal is supported under the abdomen with all of the weight on the thoracic limbs (Fig. 3–10). The normal animal can walk forward and sideways with coordinated movements of both thoracic limbs. The examiner should not lift the pelvic limbs so high that the animal's posture is grossly abnormal. If movements appear normal, the maneuver is repeated with the head lifted and the neck extended. This position prevents visual compensation, making the animal totally dependent on proprioceptive information. A tonic neck reaction, which causes slightly increased extensor tone in the forelimbs, is also elicited. *When the neck is extended, subtle abnormalities of the thoracic limbs may be seen in animals that otherwise would appear normal.*

Assessment. Weakness in the thoracic limbs may be detected when the wheelbarrowing reaction is tested, because the animal is forced to carry most of its weight on two limbs while standing and on only one limb while moving.

Slow initiation of movement may be a sign of proprioceptive deficit or of paresis that is caused by a lesion of the cervical spinal cord, the brain stem, or the cerebral cortex. Exaggerated movements (dysmetria) may indicate an abnormality of the cervical spinal cord, the lower brain stem, or the cerebellum.

HOPPING REACTION

Technique. The hopping reaction of the thoracic limbs is tested with the animal in the position for wheelbarrowing, with one thoracic limb lifted from the ground (Fig. 3–11). The entire weight of the animal is supported by one limb, and the patient is moved forward, laterally, and medially. Medial hopping is much more difficult, and more subtle abnormalities may be detected by this maneuver. Hopping of the pelvic limbs is assessed similarly, following the extensor postural thrust reaction. Large animals, such as giant-breed dogs, horses, and cows can be tested by lifting one limb and shifting the weight of the animal so that it hops on the opposite limb. Alternatively, the animal can be pulled by the tail or pushed laterally in order for movements similar to the hopping reaction to be elicited.

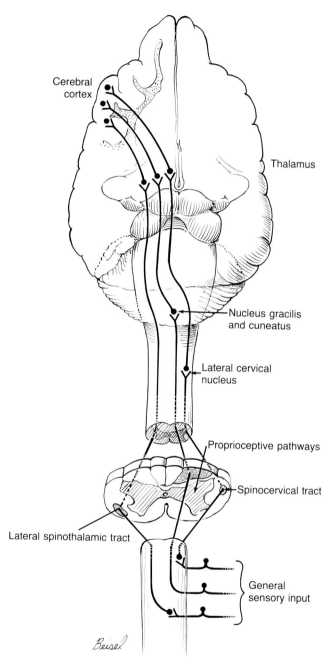

Figure 3–9. Somatic sensory innervation is transmitted to the brain through several pathways. Proprioception is a function of the spinomedullothalamic pathway (near the spinocervical tract) for the pelvic limbs and of the fasciculus cuneatus of the dorsal columns for the thoracic limbs. Pain is transmitted by several tracts (see also Fig. 3–41), including the spinothalamic, spinocervical, and spinoreticular tracts and the dorsal columns.

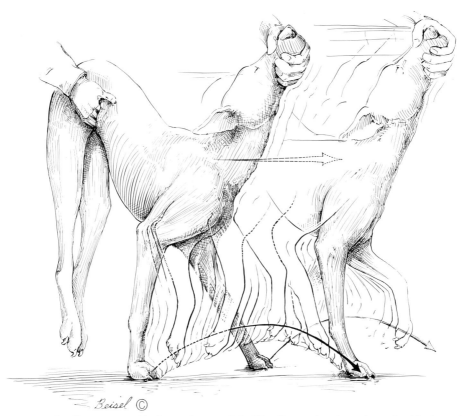

Figure 3–10. Wheelbarrowing with the neck extended. Wheelbarrowing is performed with the pelvic limbs elevated. The body should be in a position as close to normal as possible. The head may be elevated to accentuate abnormalities, as illustrated here. (From Ettinger, S. J.: Textbook of Veterinary Internal Medicine, 2nd ed. Philadelphia, W. B. Saunders Co., 1982. Used by permission.)

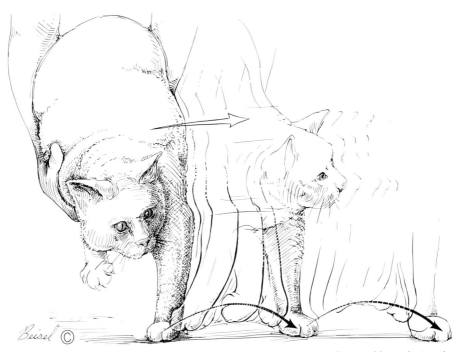

Figure 3–11. The hopping reaction. The normal animal responds to hopping by quickly replacing the limb under the body as it moves laterally. (From Ettinger, S. J.: Textbook of Veterinary Internal Medicine, 2nd ed. Philadelphia, W. B. Saunders Co., 1982. Used by permission.)

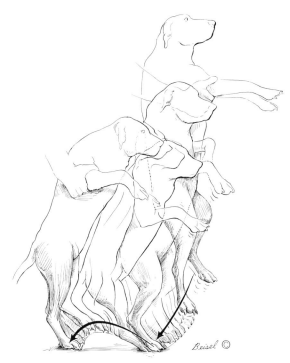

Figure 3–12. The extensor postural thrust reaction. The animal responds by stepping backward when its feet make contact with the floor (From Ettinger, S. J.: Textbook of Veterinary Internal Medicine, 2nd ed. Philadelphia, W. B. Saunders Co., 1982. Used by permission.)

Assessment. The hopping reaction is more sensitive than is the wheelbarrowing reaction for detecting minor deficits. Poor initiation of the hopping reaction suggests sensory (proprioceptive) deficits, whereas poor follow-through suggests a motor system abnormality (paresis). Asymmetry is easily seen and helps to lateralize lesions.

EXTENSOR POSTURAL THRUST REACTION

Technique. The extensor postural thrust is elicited by supporting the animal by the thorax caudal to the thoracic limb and lowering the pelvic limbs to the floor (Fig. 3–12). When the limbs touch the floor, they should move caudally in a symmetric walking movement in order for a position of support to be achieved.

Assessment. Asymetric weakness, lack of coordination, and dysmetria can be seen in the extenser postural thrust reaction as in the wheelbarrowing reaction.

HEMISTANDING AND HEMIWALKING REACTIONS

Technique. The front and rear limbs on one side are lifted from the ground, so that all of the animal's weight is supported by the op-

posite limbs. Forward and lateral walking movements then are evaluated.

Assessment. Abnormal signs may be seen in hemistanding and hemiwalking as in the other postural reactions. They are most significant in animals with cerebral cortex lesions. These animals have relatively normal gaits but have deficits of postural reactions in both the front and the rear limbs contralateral to the side of the lesion.

PLACING REACTION

Technique. Placing is evaluated first without vision (tactile placing) and then with vision (visual placing). The examiner supports the animal under the thorax and covers its eyes with one hand or with a blindfold. The thoracic limbs are brought in contact with the edge of a table at or below the carpus (Fig. 3–13). The normal response is immediate placement of the feet on the table surface in a position that will support weight. Care must be taken not to restrict the movement of either limb. When one limb is consistently slower to respond, the animal should be held in the examiner's other hand to ensure that its movements are not being restricted.

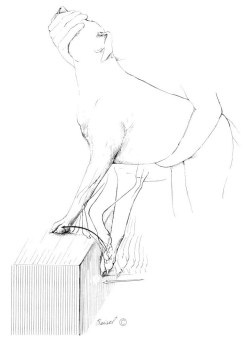

Figure 3–13. The tactile placing reaction is elicited with the eyes covered. When the carpus makes contact with the edge of the surface, the animal immediately should place its foot on the surface. (From Ettinger, S. J.: Textbook of Veterinary Internal Medicine, 2nd ed. Philadelphia, W. B. Saunders Co., 1982. Used by permission.)

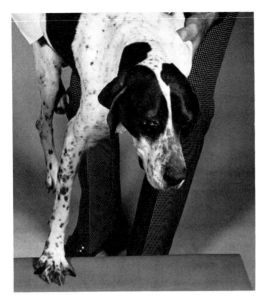

Figure 3–14. The visual placing reaction allows the animal to see the surface and to place its feet appropriately.

Visual placing is tested by allowing the animal to see the table surface. Normal animals reach for the surface before the carpus touches the table (Fig. 3–14). Peripheral visual fields can be tested by making a lateral approach to the table. The veterinarian can evaluate giant-breed dogs and large animals (e.g., horse, cow) by leading them over a curb or a step with and without vision. Some dogs and cats that are accustomed to being held may ignore the table. These animals usually will respond if they are held in a less secure or less comfortable position.

Anatomy and Physiology. Tactile placing requires touch receptors in the skin, sensory pathways through the spinal cord and the brain stem to the cerebral cortex, and motor pathways from the cerebral cortex to the LMN of the forelimbs. Visual placing requires normal visual pathways to the cerebral cortex, communication from the visual cortex to the motor cortex, and motor pathways to the LMN of the forelimbs.[15]

Assessment. A lesion of any portion of the pathway may cause a deficit in the placing reaction. Normal tactile placing with absent visual placing indicates a lesion of the visual pathways. Normal visual placing with abnormal tactile placing suggests a sensory pathway lesion. Cortical lesions will produce a deficit in the contralateral limb. Lesions below the midbrain usually will produce ipsilateral deficits.

TONIC NECK REACTION

Technique. With the animal in a normal standing position, the head is elevated and the neck is extended. The normal reaction is a slight extension of the thoracic limb and a slight flexion of the pelvic limbs. Lowering the head causes the thoracic limbs to flex and the pelvic limbs to extend. Turning the head to the side causes a slight extension of the ipsilateral thoracic limb and a slight flexion of the contralateral thoracic limb. It is easy to remember the normal reactions if one considers the usual movements of an animal. For example, a cat about to jump onto a counter extends the head and the neck, extends the front limbs, and flexes the rear limbs. A dog crawling under a bed lowers the head and the neck and flexes the front limbs as it extends the rear limbs for propulsion. A horse making a sharp turn leads with the head and the neck, plants the ipsilateral limb in extension, and flexes the contralateral limb to take a step.[16]

Tonic eye reactions also may be observed. They will be discussed with C.N. III, C.N. IV, and C.N. VI in the section on cranial nerves.

Assessment. The tonic neck reactions are initiated by receptors in the cranial cervical area and are mediated by brain stem reactions. The responses are subtle in normal animals and are often inhibited volitionally through cortical control.

Abnormalities in sensory (proprioception) or motor systems may produce abnormal reactions. Lesions in the cerebellum cause exaggerated tonic neck reactions.

Spinal Reflexes

Examination of the spinal reflexes tests the integrity of the sensory and motor components of the reflex arc and the influence of descending motor pathways on the reflex. Three kinds of responses may be seen. *Absence* or *depression* of a reflex indicates complete or partial loss of either of the sensory or motor (LMN) nerves responsible for the reflex. A *normal response* indicates that the sensory and motor nerves are intact. An *exaggerated response* indicates an abnormality in the motor pathways (UMN) that normally have an inhibitory influence on the reflex.

The examination should be performed with the animal in lateral recumbency. Muscle tone, previously evaluated with the animal in a standing position, should be tested again at this time. The pelvic limbs are evaluated first. Passive manipulation of the limb assesses the degree of muscle tone, especially in the extensor muscles. Spreading the toes with slight pressure on the foot pads will elicit the extensor thrust reflex. The myotatic (stretch) reflexes then are evaluated. Routinely, only the knee-jerk (quadriceps) reflex is tested, but the cranial tibial and gastrocnemius muscles also can be evaluated when such an assessment is indicated. The flexor reflex then is tested by gently pinching the toes. In order to maintain the cooperation of the patient, one should apply the least possible stimulus that will elicit a response. *If flexion is induced by touching the foot, there is no need to crush the toe with a hemostat!* The perineal reflex is a contraction of the anal sphincter in response to a touch, a pin prick, or a pinch in the perineal area. There may be flexion of the tail simultaneously.

The most predictable myotatic reflex in the thoracic limb is elicited when the extensor carpi radialis muscle (tendons over carpus in large animals) is struck, producing a slight extension of the carpus. The triceps and biceps reflexes are difficult to elicit in many normal animals. After examining the limbs on one side, the veterinarian turns the animal and examines the opposite limbs.

MYOTATIC (STRETCH) REFLEXES

Quadriceps (Knee-Jerk, Patellar) Reflex

Technique. With the animal in lateral recumbency, the leg is supported under the femur with the left hand (by a right-handed examiner), and the stifle is flexed slightly (Fig. 3–15). The straight patellar ligament is struck crisply with the plexor. The response is a single, quick extension of the stifle.[17] The plexor is recommended for performing myotatic reflex testing, but other instruments, such as bandage scissors, may be used. Nose tongs or similar heavy instruments are useful for testing large animals. The examiner should use the same type of instruments in each examination to obtain consistent results.

Anatomy and Physiology. The myotatic, or stretch, reflexes are basic to the regulation of posture and movement. The reflex arc is a simple, two-neuron (monosynaptic) pathway. The sensory neuron has a receptor in the muscle spindle and its cell body in the dorsal root ganglion. The motor neurons have their cell bodies in the ventral horn of the gray matter of the spinal cord. The axons form the motor components of peripheral nerves that end on the muscle (the neuromuscular junction) (Fig. 3–16).

The muscle spindle is the stretch receptor of the muscle. The spindle has three to five striated muscle fibers (intrafusal muscle) at each end, with a nonstriated portion in the middle (Fig. 3–17). The spindles are located in the belly of the skeletal muscle (extrafusal muscle). These sensory fibers are large and have a spiral ending, called the primary ending, around the nonstriated portion of each fiber. Small sensory fibers have secondary endings. Primary endings are of greatest importance in phasic responses (e.g., knee jerk),

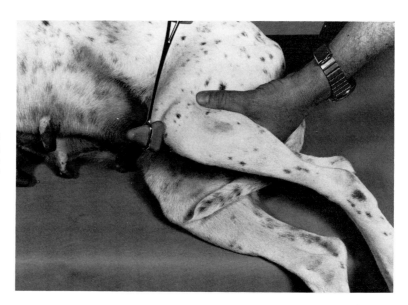

Figure 3–15. Restraining the animal in lateral recumbency with the stifle slightly flexed and relaxed is the preferred method for eliciting the quadriceps reflex.

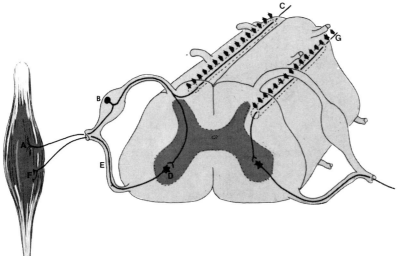

Figure 3–16. Myotatic reflex. *A.* Muscle spindle. *B.* Dorsal root ganglion. *C.* Ascending sensory pathway in the dorsal column. *D.* Ventral horn motor neuron (LMN). *E.* Ventral (motor) root. *F.* Neuromuscular junction. *G.* Descending motor pathway in the lateral column. (From Oliver, J. E., Jr.: Neurologic examination. VM/SAC 68:151–154, 1973. Used by permission.)

whereas secondary endings respond primarily to tonic activation (e.g., extensor thrust). The small intrafusal muscle fibers of the spindle are innervated by small (gamma) motor neurons.

Stretching a muscle depolarizes the nerve endings of the spindle, producing a burst of impulses in the sensory fibers. The sensory fibers monosynaptically activate the large (alpha) motor neuron in the spinal cord. The alpha motor neuron discharges impulses through its axon, causing a contraction of the extrafusal muscle fibers of the same muscle. Thus, a sudden stretch of the muscle causes a reflex muscle contraction, as seen in the knee-jerk reflex. A more tonic stretch of the muscle causes a slower discharge of sensory activity and a slower, more steady muscle contraction.

Contraction of the extrafusal muscle fibers

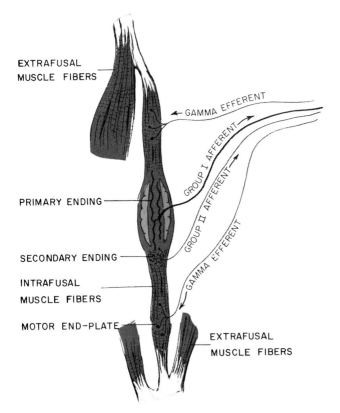

EXTRAFUSAL MUSCLE FIBERS

GAMMA EFFERENT

GROUP I AFFERENT

GROUP II AFFERENT

PRIMARY ENDING

GAMMA EFFERENT

SECONDARY ENDING

INTRAFUSAL MUSCLE FIBERS

MOTOR END-PLATE

EXTRAFUSAL MUSCLE FIBERS

Figure 3–17. Muscle spindle, the stretch receptor of skeletal muscle. (From Oliver, J. E., Jr.: Neurologic examination. VM/SAC 68:151–154, 1973. Used by permission.)

causes relaxation of the intrafusal fibers, because they are parallel (see Fig. 3–17). Loss of tension on the intrafusal fibers stops the sensory input from the spindle. To prevent this situation from occurring, gamma motor fibers adjust the length of the intrafusal fibers. Thus, tension is maintained on the spindle through the range of motion of the limb.

Gamma motor activation of the intrafusal fibers also can stretch the primary spindle endings directly and thus can elicit a response indirectly in the alpha motor neuron. Alpha and gamma motor neurons are facilitated or inhibited by a variety of segmental and long spinal pathways. The output of the motor neurons is a summation of their facilitatory and inhibitory inputs. For example, the quadriceps motor neuron responds to a sudden stretch by a quick contraction (knee jerk) but can be blocked by voluntary inhibition (Fig. 3–18).

The spindle sensory fibers also facilitate interneurons in the spinal cord, which in turn inhibit motor neurons of antagonistic muscles. This activity is called reciprocal innervation. For example, spindle sensory fibers from the quadriceps muscle inhibit antagonistic flexor motor neurons, allowing the limb to extend. Spindle sensory fibers also contribute collaterals to ascending pathways, which provide information to the brain regarding activity in the muscles.[16]

Assessment. The quadriceps reflex is the most reliably interpreted myotatic reflex. The reflex should be recorded as *absent* (0), *depressed* (+1), *normal* (+2), *exaggerated* (+3), or *exaggerated with clonus* (+4). Normal responses vary widely among species and among breeds within a species. In large dogs, the response is less brisk than in small dogs. The examiner should become familiar with these natural variations.

Absence (0) of a myotatic reflex indicates a lesion of the sensory or motor component of the reflex arc—a *lower motor neuron*, or segmental, sign (see Chapter 4). Loss of the reflex in one muscle group suggests a peripheral nerve lesion, i.e., of the femoral nerve. Bilateral loss of the reflex suggests a segmental spinal cord lesion affecting the motor neurons to both limbs located in spinal cord segments L4–L6 in the dog. Differentiation between peripheral nerve and spinal cord lesions may require assessment of the sensory examination and the presence or absence of other neurologic signs.

Depression (+1) of the reflex has the same significance as absence of the reflex, except that the lesion is incomplete. Depression of the reflex is more common with spinal cord lesions in cases in which some, but not all, of the segments (L4–L6) are affected. Other reflexes also must be tested, because generalized depression of reflexes may be seen in polyneuropathies or in abnormalities of the neuromuscular junction (botulism, tick paralysis).

Exaggerated reflexes (+3,+4) and increased tone result from loss of descending inhibitory pathways. The voluntary motor pathways are facilitatory to flexor muscles and inhibitory to extensor muscles. Damage to these pathways

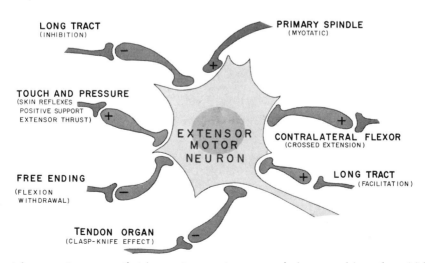

Figure 3–18. A lower motor neuron that innervates an extensor muscle (e.g., quadriceps femoris) has numerous inputs that affect the output. The monosynaptic primary spindle (myotatic) fibers facilitate discharge of the extensor motor neuron. (From Oliver, J. E., Jr.: Neurologic examination. VM/SAC 68:151–154, 1973. Used by permission.)

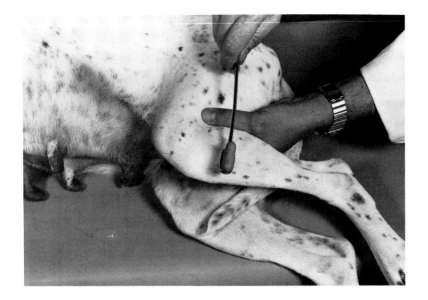

Figure 3–19. The cranial tibial reflex is elicited with the animal in the same position as that used for the quadriceps reflex. The cranial tibial muscle is percussed just below the stifle.

will *release* the myotatic reflex, causing an exaggerated reflex and increased extensor tone. Clonus (+4) is a repetitive contraction and relaxation of the muscle to a single stimulus. Clonus often is seen with chronic (weeks to months) loss of descending inhibitory pathways. Clonus has the same localizing significance as exaggerated reflexes. Bilateral exaggerated reflexes most often are associated with damage to descending inhibitory pathways rostral to the level of the reflex.

Cranial Tibial Reflex

Technique. With the animal in lateral recumbency, the examiner tests the cranial tibial reflex next. The cranial tibial reflex usually is not performed unless the quadriceps reflex is abnormal or if a lesion of the sciatic nerve is suspected. The belly of the cranial tibial muscle is struck with the plexor just below the proximal end of the tibia (Fig. 3–19). The response is flexion of the hock.

Anatomy and Physiology. The cranial tibial muscle is a flexor of the hock and is innervated by the peroneal branch of the sciatic nerve (with origin in the L6–L7 segments of the spinal cord in the dog).

Assessment. For the inexperienced, the cranial tibial reflex is difficult to elicit in a normal animal. Absent or decreased reflexes

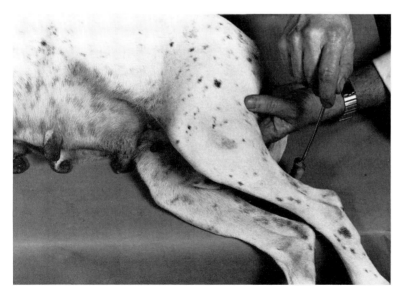

Figure 3–20. The gastrocnemius reflex is elicited with the animal in the same position as that used for the quadriceps reflex. The tendon of the gastrocnemius muscle is percussed proximal to the tarsus.

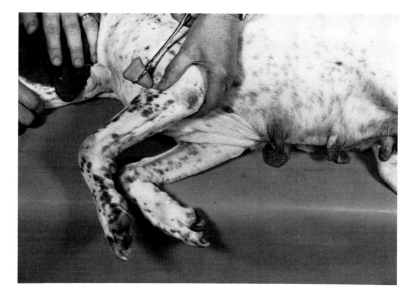

Figure 3–21. The extensor carpi radialis reflex is the most reliable myotatic reflex in the thoracic limb. With the animal in lateral recumbency and the elbow and the carpus flexed, the extensor muscle group is percussed distal to the elbow.

should be interpreted with caution. Exaggerated reflexes indicate a lesion above the spinal cord segments that are responsible for the reflex (L6–L7).

Gastrocnemius Reflex

Technique. The gastrocnemius reflex is tested after the cranial tibial reflex. The tendon of the gastrocnemius muscle is struck with the plexor just above the tibial tarsal bone (Fig. 3–20). Slight flexion of the hock is necessary in order for some tension of the muscle to be maintained. The response is extension of the hock.

Anatomy and Physiology. The gastrocnemius is primarily an extensor of the hock and is innervated by the tibial branch of the sciatic nerve (with origin in the L7–S1 segments of the spinal cord in the dog).

Assessment. The gastrocnemius reflex is interpreted in the same manner as the cranial tibial reflex.

Extensor Carpi Radialis Reflex

Technique. The animal is in lateral recumbency while the reflexes of the thoracic limb are evaluated. The limb is supported under the elbow, with flexion of the elbow and the carpus maintained. The extensor carpi radialis muscle is struck with the plexor just distal to the elbow (Fig. 3–21). The response is a slight extension of the carpus. The carpus must be

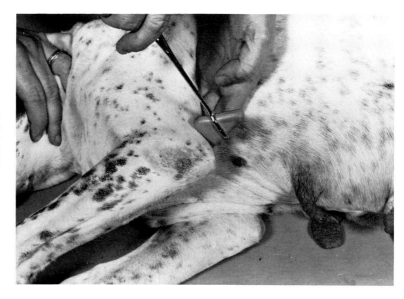

Figure 3–22. The triceps reflex is elicited with the animal in the same position as for the extensor carpi radialis reflex. The triceps tendon is percussed proximal to the elbow.

flexed and the digits must not touch the floor or the other limb, or the reflex will be mechanically inhibited.[17] The extensor tendons crossing the carpal joint are struck in large animals.

Anatomy and Physiology. The extensor carpi radialis is an extensor of the carpus and is innervated by the radial nerve (with origin in the C7, C8, and T1 segments of the spinal cord in the dog).

Assessment. The extensor carpi radialis reflex is more difficult to elicit than the quadriceps reflex but usually can be recognized in dogs. Absent or decreased reflexes should be evaluated with caution. Strong reflexes are usually exaggerated (+3) and indicate a lesion above C7.

Triceps Reflex

Technique. The animal is held in the same position as for the extensor carpi radialis reflex. The triceps brachii muscle is struck with the plexor just proximal to the olecranon (Fig. 3–22). The response is a slight extension of the elbow. The elbow must be maintained in flexion in order for a response to be elicited.

Anatomy and Physiology. The triceps brachii muscle extends the elbow and is essential for weight bearing in the forelimb. Innervation is through the radial nerve (with the origin from spinal cord segments C7–T1 in the dog).

Assessment. The triceps reflex is difficult to elicit in the normal animal. Absent or decreased reflexes should not be interpreted as abnormal. Lesions of the radial nerve can be recognized by a loss of muscle tone and an inability to support weight. Exaggerated reflexes are interpreted in the same way as for the extensor carpi radialis reflex.

Biceps Reflex

Technique. The index or middle finger of the examiner's hand that is holding the animal's elbow is placed on the biceps and the brachialis tendons cranial and proximal to the elbow. The elbow is slightly extended, and the finger is struck with the plexor (Fig. 3–23). The response is a slight flexion of the elbow. Movement of the animal's elbow must not be blocked by the examiner's restraining hand.

Anatomy and Physiology. The biceps brachii and brachialis muscles are flexors of the elbow. They are innervated by the musculocutaneous nerve (which originates from spinal cord segments C6–C8 in the dog).

Assessment. The biceps reflex is difficult to elicit in the normal animal. Absent or decreased reflexes should not be interpreted as abnormal. The flexor reflex is a better test of the musculocutaneous nerve. An exaggerated (+3) reflex is indicative of a lesion above C6.

FLEXOR (PEDAL, WITHDRAWAL) REFLEXES

Pelvic Limb

Technique. The animal is maintained in lateral recumbency, the same position as that for examination of the myotatic reflexes. A noxious stimulus is applied to the foot. The normal response is a flexion of the entire limb, including the hip, the stifle, and the hock (Fig. 3–24). The least noxious stimulus possible should be used. If an animal flexes the leg

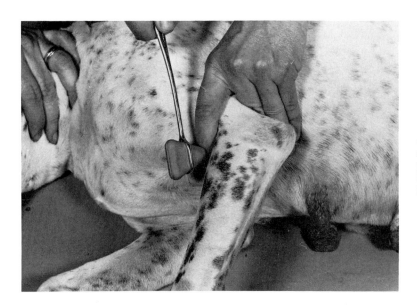

Figure 3–23. The biceps reflex is elicited with the elbow slightly extended. The examiner's finger is placed on the biceps tendon proximal to the elbow, and the finger is percussed.

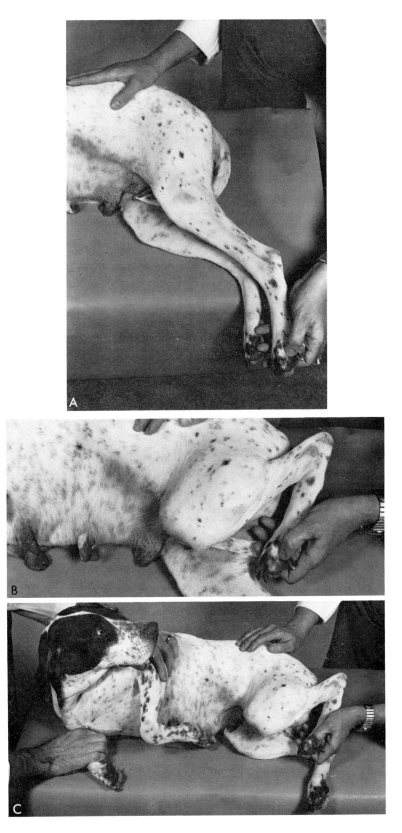

Figure 3–24. The flexor reflex is elicited with the animal in the same position as that used for the myotatic reflexes. The digits are squeezed (*A*), and the leg is flexed (*B*). Releasing the digits allows the limb to flex freely, and maintaining a grasp allows evaluation of the strength of the flexor muscles. A behavioral reaction indicates conscious perception of pain (*C*).

37

when the digit is touched, there is no need to crush the digit. If a response is not easily elicited, a hemostat should be used to squeeze across a digit. Pressure should not be so great as to injure the skin. Both medial and lateral digits should be tested on each leg. The limb should be in a slightly extended position when the stimulus is applied in order to allow the limb to flex. The opposite limb also should be free to extend.[18]

Anatomy and Physiology. The flexor reflex is less stereotyped than is the myotatic reflex. The response involves all of the flexor muscles of the limb and thus requires activation of motor neurons in several spinal cord segments.

The receptors for the flexor reflex are primarily free nerve endings in the skin and other tissues that respond to noxious stimuli such as pressure, heat, or cold. A stimulus that produces a sensory discharge in these nerves ascends to the spinal cord through the dorsal root. The sensory nerves from the digits of the pelvic limbs are primarily branches of the sciatic nerve, the superficial peroneal nerve on the dorsal surface, and the tibial nerve on the plantar surface. The sciatic nerve originates from spinal cord segments L6–S1. The medial digit is partially innervated by the saphenous nerve, a branch of the femoral nerve that originates from spinal cord segments L4–L6. Interneurons are activated at these segments and at adjacent segments both rostrally and caudally. The interneurons activate sciatic motor neu-

rons, which stimulate flexor muscle contraction (Fig. 3–25). The net result is a withdrawal of the limb from the painful stimulus. Inhibitory interneurons to the extensor motor neurons also are activated, resulting in decreased activity in the extensor muscles. Relaxation of the extensor muscles and contraction of the flexor muscles allow complete flexion of the limb.

The flexor reflex is a spinal reflex and does not require any activation of the brain. If an animal steps on a sharp piece of glass, it immediately withdraws the foot before consciously perceiving pain. If the spinal cord is completely transected above the segments that are responsible for the reflex, the reflex is present even though the animal has no conscious perception of pain.

Assessment. The pelvic limb flexor reflex primarily involves spinal cord segments L6–S1 and the sciatic nerve. Absence (0) or depression (+1) of the reflex indicates a lesion of these segments or nerves. Unilateral absence of the reflex is more likely the result of a peripheral nerve lesion, whereas bilateral absence or depression of the reflex is more likely the result of a spinal cord lesion. A normal (+2) flexor reflex indicates that the segments and the nerves are functional. An exaggerated (+3) flexor reflex rarely is seen with acute lesions of descending pathways. Chronic and severe descending pathway lesions may cause exaggeration of the reflex. This exaggeration is manifested as a sustained withdrawal after release

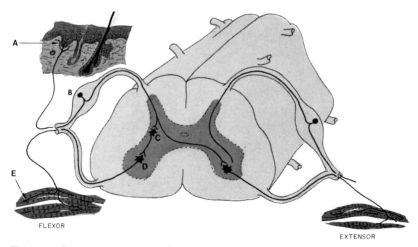

Figure 3–25. Flexion and crossed extension reflexes. *A.* Free nerve endings. *B.* Dorsal root ganglion. *C.* Interneuron. *D.* Ventral horn motor neuron (flexor). *E.* Neuromuscular junction. Only one interneuron and one flexor muscle are depicted, although the reflex involves a number of each. Note the connections to contralateral extensor motor neurons, which account for the crossed extension reflex. (From Oliver, J. E., Jr.: Neurologic examination. VM/SAC 68:383–385, 1973. Used by permission.)

of the stimulus. A mass reflex (+4) occasionally is seen as a sustained flexion of both pelvic limbs from a stimulus to only one limb. Exaggerated flexor reflexes usually reflect chronicity rather than severity of the lesion.

The crossed extensor reflex and the conscious perception of pain also are evaluated while the flexor reflex is performed, but these assessments will be discussed later.

Thoracic Limb

Technique.   The thoracic limb flexor reflex is performed in the same manner as the pelvic limb flexor reflex. Dorsal and palmar surfaces and medial and lateral digits should be tested.

Anatomy and Physiology.   Branches of the radial nerve innervate the dorsal surface of the foot and arise from spinal cord segments C7–T1. The medial palmar surface is innervated by the ulnar and median nerves, which originate from spinal cord segments C8–T1. The lateral palmar surface and most of the lateral digit are innervated by branches of the ulnar nerve. The organization of the flexor reflex of the thoracic limb is similar to that previously described for the pelvic limb (see Fig. 3–25). Flexor muscles of the thoracic limb are innervated by the axillary, musculocutaneous, median, and ulnar nerves and by parts of the radial nerve. These nerves originate from spinal cord segments C6–T1, with small contributions from C5 and T2 in some animals.

Assessment.   Depressed reflexes indicate a lesion of the C6–T1 segments of the spinal cord or of the peripheral nerves. Exaggerated reflexes indicate a lesion rostral to C6.

EXTENSOR THRUST REFLEX

Technique.   The reflex may be elicited with the animal in lateral recumbency (the same position as that for the myotatic reflex) or with the animal suspended by the shoulders with the rear limbs hanging free (Fig. 3–26). The toes are spread, and slight pressure is applied between the pads. The response is a rigid extension of the limb.[19]

Anatomy and Physiology.   The extensor thrust reflex is initiated by a stretching of the spindles in the interosseous muscles of the foot.[16] Simultaneously, the cutaneous sensory receptors are stimulated. The extensors predominate, forcing the limb into rigid extension (Fig. 3–27). The sensory fibers are in the sciatic nerve (spinal cord segments L6–S1), and the response involves both femoral and sciatic nerves (spinal cord segments L4–S1). Excessive stimulation of the flexor reflex sensory fibers (i.e., a noxious stimulus) will cause the flexor reflex to predominate, and withdrawal will occur.

The extensor thrust reflex is important for maintaining posture and is a component of more complex reactions, such as hopping.[16]

Assessment.   The extensor thrust reflex is difficult to elicit in normal animals, especially when they are in lateral recumbency. Presence of the reflex generally indicates a lesion cranial to L4.

PERINEAL (BULBOCAVERNOSUS, ANAL) REFLEX

Technique.   The perineal reflex is elicited by light stimulation of the perineum with a needle or a forceps. Painful stimuli usually are not

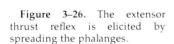

Figure 3–26. The extensor thrust reflex is elicited by spreading the phalanges.

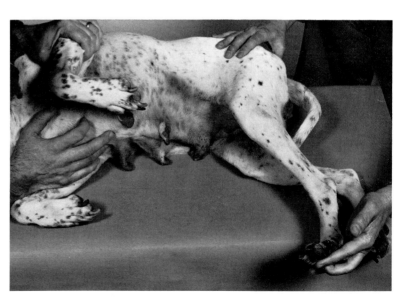

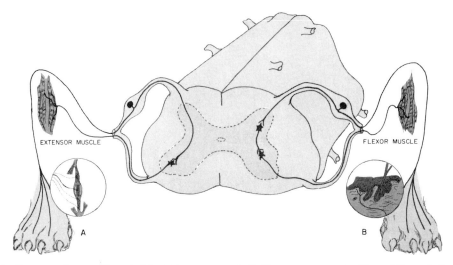

Figure 3–27. Extensor thrust reflex. *A.* Myotatic component. *B.* Flexor component. (From Oliver, J. E., Jr.: Neurologic examination. VM/SAC 68:763, 1973. Used by permission.)

necessary. The response is a contraction of the anal sphincter muscle and a flexion of the tail (Fig. 3–28). One can obtain a similar response by squeezing the penis or the vulva (bulbocavernosus reflex). If the anal sphincter appears weak or if the response is questionable, one can insert a gloved digit in the anus. Minimal responses often can be felt in this manner.

Anatomy and Physiology. Sensory innervation occurs through the pudendal nerve and spinal cord segments S1–S2 (sometimes S3) in the dog and the cat. Motor innervation of the anal sphincter also occurs through the pudendal nerve. Tail flexion is mediated through the caudal nerves. The organization of the reflex is similar to that of the flexor reflex.

Assessment. The perineal reflex is the best indication of the functional integrity of the sacral spinal cord segments and the sacral nerve roots. Evaluation of this reflex is especially important in animals with urinary bladder dysfunction (see Chapter 5). Absence (0) or depression (+1) of the reflex indicates a sacral spinal cord lesion or a pudendal nerve lesion.

CROSSED EXTENSOR REFLEX

Technique. The crossed extensor reflex may be observed when the flexor reflex is elicited. The response is an extension of the limb opposite the stimulated limb.[18]

Anatomy and Physiology. The crossed extensor reflex is a part of the normal supporting mechanism of the animal. The weight of an

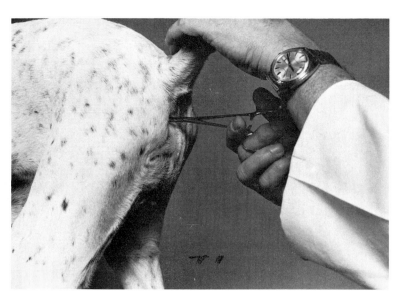

Figure 3–28. The perineal reflex is a contraction of the anal sphincter and a ventral flexion of the tail in response to tactile stimulation of the perineum.

animal in a standing position is evenly distributed among the limbs. If one leg is flexed, increased support is required of the opposite limb. The flexor reflex sensory fibers send collaterals to interneurons on the opposite side of the spinal cord, which excite extensor motor neurons (see Fig. 3–25).

Assessment. The crossed extensor reflex generally is considered an abnormal reflex, except in the standing position. The normal recumbent animal inhibits the extension response through descending pathways. Crossed extensor reflexes result from lesions in descending pathways, a sign of UMN disease. The crossed extensor reflex has been considered evidence of a severe spinal cord lesion. It is not a reliable indicator of the severity of the lesion, however. Animals that are still ambulatory may have crossed extensor reflexes, especially when the lesion is in the cervical spinal cord or in the brain stem.

EXTENSOR TOE (BABINSKI) REFLEX

Technique. The animal is positioned in lateral recumbency (the same position as that for the myotatic reflex). The rear limb is held above the hock, with the hock and the digits slightly flexed. The handle of the plexor or a forceps is used to stroke the limb on the caudolateral surface from the hock to the digits (Fig. 3–29). The normal animal will have no response or a slight flexion of the digits. The abnormal response is an extension and a fanning of the digits.[20]

Anatomy and Physiology. The extensor toe reflex has been compared with the Babinski reflex in human beings.[21] The two reflexes are not strictly analogous, because the Babinski reflex includes elevation and fanning of the large toe, which is not present in domestic animals. The Babinski reflex is reported to be a sign of pyramidal tract damage in human

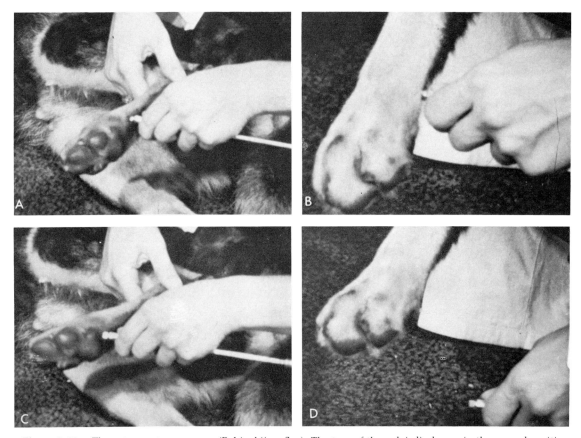

Figure 3–29. The extensor toe response (Babinski's reflex). The toes of the pelvic limbs are in the normal position. The instrument is moving down the metatarsus from the hock toward the digits (A and B). The digits extend and fan apart as the instrument completes the sweep (C and D). (Frames from a motion picture. From Kneller, S. K., Oliver, J. E., Jr., and Lewis, R. E.: Differential diagnosis of progressive caudal paresis in an aged German shepherd dog. JAAHA 11:414–417, 1975. Used by permission.)

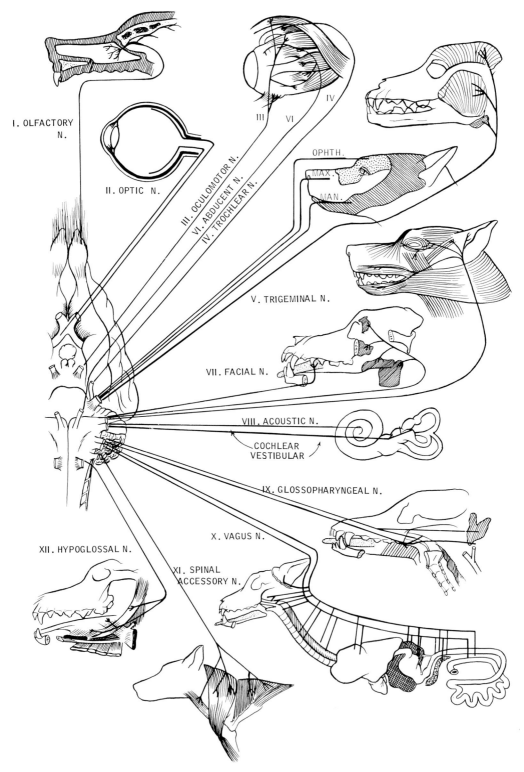

I. OLFACTORY
N.

II. OPTIC N.

III. OCULOMOTOR N.
VI. ABDUCENT N.
IV. TROCHLEAR N.

III   VI

IV

OPHTH.
MAX.
MAN.

V. TRIGEMINAL N.

VII. FACIAL N.

VIII. ACOUSTIC N.

COCHLEAR
VESTIBULAR

IX. GLOSSOPHARYNGEAL N.

X. VAGUS N.

XII. HYPOGLOSSAL N.

XI. SPINAL
ACCESSORY N.

Figure 3–30. The origin and distribution of the cranial nerves in the dog. (From Hoerlein, B. F.: Canine Neurology, 3rd ed. Philadelphia, W. B. Saunders Co., 1978. Used by permission.)

beings. The extensor toe reflex has been produced by lesions in the brain stem[21] and has been seen clinically in dogs with hypertonic pelvic limb paresis.[20] Acute experimental lesions of the sensorimotor cortex, the dorsal columns, the lateral columns, or the ventral columns of the spinal cord have not produced an extensor toe reflex. Some investigators have considered this reflex to be an abnormal form of the flexor reflex.

Assessment. The extensor toe reflex has been observed in dogs with paralysis of the pelvic limbs associated with extensor hypertonus and exaggerated myotatic reflexes. Most cases have had clinical signs for longer than 3 weeks. The reflex should be interpreted in the same manner as other exaggerated reflexes.

Cranial Nerves

Examination of the cranial nerves is an important part of the neurologic examination, especially when disease of the brain is suspected.[5] An abnormality of a cranial nerve constitutes evidence of a specific, localized area of disease not provided by postural reactions. The cranial nerve examination is not difficult, and the most frequently affected cranial nerves can be evaluated quickly (see Table 3–1 and Fig. 3–30).

Portions of the examination are completed during *observation* and *palpation* of the animal. The head is observed for posture. Head tilts commonly are associated with vestibular (C.N. VIII) disorders. Symmetry of the face, the ears,

and the musculature is evaluated. The muscles of facial expression are innervated by the facial nerve (C.N. VII). Abnormalities may include drooping of the ears, the lips, or the eyelids; deviation of the nasal philtrum; or inability of the animal to move these structures. Atrophy of the temporal or the masseter muscles (C.N. V—trigeminal) may be observed or palpated. While palpating the head, the examiner tests the palpebral reflex (C.N. V and C.N. VII) and the menace response (C.N. II and C.N. VII) (Figs. 3–31 and 3–32). The examiner also tests the animal's vision by assessing the visual placing reaction. The symmetry of the pupils and the pupillary light reflexes are evaluated (C.N. II and C.N. III—oculomotor). The eyes are observed for symmetry in the palpebral fissure (C.N. III, C.N. IV—trochlear, and C.N. VI—abducent), retraction of the globe (enophthalmos; usually sympathetic nerve damage [Horner's syndrome]), or abnormal eye movements (nystagmus, usually involving C.N. VIII). The head is moved first from side to side, then dorsally and ventrally in order to elicit vestibular eye movements (C.N. III, C.N. IV, C.N. VI, and C.N. VIII) (Fig. 3–33). At each extreme position of the head, the eyes are observed for positional nystagmus (C.N. VIII). The examiner evaluates the sensation of the face (C.N. V) by tapping the temporal area and the muzzle with a finger. Most animals will blink in response to this stimulus. If no response occurs, a slightly blunted 18G needle or a hemostat can be used. The temporal area (the ophthalmic branch of C.N. V), the nose (the maxillary

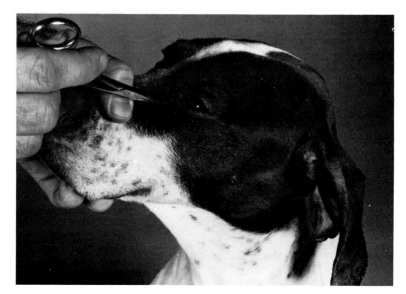

Figure 3–31. The palpebral reflex is performed by touching the eyelid and observing for a blink. The sensory pathway is in the trigeminal nerve; the motor pathway is in the facial nerve.

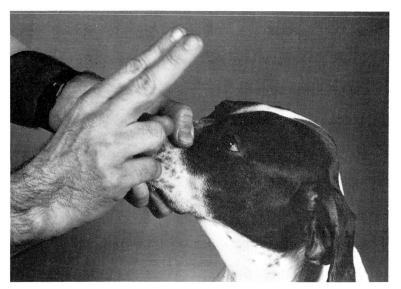

Figure 3–32. The menace reaction is elicited by making a threatening gesture at the eye, which should result in a blink. The examiner must avoid creating wind currents or touching the hairs around the eyes, which will cause a palpebral reflex. The sensory pathway is in the optic nerve and the visual pathway. The motor pathway is in the facial nerve.

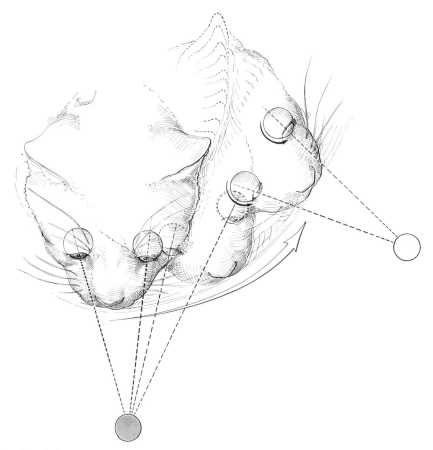

Figure 3–33. Vestibular eye movements are elicited by turning the animal's head from side to side. The eyes will lag behind the head movement and then will rotate to return to the center of the palpebral fissure. Both visual (opticokinetic nystagmus) and vestibular pathways are active in this response, but vestibular pathways predominate and will produce these movements in the absence of vision.

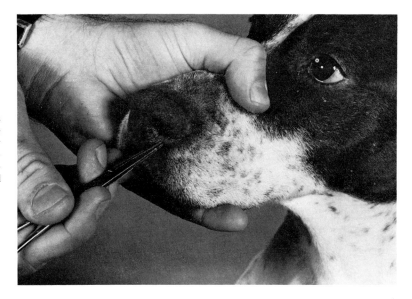

Figure 3–34. Tactile stimulation on the head rostral to the ears tests the sensory branches of the trigeminal nerve. The reactions may be behavioral or reflex. Even depressed or stoic animals will respond to stimulation of the nasal mucosa.

branch of C.N. V), and the lower lip (the mandibular branch of C.N. V) are tested for a blink or a behavioral response (Fig. 3–34). The nasal mucosa is extremely sensitive and is tested in those animals with questionable response to other stimuli. By opening and closing the animal's mouth, the examiner can assess the tone of the muscles of mastication (C.N. V). Licking movements of the tongue are induced by stimulation of the tip of the nose. The position and symmetry of the tongue are evaluated (C.N. XII—hypoglossal) (Fig. 3–35). Gentle traction of the tongue is used to test its strength. The positions of the soft palate and the larynx are observed. A gag reflex is tested with the finger or with a tongue depressor (C.N. IX—glossopharyngeal and C.N. X—vagus). The trapezius and brachiocephalicus muscles are palpated for symmetry and atrophy (C.N. XI—accessory).

It takes less time to perform this examination than to read these instructions. The examination tests every cranial nerve but the olfactory nerve (C.N. I). A history of anorexia may support a diagnosis of olfactory deficits. The olfactory nerve can be tested by presenting the animal with a noxious odor that is not irritating (irritating materials may stimulate C.N. V), such as alcohol (Fig. 3–36).

The detection of any abnormalities on the

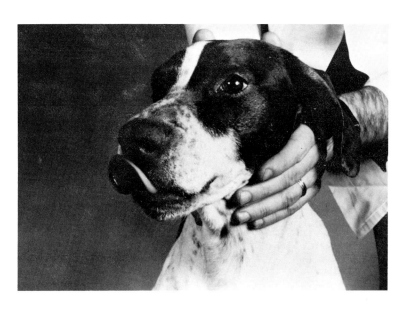

Figure 3–35. Most animals can be induced to lick if their noses are moistened. The tongue should extend without forced deviation to the side.

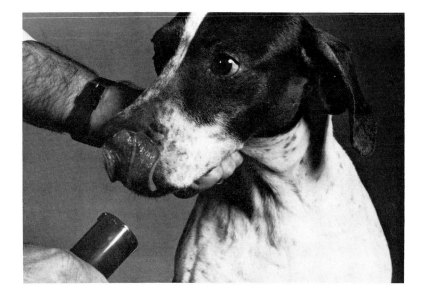

Figure 3–36. Noxious odors that are nonirritating will cause an aversion, or licking reaction.

screening examination may be followed by a more complete examination in order to define the abnormality further.

OLFACTORY NERVE (C.N. I)

The olfactory nerve is the sensory path for the conscious perception of smell.

Technique. A behavioral response to a pleasurable or a noxious odor, either inferred from the history or assessed by direct testing, may be used. Alcohol, cloves, xylol, benzol, or cat food containing fish appears to stimulate the olfactory nerves. Irritating substances, such as ammonia or tobacco smoke, cannot be used because they stimulate the endings of the trigeminal nerve in the nasal mucosa.

Anatomy and Physiology. Chemoreceptors in the nasal mucosa give rise to axons, which pass through the cribriform plate to the synapse in the olfactory bulb. Axons from the olfactory bulb course through the olfactory tract to the ipsilateral olfactory cortex. Behavioral reactions to smell are controlled by connections to the limbic system (see Fig. 3–3).[4]

Assessment. Deficiencies in the sense of smell are difficult to evaluate. Rhinitis is the most common cause of anosmia (loss of olfaction). Tumors of the nasal passages and diseases of the cribriform plate also must be considered.

OPTIC NERVE (C.N. II)

The optic nerve is the sensory path for vision and pupillary light reflexes (see Figs. 13–1 and 13–2).

Technique. The optic nerve is tested in conjunction with the oculomotor nerve (C.N.

III), which provides the motor pathway for the pupillary light reflex, and the facial nerve, which provides the motor pathway for the blink reflex. Vision may be assessed by observation of the animal's movements in unfamiliar surroundings. More objective evaluation requires three tests. The examiner elicits the menace reaction by making a threatening gesture with the hand at one eye. The normal response is a blink and, sometimes, an aversive movement of the head (see Fig. 3–32). The visual placing reaction (see the section on postural reactions) is an excellent method of assessing vision (see Fig. 3–14). The examiner induces the pupillary light reflex by shining a light in each eye and observing for pupillary constriction in both eyes.

Assessment. See Chapter 13.

OCULOMOTOR NERVE (C.N. III)

The oculomotor nerve contains the parasympathetic motor fibers for pupillary constriction and is the motor pathway for the following extraocular muscles: dorsal, medial and ventral recti, and ventral oblique. It is also the motor pathway for the levator palpebrae muscle of the upper lid (see Fig. 13–4).

Technique. The examiner tests the pupillary light reflex by shining a light in the animal's eye and observing for pupillary constriction in both eyes. One can assess eye movement by observing the eyes as the animal looks in various directions voluntarily or in response to movements in the peripheral fields of vision. A more direct method is to elicit vestibular eye movements (normal nystagmus). The fast beat of the nystagmus will be in the direction of the head movement. The eyes should move in coordination with each other (conjugate movements). One can easily test the rectus muscles by this method. A drooping upper lid (ptosis) is indicative of paresis of the levator palpebrae muscle. Lesions of the oculomotor nerve cause a fixed ventrolateral deviation (strabismus) of the eye and a dilated pupil. In cattle, the eye usually remains horizontal regardless of the head position. The function of each of the extraocular muscles can be assessed in the same manner if the examiner bears this difference in mind. The functions of the extraocular muscles of large animals have not been directly established, but it is assumed that they are similar to the functions of the corresponding muscles in other species.

Anatomy and Physiology. See Chapter 13.
Assessment. See Chapter 13.

TROCHLEAR NERVE (C.N. IV)

The trochlear nerve is the motor pathway to the dorsal oblique muscle of the eye.

Technique. The trochlear nerve is difficult to assess. Lesions may cause a lateral rotation of the eye, which can be seen most clearly in animals with a horizontal (cow) or a vertical (cat) pupil or by ophthalmoscopic examination of the dorsal retinal vein (see Fig. 13–4). There is a slight deficit in dorsomedial gaze.

Anatomy and Physiology. See Chapter 13.
Assessment. See Chapter 13.

TRIGEMINAL NERVE (C.N. V)

The trigeminal nerve is the motor pathway to the muscles of mastication and the sensory pathway to the face.

Technique. The motor branch of the trigeminal nerve is in the mandibular nerve and innervates the masseter, temporal, rostral digastric, pterygoid, and mylohyoid muscles.[4] Bilateral paralysis produces a dropped jaw that cannot be closed voluntarily. Unilateral lesions may cause decreased jaw tone. Atrophy of the temporal and masseter muscles is recognized by careful palpation approximately 1 week after the onset of paralysis. Sensation should be tested over the distribution of all three branches. A touch of the skin may be an adequate stimulus in some animals, whereas a gentle pinch with a forceps may be needed in others. The palpebral reflex is a blink response to a touch at the medial canthus of the eye, which tests the ophthalmic branch (see Fig. 3–31). Touching the lateral canthus tests the maxillary branch. The blink response is

dependent on the innervation of the muscles by the facial nerve. Stimulation of the nasal mucosa tests the maxillary branch and should elicit a response even in depressed or stoic animals (see Fig. 3–34). Pinching the jaw tests the mandibular branch.

Anatomy and Physiology. See Chapter 12.
Assessment. See Chapter 12.

ABDUCENT NERVE (C.N. VI)

The abducent nerve innervates the lateral rectus and the retractor bulbi muscles.

Technique. Eye movements are tested by the method described for the oculomotor nerve. The retractor bulbi muscles can be tested with a palpebral or a corneal reflex. Normally, the globe is retracted, allowing extrusion of the third eyelid. Lesions of the abducent nerve cause a loss of lateral (abducted) gaze and medial strabismus combined with an inability to retract the globe (see Fig. 13–4).

Anatomy and Physiology. See Chapter 13.
Assessment. See Chapter 13.

FACIAL NERVE (C.N. VII)

The facial nerve is the motor pathway to the muscles of facial expression and the sensory pathway for taste to the palate and the rostral two thirds of the tongue.

Technique. Asymmetry of the face usually is seen in cases of facial paralysis. The lips, the eyelids, and the ears may droop. The nose may be slightly deviated to the normal side, and the nostril may not flare on inhalation. The palpebral fissure may be slightly widened and will fail to close when a palpebral or a corneal reflex is attempted. Pinching the lip will produce a behavioral response, but the lip may not retract. The examiner can test the animal's sense of taste by moistening a cotton-tipped applicator stick with atropine and touching it to the rostral part of the tongue. The affected side is tested first. Normal dogs will react immediately to the bitter taste. Delayed reactions may occur as the atropine spreads to normal areas of the tongue.

Anatomy and Physiology. See Chapter 12.
Assessment. See Chapter 12.

VESTIBULOCOCHLEAR NERVE (C.N. VIII)

The vestibulocochlear nerve has two branches: the cochlear division, which mediates hearing, and the vestibular division, which provides information about the orientation of the head with respect to gravity.

Technique

COCHLEAR DIVISION. Most tests for hearing are dependent upon behavioral reactions to sound and therefore are subject to misinterpretation. There is no good test for unilateral deficits other than those involving electrophysiologic systems. Crude tests involve startling the animal with a loud noise (clap, whistle). Similar responses may be monitored on an electroencephalogram (EEG) or by observation or direct measurement of the respiratory cycle. Human audiometry equipment also can be adapted for animal use. The most precise measurement involves the use of a signal-averaging computer, which measures electrical activity of the brain stem in response to auditory stimuli (brain stem auditory-evoked response—*BAER*).[22] BAER not only detects deafness but also indicates the location of the lesion (see Chapter 6).

VESTIBULAR DIVISION. Abnormalities of the vestibular system produce several characteristic signs. Most vestibular lesions are unilateral, except in congenital anomalies and, occasionally, in inflammatory diseases. Unilateral vestibular disease usually produces ataxia, nystagmus, and a head tilt to the side of the lesion.[23]

The head tilt should be apparent on observation (see Fig. 3–4). The examiner can accentuate the head tilt by removing visual compensation or by removing tactile proprioception. Ataxia (an uncoordinated, staggering gait) usually is accompanied by a broad-based stance and a tendency to fall or to circle to the side of the lesion.

Nystagmus should be observed with the head held in varying positions. The direction of the fast component is noted (for example, left horizontal nystagmus). Forced deviation of the globe (strabismus) also may be seen when the head is elevated or lowered. Producing eye movements by moving the animal's head from side to side (see the section on C.N. III) also tests the vestibular system (see Fig. 3–33). Vestibular lesions may alter the direction or may abolish the response. In some cases, the eyes will not move together (dysconjugate movement).

Postrotatory nystagmus may help to evaluate vestibular disease. As an animal is rotated rapidly, physiologic nystagmus is induced. When rotation is stopped, nystagmus (postrotatory) occurs in the opposite direction and is observed for a short time. The receptors opposite the direction of rotation are stimulated more than the ipsilateral receptors, because they are farther from the axis of rotation. Unilateral lesions will produce a difference in the rate and the duration of postrotatory nystagmus when the animal is tested in both directions. The test is performed in the following manner: The animal is held by an assistant, who rapidly turns 360 degrees ten times and then stops. The examiner counts the beats of nystagmus. After several minutes, the test is repeated in the opposite direction. Normal animals will have three to four beats of nystagmus with the fast phase opposite the direction of rotation. Peripheral lesions usually depress the response when the animal is rotated away from the side of the lesion. Central lesions may depress or prolong the response.

The caloric test is a specific test for vestibular function. This test has the advantage of assessing each side independently. It is difficult to perform in many animals, however, and may be unreliable if the patient is uncooperative. Negative responses occur in many normal animals. The examiner performs the test by holding the animal's head securely in one position, irrigating the ear canal with ice water, and observing for nystagmus. A rubber ear syringe should be used for the irrigation. Usually, 50 to 100 ml of cold water is adequate, and the infusion takes approximately 3 minutes. The test should not be performed if the tympanic membrane is ruptured or if the ear canal is plugged. Nystagmus is induced, with the fast phase away from the side being tested. Warm water also will produce the same effect, except that the nystagmus will be in the opposite direction. The use of warm water is even less reliable. If the animal resists and shakes its head, the response usually is abolished. The test is useful for the evaluation of brain stem function in comatose animals.

Anatomy and Physiology. See Chapter 11.

Assessment. See Chapters 4 and 11.

GLOSSOPHARYNGEAL NERVE (C.N. IX) AND VAGUS NERVE (C.N. X)

C.N. IX and X will be considered together because of their common origin and their common intracranial pathway. The glossopharyngeal nerve is the motor pathway to the muscles of the pharynx along with some fibers from the vagus nerve. The glossopharyngeal nerve also supplies parasympathetic motor fibers to the zygomatic and parotid salivary glands. It is sensory to the caudal one third of the tongue and the pharyngeal mucosa, including the sensation of taste. The vagus nerve is the motor pathway to the pharynx, the larynx, and the palate and supplies parasympathetic motor fibers to the viscera of the body, except for the pelvic viscera (which is innervated by sacral parasympathetic nerves). The vagus nerve is the sensory pathway to the caudal pharynx, the larynx, and the viscera of the body.

Technique. Evaluation of taste can be accomplished by the method described for C.N. VII, although it is more difficult to make an accurate assessment of the caudal part of the tongue. The simplest test for function is to observe the palate and the larynx for asymmetry and to elicit a gag or a swallowing response by inserting a tongue depressor to the pharynx. Historical evidence of an inability to swallow may be suggestive of an abnormality in C.N. IX and X. The clinician should be cautious when examining animals with swallowing problems, since dysphagia is one of the signs of rabies.

Anatomy and Physiology. See Chapter 12.
Assessment. See Chapter 12.

ACCESSORY NERVE

The accessory nerve is the motor pathway to the trapezius muscle and parts of the sternocephalicus and brachiocephalicus muscles.

Technique. The detection of an abnormality in an accessory nerve injury may be difficult, except by careful palpation for atrophy of the affected muscles (Fig. 3–37). Passive movement of the head and the neck may demonstrate a loss of resistance to lateral movements in a contralateral direction.

Anatomy and Physiology. The accessory nerve arises from fibers in the ventral roots of C1–C7 spinal cord segments and from the medulla. The fibers course cranially as the spinal root of the accessory nerve, which lies between the dorsal and the ventral spinal nerve roots. It emerges from the skull by way of the jugular foramen and the petro-occipital fissure. It then courses caudally in the neck to innervate the trapezius and portions of the sternocephalicus and brachiocephalicus muscles. These muscles elevate and advance the limb and fix the neck laterally.[4]

Assessment. Lesions of the accessory nerve either are rare or are rarely recognized. An injury to the nerve in the spinal canal or the cranium probably would be masked by other, more severe signs of paresis. The course of the nerve in the neck is well-protected by muscle but could be damaged by deep penetrating wounds or contusion. Atrophy of the affected muscles would be the most obvious sign of injury. Lesions in the spinal canal should produce other signs of spinal cord dysfunction.

HYPOGLOSSAL NERVE

The hypoglossal nerve is the motor pathway to the intrinsic and extrinsic muscles of the tongue and the geniohyoideus muscle.

Technique. The muscles of the tongue protrude and retract it. Each side is innervated independently. The protrusion of the tongue is tested by wetting the animal's nose and observing the ability to extend the tongue forward (see Fig. 3–35). The strength of retraction

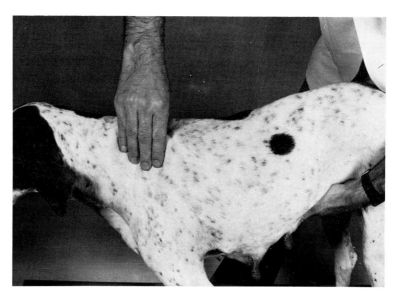

Figure 3–37. Palpation of the trapezius muscle for atrophy evaluates the accessory nerve.

can be tested by grasping the tongue with a gauze sponge. Atrophy can be observed if the lesion has been present for 5 to 7 days.

Anatomy and Physiology. See Chapter 12.
Assessment. See Chapter 12.

Sensation

The sensory examination provides information relative to the anatomic location and the severity of the lesion. At this point in the neurologic examination, sensation has been tested by assessment of the cranial nerves, the spinal reflexes, and proprioceptive positioning. Sensory modalities still to be tested include touch, superficial pain, and deep pain from the limbs and the trunk.

Technique. The evaluation of sensation begins caudally and progresses cranially. The severity of the stimulus is increased from light touch to a deep palpation. If no response occurs, a sharp pin prick and then a hard pinch are used. A significant behavioral response at any step indicates the presence of sensation, and more severe stimuli are not needed once sensation has been established. If a dog turns and snaps when its toe is touched, there is no need to squeeze the toe with a hemostat![24]

During palpation of the animal, areas of increased sensitivity (hyperesthesia) are noted. The rear limbs are palpated first, followed by the spinal column. Beginning with L7 and progressing cranially, the examiner squeezes the transverse processes. Alternatively, one can press each dorsal spinous process firmly. While palpating the spine, it is useful for the examiner to place the other hand on the animal's abdomen in order to detect increased tension in the abdominal muscles as sensitive areas are palpated (Fig. 3–38). Localized areas of hyperesthesia are detected in this manner.

The area of hyperesthesia may be defined more precisely by gently pricking or pinching the skin with an 18G needle or a hemostat. Again, pin pricking should be performed systematically, in a caudal to cranial direction (Fig. 3–39). Two responses may be observed: a twitch of the skin (the panniculus reflex) or a behavioral response, such as a display of anxiety, an attempt to escape, a turning of the head, or a vocalization. When evaluating spinal cord disorders, the examiner tests the skin just lateral to the midline. The test is repeated on a line lateral to the site of the first evaluation and then is repeated on the opposite side. The cranial and caudal margins of a hyperesthetic area can be determined bilaterally. Spinal cord or nerve root lesions produce an area of hyperesthesia, or a transition from decreased to normal sensation, in a pattern conforming to the dermatomal distribution of the nerves (Fig. 3–40). Pin pricking the neck is unreliable for localizing cervical lesions. Manipulation of the head and the neck and deep palpation of the cervical vertebrae are more useful for localizing pain in this area.

A noxious stimulus that elicits any behavioral response is adequate for determining the presence of deep pain. When a response is difficult to elicit, a hemostat is used to squeeze a digit. *Withdrawal of the limb is not a behavior-*

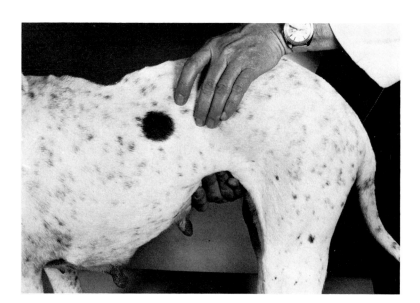

Figure 3–38. Deep palpation may elicit areas of hyperesthesia. Minimal response may be detected by simultaneously palpating adjacent areas for changes in muscle tone (guarding reaction).

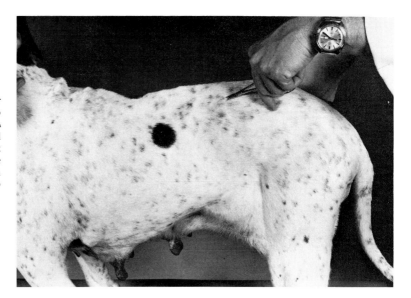

Figure 3–39. Gentle pricking or pinching of the skin can be used to outline the area of hyperesthesia more precisely. Both behavioral reactions and the panniculus reflex may be elicited. The skin should be stimulated dorsally and laterally in order for the examiner to develop a map of abnormal reaction.

ial response (see the section on the flexor reflex in this chapter).

Anatomy and Physiology. Newer concepts emphasize the integration and interaction of all sensory systems. Descending motor pathways have been found to modify sensation. The concepts presented in this section are in general agreement with current research and are adequate for the clinical interpretation of sensory signs.[24–32]

Sensory fibers from the skin, the muscles, the joints, and the viscera enter the spinal cord at each segment by way of the dorsal nerve root. Fibers that innervate the skin are arranged in regular patterns called *dermatomes* (see Fig. 3–40). A dermatome is the area of skin

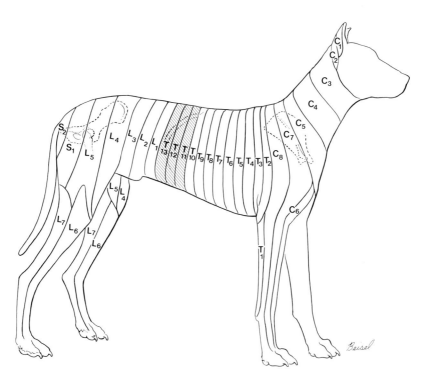

Figure 3–40. Dermatomes of the dog. This illustration is a composite interpretation of several studies.[29–31,33] Dermatomes vary slightly among individuals, and overlapping innervation of approximately three segments is present, as indicated in T11–T13.

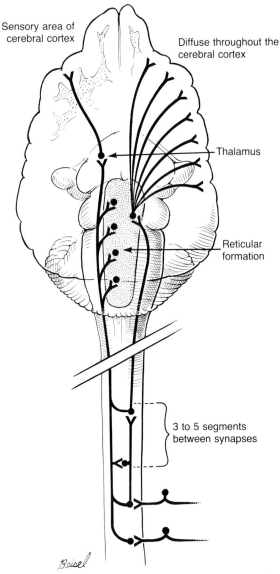

scious proprioception and sensitivity to touch, temperature, and superficial pain.[32]

The deep pain pathway (spinoreticular and propriospinal tracts) is interrupted at three- to five-segment intervals to synapse on neurons in the spinal cord gray matter. These neurons give rise to axons, which rejoin the pathway on the same side or on the opposite side. The deep pain system is bilateral and multisynaptic and is composed of small diameter fibers (Fig. 3–41).[26,27]

The *panniculus reflex* is a twitch of the cutaneous muscle in response to a cutaneous stimulus.[25] The sensory nerves from the skin enter by way of the dorsal root. The ascending pathway is probably the same as that for superficial pain. The synapse occurs at the C8, T1 segments with motor neurons of the lateral thoracic nerve that innervates the cutaneous trunci muscle (Fig. 3–42).[25]

Assessment. Alterations in a sensory modality are described as absent (0), decreased (+1), normal (+2), or increased (hyperesthesia, +3). Absent or decreased sensation indicates that there is damage to a sensory nerve or a pathway. Increased sensitivity may indicate irritation of a nerve or, more commonly, irritation of adjacent structures (e.g., disk herniation with irritation of meninges).

The panniculus reflex is most prominent in the "saddle" area of the trunk. It cannot be elicited from stimulation over the sacrum or the neck. The response is absent caudal to the level of a lesion that disrupts the superficial pain pathway. For example, a compression of spinal cord segment L1 results in a normal panniculus response when stimulation is applied to the T13 dermatome but no response caudal to that point.

When alterations in touch, superficial pain, or areas of hyperesthesia are found, the pattern of abnormality is carefully mapped. The pattern generally conforms to one of three possibilities: (1) Transverse spinal cord lesions cause an abnormality in all areas caudal to the lesion. The line of demarcation between normal and abnormal areas follows the pattern of a dermatome (see Fig. 3–40). (2) Hyperesthesia, reflecting an irritation at a spinal cord segment or a nerve root, has the distribution of one or more dermatomes (usually no more than three). (3) Lesions of a peripheral nerve produce a pattern of abnormality conforming to the distribution of that peripheral nerve (Fig. 3–43). One of these three patterns localizes the lesion to a peripheral nerve (e.g., sciatic nerve, radial nerve) or to a spinal cord segment (accurate to within three segments, e.g., L1–L3).

Figure 3–41. The pain pathway in animals is bilateral and multisynaptic (see also Fig. 3–9). The deep pain pathway apparently has synapses every three to five segments, with projections continuing cranially on both sides of the spinal cord.

innervated by one spinal nerve root. Because of overlap, each strip of skin has some innervation from three segments.[29–31]

Proprioceptive fibers entering the spinal cord may ascend in the dorsal columns and the spinomedullothalamic tract to relay nuclei in the medulla (see Fig. 3–9). Other fibers synapse on neurons in the dorsal horn of the gray matter. The neurons then send axons cranially as one of several named pathways both ipsilaterally and contralaterally (see Fig. 3–9). The primary functions of these pathways include uncon-

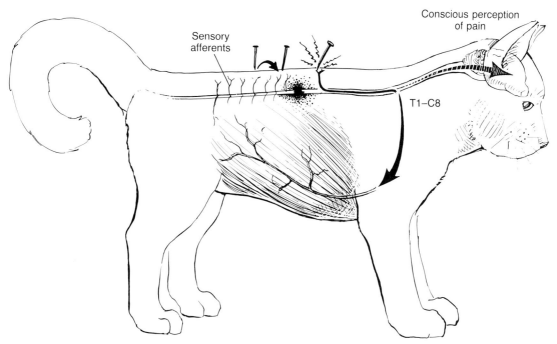

Figure 3–42. The panniculus reflex is the contraction of cutaneous trunci muscle, producing a skin twitch from stimulation of cutaneous sensory fibers (From Ettinger, S. J.: Textbook of Veterinary Internal Medicine, 2nd ed. Philadelphia, W. B. Saunders Co., 1982. Used by permission.)

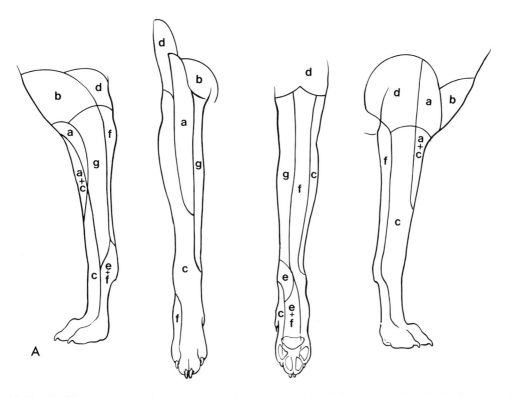

Figure 3–43. *A.* Schema of approximate cutaneous innervation of the right thoracic limb of the dog: *a.* axillary nerve (C6, 7, 8), *b.* brachiocephalic nerve (C5, 6), *c.* radial nerve (C7, 8, T1, 2), *d.* thoracic nerve (T2–T4), *e.* median nerve (includes the branch from the musculocutaneous nerve) (C6, 7, 8, T1, 2), *f.* ulnar nerve (C8, T1, 2), *g.* musculocutaneous nerve (C6, 7, 8).

Illustration continued on following page

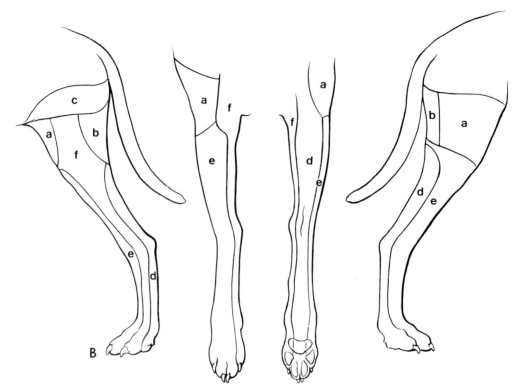

Figure 3–43 *Continued* B. Schema of approximate cutaneous innervation of right pelvic limb of the dog: *a.* lateral cutaneous femoral nerve (L3, *4*, 5), *b.* caudal cutaneous femoral nerve (L7–S1, *2*), *c.* genitofemoral nerve (*L3, 4*), *d.* tibial nerve (L6, *7*, S1), *e.* peroneal nerve (L6, *7*, S1), *f.* saphenous nerve (femoral) (L4, *5*). (Modified from Evans, H. E., and deLahunta, A.: Miller's Guide to the Dissection of the Dog. Philadelphia, W. B. Saunders Co., 1971 and Kitchell, R. W., et al.: Electrophysiologic studies of cutaneous nerves of the thoracic limb of the dog. Am. J. Vet. Res. 41:61–76, 1980.)

The presence or absence of sensation provides an important assessment of the extent of neural damage, especially in compressive lesions. When nerves are compressed, large nerve fibers are the first to lose function. With greater compression, small nerve fibers may be affected. In the spinal cord, loss of function develops in the following sequence: (1) loss of proprioception, (2) loss of voluntary motor function, (3) loss of superficial pain sensation, (4) loss of deep pain sensation. Therefore, an animal with a spinal cord compression that has lost proprioception and voluntary motor function (paralyzed) but still has superficial and deep pain sensation has less spinal cord damage than one that has lost all four functions (see Chapter 2). A loss of deep pain sensation indicates a severely damaged spinal cord and a poor prognosis.

CASE HISTORIES

Learning to assess the findings of the neurologic examination requires practice. Practice with immediate feedback from an experienced examiner is best but is not always possible. The cases presented here are designed to point out the kinds of abnormalities that may be present in the various reactions and reflexes and to assist you in making decisions regarding normality or abnormality. The history for these cases was presented in Chapter 2.

Case History 3A

Signalment. Canine, West Highland white terrier, female, 6 years old.
History. See Case History 2A (Chapter 2).
Physical Examination. No abnormalities are found other than those detected on the neurologic examination.
Neurologic Examination. The dog is bright, alert, and responsive. She is unable to walk. When placed in a standing position, she falls to the right. The proprioceptive positioning is good on the left thoracic limb, slightly delayed on the left pelvic limb, and absent in the limbs on the right. The hopping reactions appear good in the left thoracic limb, with quick initiation of movement and accurate placement of the limb to support weight. The left pelvic limb has a slow initiation of movement, but the limb is accurately placed. The right

limbs do not initiate movement at all. The tactile and visual placing reactions are prompt and accurate in the left thoracic limb, somewhat delayed and inconsistent in the left pelvic limb, and absent in the right limbs. The quadriceps reflex is a single, brisk response, and withdrawal is present when the toes are touched in the left pelvic limb. The extensor carpi radialis reflex is small but present in the left thoracic limb. Attempts to elicit a triceps or a biceps reflex in the left thoracic limb are unsuccessful, but withdrawal is strong with a weak pinch of the digits. The right pelvic limb has a quadriceps reflex that is slightly more brisk than that of the left pelvic limb. Withdrawal is strong. The extensor carpi radialis reflex is small but present. Withdrawal is weak compared with that of the left thoracic limb. The biceps and triceps reflexes cannot be elicited. The cranial nerves are normal. Sensation is present, except that pinching the skin of the right thoracic limb produces no reaction, and pinching a digit on this limb requires considerably more force to produce a behavioral response than does pinching a digit on the other limbs.

Case History 3B

Signalment. Canine, German shepherd, female, 7 years old.
History. See Case History 2B (Chapter 2).
Physical Examination. There are no significant physical abnormalities other than neurologic dysfunction.
Neurologic Examination. The dog is alert and responsive. She has some difficulty in getting up, especially on a slick surface. When she walks on the grass, there is some swaying of the rear quarters from side to side. Occasionally, she knuckles one of the pelvic limbs and stumbles but does not fall. The pelvic limbs cross at times, but generally they are set wide apart. The thoracic limbs seem normal, but she carries much of her weight on them. The hopping and proprioceptive positioning reactions are good in the thoracic limbs. Hopping on the pelvic limbs is poor. When the dog's weight is shifted laterally, there is a long delay before the leg is moved. When she shifts the leg, it is not moved far enough to support her weight adequately, so that after approximately two hops she falls over. When the digits are knuckled over, she stands in that position without attempting to replace them in a normal position. Both pelvic limbs have similar reactions.

The spinal reflexes are considered normal in the thoracic limbs. The quadriceps reflex is more brisk in the left pelvic limb than in the right. The flexor reflexes are present in both pelvic limbs. The cranial nerves are normal. There are no areas of hyperesthesia on deep palpation of the limb and trunk. The panniculus reflex is present, beginning at approximately L7. The dog immediately reacts to a pinching of the skin of the pelvic limbs in all areas.

Case History 3C

Signalment. Feline, domestic short hair, female, 3 months old.

History. See Case History 2C (Chapter 2).
Physical Examination. No abnormalities are found other than those detected on the neurologic examination.
Neurologic Examination. The kitten is alert and eager to play. The gait is characterized by jerky, exaggerated steps and a swaying of the body. The limbs are picked up rapidly and slapped on the floor. At times, it appears that she stops the step before reaching the floor and lurches to one side. She tries to grab a piece of string with the thoracic limbs but is seldom successful. A tremor of the head is noticed at times. All postural reactions can be performed, but the movements are exaggerated. Initiation of hopping is slightly delayed, and the response is often too far or too short for proper support of weight. Proprioceptive positioning is present, but the foot is often placed more laterally than expected.

Myotatic reflexes are difficult to perform because the kitten is so excited. Flexor reflexes are present in all four limbs.

The menace reaction is absent in both eyes, although the kitten can follow movements of objects, such as the piece of string. At times, there is a slight side-to-side oscillation of the eyes. There do not appear to be fast and slow components to the eye movements. The pupillary light reflexes and the palpebral reflex are normal.

There is no hyperesthesia, and the kitten feels a weak pinch of the skin on all four limbs. The panniculus reflex is present, starting at approximately S1.

Case History 3D

Signalment. Feline, Siamese, male, 2 years old.
History. See Case History 2D (Chapter 2).
Physical Examination. An ophthalmic examination confirms the diagnosis of anterior uveitis in the right eye. The cat is slightly depressed. No other abnormalities are found other than those detected on the neurologic examination.
Neurologic Examination. The cat is slightly depressed but responsive. The left thoracic limb knuckles over when he walks. A tremor of the head is evident when the cat is active, but it tends to disappear when he is at rest. Palpation reveals atrophy of the triceps and all of the muscles below the elbow of the left thoracic limb. The postural reactions are normal on the right side. The hopping reaction is poor (+1) in the left thoracic limb and absent (0) in the left pelvic limb. The proprioceptive positioning reaction is absent in both limbs on the left side. The extensor carpi radialis and flexor reflexes are absent in the left thoracic limb. The quadriceps reflex is exaggerated (+3) in the left pelvic limb as compared with the right pelvic limb. The flexion reflex is present and of approximately the same strength on the left pelvic limb as on the right pelvic limb. Perineal reflexes are present. The cranial nerves are normal, except for miosis of the left eye, which presumably is related to the uveitis. There are no areas of hyperesthesia, and sensation is intact, including superficial and deep pain sensation in the left thoracic limb.

Case History 3E

Signalment. Canine, Yorkshire terrier, male, 8 months old.

History. See Case History 2E (Chapter 2).

Physical Examination. The dog is very thin but otherwise normal.

Neurologic Examination. At the time of the initial examination, the dog is normal. Because of the history and the suspicion of metabolic disease, the dog is hospitalized for further evaluation. Food is withheld for 12 hours, blood and urine are collected for laboratory examination, and the dog is given a meal of cat food. Six hours later, the dog is re-examined. At this time, he seems depressed. Although his gait seems relatively normal, he walks continually around the room. The movement of the limbs is somewhat jerky, and he occasionally bumps into a chair or a table. Postural reactions are present, but they all appear to be somewhat slow in all limbs. The dog becomes agitated during these reactions. If he is restrained on the table, he becomes quiet and almost goes to sleep. The spinal reflexes are normal. The menace response is present at times but is not consistent. Other cranial nerve responses are normal. The dog's reaction to painful stimuli is somewhat slow but present.

ASSESSMENT 3A

The dog's mental status suggests that the cerebrum, the diencephalon, and the rostral brain stem are relatively normal. The dog cannot support weight and cannot move the right limbs voluntarily—a hemiparesis. Is the problem strictly unilateral? This question is answered by the assessment of postural reactions. The right side is obviously abnormal. The left thoracic limb has normal postural reactions, but there is some delay in the initiation of the hopping reaction in the left pelvic limb. Is that finding abnormal? The answer is maybe. If the hopping reaction is only slightly delayed, you should be cautious in calling it abnormal. Most dogs do not hop as well on the pelvic limbs as on the thoracic limbs. Placing reactions also are difficult to assess in the pelvic limbs. Proprioceptive positioning is more reliable, and this reaction is normal in the pelvic limb. The extensor postural thrust reaction also can be helpful. In this dog, it appears to be somewhat slow in initiation. We assessed the postural reactions as absent on the right, normal in the left thoracic limb, and questionable in the left pelvic limb.

The quadriceps reflex in the left pelvic limb is brisk but not abnormal for this breed. Smaller dogs have relatively brisk reflexes. The significant finding is that the right quadriceps reflex is stronger than the left. Comparing the two sides gives the examiner a built-in control. We assessed the left quadriceps reflex as normal (+2) and the right as exaggerated (+3). Withdrawals (flexor reflex) are present and strong in both pelvic limbs. The extensor carpi radialis reflex is small, but present and approximately equal, in both thoracic limbs. This reflex is rarely strong and usually is abnormal if it is strong. The triceps and biceps reflexes are absent in both thoracic limbs. Is this finding abnormal? Not in our

assessment. These reflexes are so difficult to elicit that we rarely use them. The flexor reflex is markedly weaker on the right than on the left. This is the most significant finding. Either the sensory or motor neurons (or both) of the reflex are damaged. The sensory examination is useful for deciding which are involved.

Sensation, both superficial and deep, is normal, except in the right thoracic limb. No response is obtained to pinching or to pin pricking the skin distal to the elbow. The rostral, caudal, medial, and lateral surfaces are similar. The dog does not respond to a forceful pinch of the digits. The mapping of the distribution of sensory deficits is important for differentiating peripheral nerve lesions from spinal cord lesions.

The localization of the lesion in this case will be discussed at the end of Chapter 4.

ASSESSMENT 3B

The gait can be described as pelvic limb ataxia and paresis. The swaying movements of the rear quarters indicate some loss of function in paraspinal muscles. The hopping reactions are indicative of both sensory and motor deficits. The slow initiation of the reaction usually means that proprioception is poor. This finding is also confirmed by the complete absence of proprioceptive positioning. The inadequate movement of the limb as the weight is shifted indicates some paresis and loss of motor function. This dog also has some asymmetry in the quadriceps reflex, with the left slightly more brisk than the right. The dog's cranial nerves and sensation are considered normal.

The localization of the lesion in this case will be discussed at the end of Chapter 4.

ASSESSMENT 3C

The gait can be described as truncal ataxia with dysmetria of all four limbs. There is no paresis at gait or on postural reactions. Dysmetria is caused by a loss of coordination between the initiation and the follow-through of a movement. The movement overshoots or undershoots its target. The head tremor was most apparent when the kitten initiated a movement and disappeared at rest. This is an intention tremor. Postural reactions can be difficult to induce when an animal is uncoordinated, but it is important to determine the presence of any paresis. Spinal reflexes also may be difficult to elicit, especially in a young, excited animal. Flexor reflexes always can be tested. The absent menace reaction ordinarily indicates an abnormality in the visual pathways (afferent) or in the facial nerve (efferent). The animal can see and can follow moving objects, however, and the palpebral reflex is intact.

The localization of the lesion will be discussed at the end of Chapter 4.

ASSESSMENT 3D

The slight depression and the head tremor suggest that this cat has brain disease, although it is possible that these findings are merely manifestations of generalized disease. The lameness of the left thoracic limb suggests a more focal abnormality. The postural reactions confirm the diagnosis of an abnormality in this limb and in the left pelvic limb; therefore, this is a hemiparesis. The spinal reflexes are absent in the left thoracic limb and present (flexion) to exaggerated (quadriceps reflex) in the left pelvic limb. Atrophy of the muscles of the left thoracic limb is also significant. You immediately should wonder whether the atrophy is a result of disuse or denervation. The history does not give a clear indication of the duration of the lameness. (Disuse atrophy is slow, whereas denervation atrophy is rapid.) You should note, however, that the triceps and the muscles below the elbow are atrophied, but the flexors of the elbow and the scapular muscles are not. This finding is strongly indicative of denervation rather than disuse. The sensory examination indicates that the afferent nerves of the limb are intact. With a peripheral nerve lesion, one would expect both motor and sensory loss. Atrophy, loss of reflexes, and intact sensation indicate a lesion in the ventral spinal nerve roots or the motor neurons in the spinal cord. The postural reaction deficits in the pelvic limb on the same side indicate spinal cord disease.

The localization of the lesions will be discussed at the end of Chapter 4.

ASSESSMENT 3E

In addition to being depressed, the dog makes inappropriate responses. He becomes agitated during postural reaction testing but then dozes off when restrained on the table. The menace reaction is not always present. A sharp tap on the eyelid (palpebral reflex) followed by a menacing gesture almost always elicits a response. Menacing gestures at other times may not produce a reaction. This finding is suggestive of inattention rather than a loss of vision and may be seen in animals that are severely depressed, disoriented, or demented. The reaction to painful stimuli is interpreted similarly.

The localization of the lesion will be discussed at the end of Chapter 4.

REFERENCES

1. Oliver, J. E., Jr.: Neurologic examinations: Observations on mental status. VM/SAC 67:654–659, 1972.
2. Oliver, J. E., Jr.: Neurologic examinations: Observations on posture. VM/SAC 67:882–884, 1972.
3. Oliver, J. E., Jr.: Neurologic examinations: Observations on movement. VM/SAC 67:1105–1106, 1972.
4. deLahunta, A: Veterinary Neuroanatomy and Clinical Neurology. Philadelphia, W. B. Saunders Co., 1977.
5. Hoerlein, B. F.: Canine Neurology: Diagnosis and Treatment. Philadelphia, W. B. Saunders Co., 1978.
6. Grillner, S.: Locomotion in vertebrates: Central mechanisms and reflex interaction. Physiol. Rev. 55:247–303, 1975.
7. Shik, M. L., and Orlovsky, G. N.: Neurophysiology of locomotor automatism. Physiol. Rev. 56:465–501, 1976.
8. Stein, P. S. G.: Motor systems with specific reference to control of locomotion. Annu. Rev. Neurosci. 1:61–81, 1978.
9. Adams, R. D., and Victor, M.: Principles of Neurology. New York, McGraw-Hill Book Co., 1977.
10. Few, A. B.: The study of the clinical signs and necropsy findings resulting from experimentally produced intracranial lesions in the dog. Thesis, Auburn University, Auburn, AL, 1964.
11. Breazile, J. E., Blaugh, B. S., and Nail, N.: Experimental study of canine distemper myoclonus. Am. J. Vet. Res. 27:1375–1379, 1966.
12. Oliver, J. E., Jr.: Neurologic examinations: Palpation and inspection. VM/SAC 67:1327–1328, 1972.
13. Oliver, J. E., Jr.: Neurologic examinations—sensation: Proprioception and touch. VM/SAC 69:295–298, 1974.
14. Palmer, A. C.: Introduction to Animal Neurology, 2nd ed. Oxford, Blackwell Scientific Publications, 1976.
15. Woolsey, C. N.: Postural regulation of the frontal and motor cortex of the dog. Brain 56:353–370, 1933.
16. Roberts, T. D. M.: Neurophysiology of Postural Mechanisms. New York, Plenum Press, 1967.
17. Oliver, J. E., Jr.: Neurologic examinations—spinal reflexes: Myotatic reflex. VM/SAC 68:151–154, 1973.
18. Oliver, J. E., Jr.: Neurologic examinations: Flexion and crossed extension reflexes. VM/SAC 68:383 385, 1973.
19. Oliver, J. E., Jr.: Neurologic examinations—spinal reflexes: Extensor thrust reflex. VM/SAC 68:763, 1973.
20. Kneller, S. K., Oliver, J. E., Jr., and Lewis, R. E.: Differential diagnosis of progressive caudal paresis in an aged German shepherd dog. JAAHA 11:414–417, 1975.
21. Hoff, H. E., and Breckenridge, C. G.: Observations on the mammalian reflex prototype of the sign of Babinski. Brain 79:155, 1956.
22. Marshall, A. E., Byars, T. D., Whitlock, R. H., and George, L. W.: Brainstem auditory evoked response in the diagnosis of inner ear injury in the horse. JAVMA 178:282–286, 1981.
23. Chrisman, C. L.: Disorders of the vestibular system. Comp. Cont. Ed. Pract. Vet. 1:744–752, 1979.
24. Oliver, J. E., Jr.: Neurologic examinations—sensation: Pain. VM/SAC 69:607–610, 1974.
25. Fox, M. W.: Clinical observations on the panniculus reflex in the dog. JAVMA 142:1296–1299, 1963.
26. Breazile, J. E., and Kitchell, R. L.: A study of fiber systems within the spinal cord of the domestic pig that subserve pain. J. Comp. Neurol. 133:373–382, 1968.
27. Kennard, M. A.: The course of ascending fibers in the spinal cord of the cat essential to the recognition of painful stimuli. J. Comp. Neurol. 100:511–524, 1954.
28. Vierck, C. J., Jr., and Luck, M. M.: Loss and recovery of reactivity to noxious stimuli in monkeys with primary spinothalamic cordotomies, followed by secondary and tertiary lesions of other cord sectors. Brain 102:232–248, 1979.
29. Fletcher, T. F., and Kitchell, R. L.: The lumbar, sacral and coccygeal tactile dermatomes of the dog. J. Comp. Neurol. 128:171–180, 1966.
30. Hekmatpanah, J.: Organization of tactile dermatomes C-1 through L-4 in the cat. J. Neurophysiol. 24:129–140, 1961.
31. Kitchell, R. L., Whalen, L. R., Bailey, C. S., and Lohse, C. L.: Electrophysiologic studies of cutaneous nerves of the thoracic limb of the dog. Am. J. Vet. Res. 41:61–76, 1980.
32. Willis, W. D., and Coggeshall, R. E.: Sensory Mechanisms of the Spinal Cord. New York, Plenum Press, 1978.
33. Bailey, C. S., Kitchell, R. L., and Johnson, R. D.: Spinal nerve root origins of the cutaneous nerves arising from the canine brachial plexus. Am. J. Vet. Res. 43:820–825, 1982.

4

CHAPTER

LOCALIZATION OF LESIONS IN THE NERVOUS SYSTEM

INTRODUCTION

The complex combination of clinical signs, the history, and laboratory data compiled on an individual patient can make the diagnosis of a disease seemingly impossible. L. L. Weed has demonstrated the value of independently listing and analyzing all of the patient's problems.[1] A minimum set of data is necessary in order to solve any medical problem. The actual amount of data to be gathered in order to solve a problem may be modified because of risk, cost, or accessibility, as balanced against the severity of the disease. Priorities can be established for collecting data that will rule out the most probable causes of a given clinical sign early. Tests for rare diseases are reserved until last.

Weed's problem-oriented system is eminently suited for neurologic diagnosis. The steps necessary for the management of a neurologic problem are listed in Table 4–1.

Table 4–1. PLAN FOR NEUROLOGIC DIAGNOSIS *

Collect a minimum data base
Identify the problems
Identify one or more problems related to the nervous system
Localize the level of the lesion
Estimate the extent of the lesion within that level
Determine the cause or the pathology
Determine the prognosis with and without therapy

*Modified from Oliver, J. E., Jr.,: Localization of lesions in the nervous system. *In* Hoerlein, B. F.: Canine Neurology, 3rd ed. Philadelphia, W. B. Saunders Co., 1978.

MINIMUM DATA BASE

The initial evaluation of a patient, including a history and a physical examination, usually will provide evidence that a neurologic problem is present (Tables 4–2 and 4–3). Some problems are difficult to classify, for example, syncope versus convulsions or weakness (loss of muscle strength) versus paresis (loss of neural control). The initial physical examination of every patient should include a screening neurologic examination designed to detect the presence of any neurologic abnormality. It should include (1) an observation of the animal's mental status, gait, and posture; (2) a superficial examination of C.N. II (vision), C.N. III (pupils), C.N. V (sensation in the face, the ability to open and close the mouth), C.N. VII (facial expression, the palebral reflex), and C.N. XII (movement of the tongue); (3) an examination of the proprioception of all four limbs; (4) an evaluation of the hopping reactions; and (5) an assessment of sensation (hyperesthesia). Most of these tests are performed in the course of a routine physical examination. For example, the routine assessment of a dog or a cat almost always includes an inspection of the mouth, the pharynx, and the tonsils. The examiner who is conscious of the cranial nerves evaluates C.N. IX and C.N. X (the gag reflex) and C.N. XII (tongue movement) at this time. Similarly, when the face and the eyes are evaluated, C.N. II, C.N. III, C.N. V, C.N. VI, and C.N. VII are tested (see Chapter 3 for a clarification). Animals that have no deficits on this examination rarely have other neurologic deficits.

The minimum data base recommended for an animal with a neurologic problem is listed in Table 4–3. If automated analysis is available, the chemistry profile is recommended so that the cost will not be a major factor. Otherwise, the selection of chemistry profiles should be based on the problems presented. Additions to the data base are recommended for specific problems.

PROBLEM LIST

A problem list is formulated from information obtained for the minimum data base. For each problem, a diagnostic plan is formulated. A diagnostic plan for a neurologic problem includes the following steps: (1) The level of the lesion is localized with a neurologic examination. Confirmation of the lesion may require survey or contrast radiography. (2) The extent of the lesion is estimated both longitudinally and transversely. The neurologic examination

Table 4-2. CLINICAL PROBLEMS IN THE NERVOUS SYSTEM*

Usually of CNS Origin	
Problem	*Localization*
Convulsions	Cerebrum, diencephalon
Altered mental status	Cerebrum, limbic system
Stupor or coma	Brain stem reticular formation
Abnormal behavior	Limbic system
Paresis, paralysis	See Tables 4–5, 4–6, and 4–7
Proprioceptive deficit	Similar to UMN—see Tables 4–5, 4–6, and 4–7
Ataxia	
Head tilt, nystagmus	Vestibular system
Intention tremor, dysmetria	Cerebellum
Proprioceptive deficit, no head involvement	Spinal cord
Hypesthesia, analgesia	See Figure 4–7 or Figure 4–10, C.N. V
Possibly of CNS Origin	
Problem	*Localization*
Syncope	Usually cardiovascular, metabolic
Weakness	See Figure 4–7 and Table 4–6; metabolic or muscular
Lameness	Orthopedic—see Table 4–4
Pain, hyperesthesia	
Generalized	Thalamus, meningitis
Localized	See Figure 4–7 or Figure 4–10, C.N. V
Blindness	
Pupils normal	Occipital cortex (contralateral)
Pupils abnormal	See Chapter 13
Hearing deficit	
No vestibular signs	Cochlea
Vestibular signs	C.N. VIII, labyrinth
Anosmia	Nasal passages, C.N. I
Visceral dysfunction	See Chapter 5

*Modified from Oliver, J. E., Jr.: Localization of lesions in the nervous system. *In* Hoerlein, B. F.: Canine Neurology, 3rd ed. Philadelphia, W. B. Saunders Co., 1978.

provides most of this information, but ancillary diagnostic procedures may be of assistance. (3) The cause of the pathologic process is determined. The history is most useful for

Table 4-3. MINIMUM DATA BASE: NEUROLOGIC PROBLEM*

History
Physical examination
Neurologic examination
Clinical pathology
  CBC   Urinalysis
  Chemistry profile
    BUN levels   Calcium levels
    SGPT levels   Alkaline phosphatase levels
    Fasting blood glucose levels
    Total serum protein levels
    Albumin levels

*Modified from Oliver, J. E., Jr.: Localization of lesions in the nervous system. *In* Hoerlein, B. F.: Canine Neurology, 3rd ed. Philadelphia, W. B. Saunders Co., 1978.

establishing the class of disease (neoplasia, infectious disease, trauma, and so forth). Laboratory, radiographic, or electrophysiologic tests may be necessary in order for the cause of the problem to be substantiated. From this information, the clinician can establish a prognosis with and without appropriate therapy based on information available about the disease (see Table 4–1).

FUNCTIONAL ORGANIZATION OF THE NERVOUS SYSTEM

Comprehensive knowledge of the anatomy and physiology of the nervous system is very useful in clinical neurology; however, the majority of neurologic problems in clinical practice can be diagnosed and managed without knowing the names of tracts or nuclei. This section is intended to provide a guide to local-

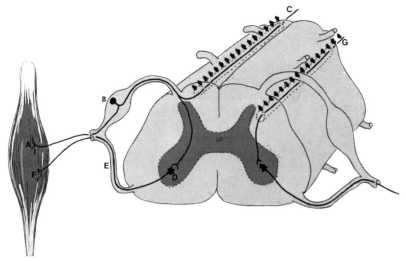

Figure 4–1. Components of the spinal reflex. *A.* Muscle spindle. *B.* Dorsal root ganglion. *C.* Ascending sensory pathway in the dorsal column. *D.* Ventral horn motor neuron (LMN). *E.* Ventral (motor) root. *F.* Neuromuscular junction. *G.* Descending motor pathway in the lateral column (UMN). The dorsal and the ventral roots join to form the peripheral nerve. (From Oliver, J. E., Jr.: Neurologic examination. VM/SAC 68:151–154, 1973. Used by permission.)

ization of lesions for those with minimal knowledge of neuroanatomy.[2]

Motor System

LOWER MOTOR NEURON

Definition

The lower motor neuron (LMN) is an efferent neuron connecting the central nervous system (CNS) to an effector (muscle or gland). Any activity of the nervous system ultimately must be expressed through LMNs located in all spinal segments in the intermediate and ventral horns of the gray matter and in cranial nerve nuclei (C.N. III, C.N. IV, C.N. VI, C.N. VII, C.N. IX, C.N. X, and C.N. XII) in the brain stem. The axons extending from these cells form the peripheral and the cranial nerves (Fig. 4–1).

The nervous system is arranged in a segmental fashion. A spinal cord segment is demarcated by a pair of spinal nerves. Each spinal nerve has a dorsal (sensory) and a ventral (motor) root (Fig. 4–2). The segmentation of the brain is less uniform, but anatomically and functionally distinct sections can be identified (Fig. 4–3). The muscle or group of muscles innervated by one spinal nerve is called a *myotome.* Myotomes are arranged segmentally in the paraspinal muscles but are more irregular in the limbs. A specific muscle dysfunction is detected in order for a lesion to be localized to a spinal nerve or a ventral root (Fig. 4–4).

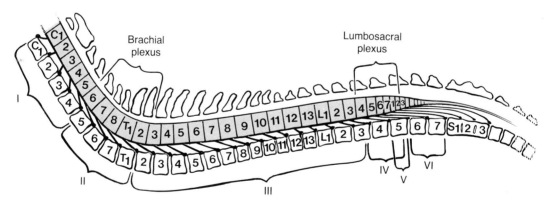

Figure 4–2. The spinal cord has a segmental arrangement; each segment has a pair of spinal nerves. The approximate relationship of spinal cord segments and vertebrae in the dog is illustrated here. Regions of the spinal cord that give rise to characteristic clinical signs when damaged are labeled. *I.* C1–C5, upper motor neuron (UMN) to all limbs. *II.* C6–T2, lower motor neuron (LMN) to thoracic, UMN to pelvic limbs. *III.* T3–L3, normal thoracic, UMN to pelvic limbs. *IV.* L4–S2, normal thoracic, LMN to pelvic limbs. *V.* S1–S3, partial LMN to pelvic limbs, absent perineal reflex, atonic bladder. *VI.* caudal nerves, atonic tail.

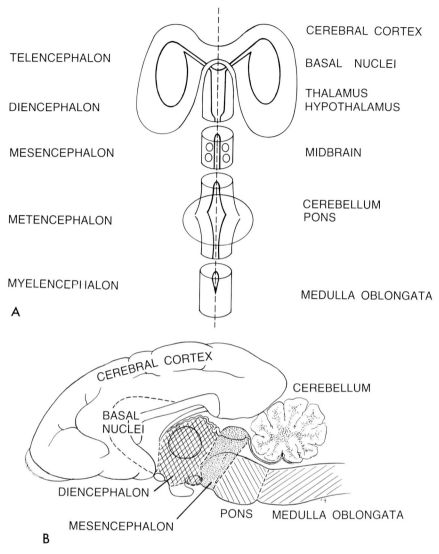

Figure 4–3. Segmental organization of the brain. Five major regions are significant clinically: the cerebrum, including the cerebral cortex and the basal nuclei; the diencephalon, including the thalamus and the hypothalamus; the brain stem, including the midbrain, the pons, and the medulla oblongata; the vestibular system, including the labyrinth (peripheral) and the vestibular nuclei (central) in the rostral medulla; and the cerebellum. (From Hoerlein, B. F.: Canine Neurology, 3rd ed. Philadelphia, W. B. Saunders Co., 1978. Used by permission.)

Signs

Lesions of the LMN, whether of the cell body or the axon, produce a characteristic group of clinical signs summarized in Table 4–4. LMN signs are easily recognized on neurologic examination. Paralysis, loss of tone, and loss of reflexes occur immediately after the neuron is damaged. Proper interpretation of LMN signs allows the clinician to localize accurately lesions to a peripheral nerve, a nerve root, or a motor neuron within the brain or the spinal cord.

Most muscles are innervated by nerves that originate in more than one spinal cord segment. For example, the quadriceps muscle is innervated by neurons originating in segments L4–L6. Loss of one segment or one root causes partial loss of the innervation of the muscle. The clinical sign is paresis, but not paralysis, of the affected muscles. The reflexes may be depressed. Lesions of peripheral nerves cause a more severe loss of function, and all muscles innervated by the nerve are affected. The reflexes are usually absent in this case (see Fig. 4–4).

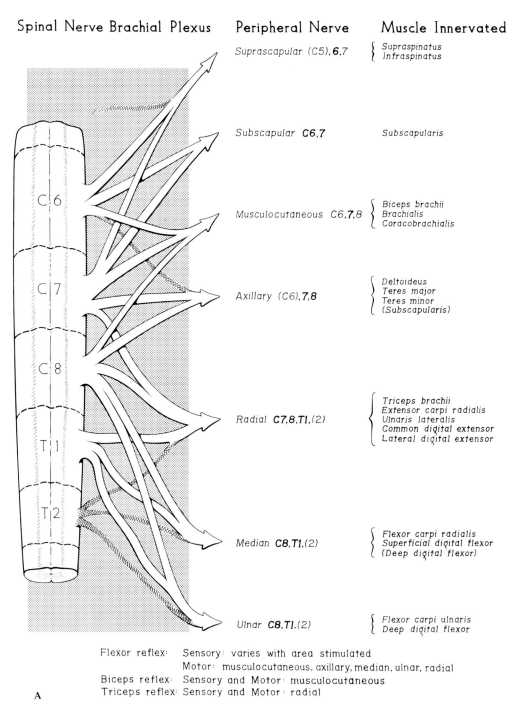

Spinal Nerve Brachial Plexus · Peripheral Nerve · Muscle Innervated

Suprascapular (C5),**6,7**
{ Supraspinatus
  Infraspinatus

Subscapular **C6,7**
  Subscapularis

Musculocutaneous C6,7,8
{ Biceps brachii
  Brachialis
  Coracobrachialis

Axillary (C6),**7,8**
{ Deltoideus
  Teres major
  Teres minor
  (Subscapularis)

Radial **C7,8,T1**,(2)
{ Triceps brachii
  Extensor carpi radialis
  Ulnaris lateralis
  Common digital extensor
  Lateral digital extensor

Median **C8,T1**,(2)
{ Flexor carpi radialis
  Superficial digital flexor
  (Deep digital flexor)

Ulnar **C8,T1**.(2)
{ Flexor carpi ulnaris
  Deep digital flexor

Flexor reflex: Sensory: varies with area stimulated
Motor: musculocutaneous, axillary, median, ulnar, radial
Biceps reflex: Sensory and Motor: musculocutaneous
Triceps reflex: Sensory and Motor: radial

A

Figure 4–4. *A.* Segmental innervation from cervical intumescence of thoracic limb muscles in the dog. *B.* Segmental innervation from lumbosacral intumescence of pelvic limb muscles in the dog. (From deLahunta, A.: Veterinary Neuroanatomy and Clinical Neurology. Philadelphia, W. B. Saunders Co., 1977. Used by permission.)

Illustration continued on opposite page

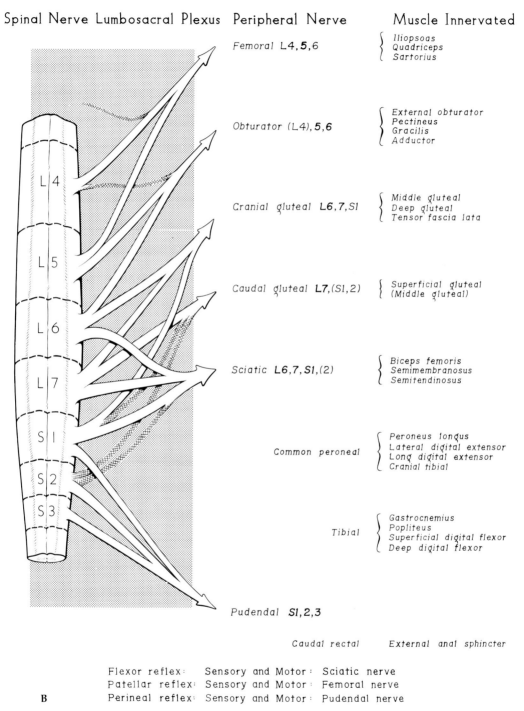

Spinal Nerve Lumbosacral Plexus   Peripheral Nerve   Muscle Innervated

Femoral L4,**5**,6
{ Iliopsoas
Quadriceps
Sartorius

Obturator (L4),**5,6**
{ External obturator
Pectineus
Gracilis
Adductor

Cranial gluteal L6,7,S1
{ Middle gluteal
Deep gluteal
Tensor fascia lata

Caudal gluteal L7,(S1,2)
{ Superficial gluteal
(Middle gluteal)

Sciatic L6,7,S1,(2)
{ Biceps femoris
Semimembranosus
Semitendinosus

Common peroneal
{ Peroneus longus
Lateral digital extensor
Long digital extensor
Cranial tibial

Tibial
{ Gastrocnemius
Popliteus
Superficial digital flexor
Deep digital flexor

Pudendal S1,2,3

Caudal rectal   External anal sphincter

Flexor reflex: Sensory and Motor: Sciatic nerve
Patellar reflex: Sensory and Motor: Femoral nerve
Perineal reflex: Sensory and Motor: Pudendal nerve

B

Figure 4–4. *See legend on opposite page*

UPPER MOTOR NEURON

Definition

Upper motor neuron (UMN) is a collective term for motor systems in the brain that control lower motor neurons. The UMN systems are responsible for the initiation and maintenance of normal movements and the maintenance of tone in the extensor muscles for the support of the body against gravity. The cell bodies are located in the cerebral cortex, the basal nuclei, and the brain stem. The pathways include the corticospinal and corticorubrospinal tracts, primarily responsible for voluntary motor activity, and the reticulospinal and vestibulospinal tracts, responsible for muscle tone and posture (Fig. 4–5).

Signs

UMN lesions produce a characteristic set of clinical signs caudal to the level of the injury. These signs are summarized in Table 4–4 and are compared with signs of LMN lesions. The primary sign of motor dysfunction is paresis. With UMN disease, the paresis or paralysis is associated with increased extensor tone and normal or exaggerated reflexes. Abnormal reflexes (e.g., a crossed extensor) may be seen in some cases. Loss of descending inhibition on the LMN produces these findings. UMN signs

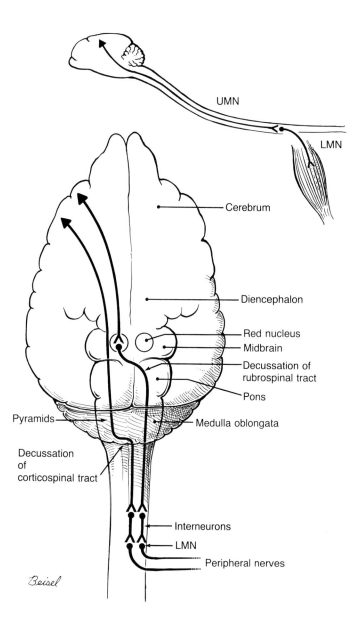

UMN

LMN

Cerebrum

Diencephalon

Red nucleus

Midbrain

Decussation of rubrospinal tract

Pons

Pyramids

Medulla oblongata

Decussation of corticospinal tract

Interneurons

LMN

Peripheral nerves

Beisel

Figure 4–5. Neurons in the cerebral cortex and the brain stem send axons to the lower motor neurons (LMN) in the brain stem and the spinal cord. The upper motor neurons (UMN) provide voluntary control of movement. Two of the major voluntary motor pathways, the corticospinal (pyramidal) pathway and the corticorubrospinal pathway, are illustrated.

Table 4–4. SUMMARY OF LMN AND UMN SIGNS

	LMN: Segmental Signs	UMN: Long Tract Signs
Motor function	Paralysis—loss of muscle power, flaccidity.	Paresis to paralysis—loss of voluntary movements.
Reflexes	Hyporeflexia to areflexia.	Normal to hyperreflexia (especially myotatic reflexes).
Muscle atrophy	Early and severe: neurogenic. Contracture after several weeks.	Late and mild: disuse.
Muscle tone	Decreased.	Normal to increased.
Electromyographic (EMG) changes	Abnormal potentials (fibrillation, positive sharp waves) after 5 to 7 days.	No changes.
Associated sensory signs	Anesthesia of innervated area (dermatome); paresthesia or hyperesthesia of adjacent areas.	Decreased proprioception; decreased perception of superficial and deep pain.

are more common than LMN signs in clinical patients. Because a lesion at many different levels of the CNS may produce UMN signs, localization of a lesion to a specific segment usually is not possible when only UMN signs are considered. Proper interpretation of UMN signs and other associated signs, however, allows one to localize a lesion to a region. For example, UMN paresis of the pelvic limbs indicates that there is a lesion cranial to L4. If the lesion were L4–S2, there would be LMN paresis. If the thoracic limbs are normal, the lesion must be caudal to T2. Therefore, pelvic limb paresis (UMN) with normal thoracic limbs indicates a lesion between T3 and L3.

Sensory System

SEGMENTAL SENSORY NEURONS

Definition

Sensory neurons are located in the ganglia of the dorsal roots along the spinal cord (see Fig. 4–1) and in the ganglia of some cranial nerves. Exceptions are the special sensory pathways (olfaction, vision, hearing, balance).

The area of skin innervated by one spinal nerve is called a *dermatome*. Dermatomes also are arranged in regular, segmental fashion, except for some variation in the limbs (Fig. 4–6). Alterations in the sensation of a dermatome can be used to localize a lesion to a spinal nerve or a dorsal root.

Signs

Lesions of the sensory neurons also produce characteristic clinical signs. Segmental sensory signs include (1) anesthesia (complete le-

sion), (2) hypesthesia (decreased sensation, partial lesion), (3) hyperesthesia (increased sensation of pain, irritative lesion), and (4) loss of reflexes. Increased or decreased sensation of a dermatome can be mapped by pin pricking the skin. Mapping the distribution of sensory loss is accurate to within three spinal cord segments (see Chapter 3).

LONG TRACT SENSORY SIGNS

Definition

Sensory pathways of clinical significance include those responsible for proprioception (position sense) and pain. Sensory neurons from the body are located in the dorsal root ganglia and synapse in the gray matter of the spinal cord (see Fig. 4–1). Proprioceptive pathways are located in the dorsal and the dorsolateral portions of the spinal cord. They project to the cerebral cortex and the cerebellum by relays in the brain stem and the thalamus. Superficial pain pathways (for perception of discrete pain in the skin, e.g., a pin prick) are located primarily in the ventrolateral portion of the spinal cord with a relay in the thalamus.[3] The pathway primarily projects to the contralateral cerebral cortex for conscious recognition of pain. The deep pain pathway (for perception of severe pain in the bones, the joints, or the viscera, e.g., a crushing pain) is a bilateral, multisynaptic system that projects to the reticular formation, the thalamus, and the cerebral cortex.[4,5]

Signs

The signs of sensory long tract lesions are valuable for the formulation of a prognosis of CNS disorders, although they are less useful

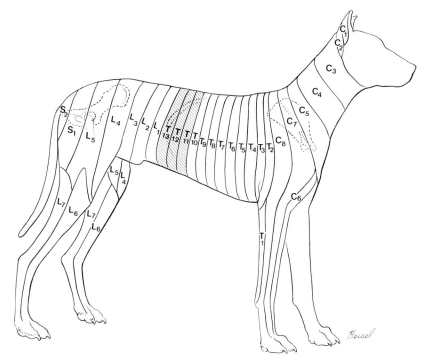

Figure 4–6. Dermatomes of the dog. This illustration is a composite interpretation of several studies (see references 29 through 32 in Chapter 3). Dermatomes may vary slightly among individuals, and overlapping innervation of most areas is present.

for localization. Proprioceptive deficits usually are the first signs observed with compressive lesions of the spinal cord. Abnormal positioning of the feet and ataxia may be present before there is any significant loss of voluntary motor activity. Superficial pain sensation (the conscious perception of a pin prick) and voluntary motor activity often are lost at the same time. Deep pain sensation (perception of a strong pinch of a bone or a joint) is the last neurologic function to be lost during spinal cord compression.[6] Sensation is depressed or absent caudal to the level of the lesion.

LOCALIZATION OF LESIONS

Localization to a Region of the Spinal Cord or the Brain

UMN AND LMN SIGNS

The examination of the motor system should allow the clinician to localize the lesion to one of five levels of the spinal cord or to the brain (see Figs. 4–2 and 4–3). The thoracic and pelvic limbs should be classified as normal or as having LMN or UMN signs (see Table 4–4). Briefly, LMN signs are paresis, a loss of reflexes, and a loss of tone. UMN signs are a loss of volun-

tary motor activity, an increase in tone, and an exaggeration of reflexes. The examiner can localize a lesion to a region of the spinal cord or the brain by using these findings and the material presented in Figure 4–7. For example, UMN signs in both the thoracic and the pelvic limbs indicate a lesion in the brain or in segments C1–C5. Other findings are used to localize the lesion further. In this case, one should examine the cranial nerves in order to rule out brain stem disease. The sensory examination is reviewed for possible signs related to the neck (i.e., C1–C5).

Using only the information related to LMN and UMN signs of the limbs, the examiner can localize the lesion to one of the following regions: (a) the brain, (b) C1–C5, (c) C6–T2—brachial plexus (thoracic limb), (d) T3–L3, (e) L4–S2—lumbosacral plexus (pelvic limb), or (f) S3–Cd5.

PROPRIOCEPTION

For the purpose of localization, abnormalities of proprioception are interpreted in the same way as UMN signs. For example, loss of proprioception in the pelvic limbs with normal thoracic limbs indicates a lesion in the region T3–L3 (Table 4–5). Spinal nerve or peripheral nerve lesions may cause a loss of

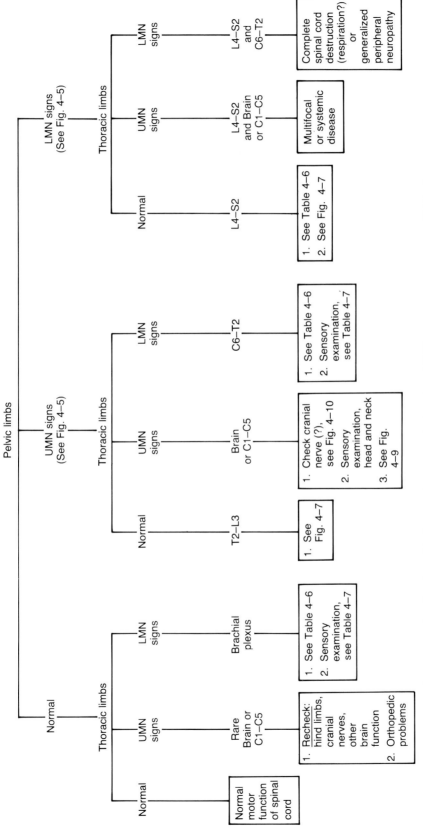

Figure 4–7. Localization of lesion causing motor dysfunction. UMN = upper motor neuron, LMN = lower motor neuron, C = cervical, T = thoracic, L = lumbar, S = sacral spinal cord segments. (Modified from Oliver, J. E., Jr.: Localization of lesions in the nervous system. *In* Hoerlein, B. F.: Canine Neurology, 3rd ed. Philadelphia, W. B. Saunders Co., 1978, pp. 71–102.)

Table 4–5. SPINAL REFLEXES*

Reflex	Muscle(s)	Peripheral Nerve	Spinal Cord Segments†
Myotatic (stretch)	Biceps brachii	Musculocutaneous	(C6), C7–C8, (T1)
	Triceps brachii	Radial	C7–C8, T1, (T2)
	Extensor carpi radialis	Radial	C7–C8, T1, (T2)
	Quadriceps	Femoral	(L3), L4–L5, (L6)
	Cranial tibial	Peroneal (sciatic)	L6–L7, S1
	Gastrocnemius	Tibial	L6–L7, S1
Flexor (withdrawal)	Thoracic limb	Radial, ulnar, median, musculocutaneous	C6–T2
	Pelvic limb	Sciatic	L6–S1, (S2)
Perineal	Anal sphincter	Pudendal	S1–S2, (S3)

*Modified from Oliver, J. E., Jr.: Localization of lesions in the nervous system. In Hoerlein, B. F.: Canine Neurology, 3rd ed. Philadelphia, W. B. Saunders Co., 1978.

†Parentheses indicate segments that sometimes contribute to a nerve.

proprioceptive positioning, but the LMN signs are obvious.

Localization to a Segmental Level of the Spinal Cord

LMN SIGNS

If LMN signs are present in the limbs, the examiner can localize the lesion further by identifying the affected muscles. Table 4–5 lists spinal cord segments (roots) and peripheral nerves for the most commonly tested reflexes. It is possible to localize within two to four segments or to a peripheral nerve if LMN signs are present. Spinal cord segments do not correlate directly with vertebral levels. When you have determined the spinal cord level, refer to Figure 4–2 for an estimation of the vertebral level.

Peripheral nerve lesions usually cause monoparesis (paresis of one limb) because the most common lesions are the result of trauma. Localization of lesions in monoparesis will be reviewed in Chapter 8. The primary exception is generalized peripheral neuropathies, which affect all of the limbs. These conditions will be discussed in Chapter 10.

PAIN

Hyperesthesia (increased sensitivity) is a very useful localizing sign and may be present when there is little or no motor deficit. The animal's limbs and trunk, especially the vertebral column, are palpated and manipulated while the examiner observes for signs of pain.

Obvious reactions may include resistance to movement and tensing of the muscles. If the clinician places one hand on the animal's abdomen while squeezing each vertebral segment with the other hand, increased tension of the abdominal muscles may be elicited as painful areas are palpated. The skin is pricked with an 18G needle after palpation is completed. The skin is pricked lightly so that no significant behavioral reaction is elicited from normal areas. Pin pricking areas of hyperesthesia will elicit an exaggerated skin twitch or a behavioral response.

Pin pricking should be performed in a caudal to cranial direction, because areas caudal to a lesion usually will have decreased skin sensation. A level of normal or increased sensation can be ascertained by this method. If a spinal lesion is present, the sensory level should have the conformation of a dermatome (see Fig. 4–6). Peripheral nerves have a different pattern of sensory distribution (see Fig. 3–43).

The panniculus (cutaneous muscle) reflex is elicited with a needle in the same manner as that just described for detecting hyperesthesia. Cutaneous sensation enters the spinal cord at each segment (dermatomes) and ascends to the brachial plexus (C8–T1) to the *lateral thoracic* nerve, which innervates the cutaneous trunci (panniculus carnosus) muscle. Contraction of the cutaneous muscle causes a skin twitch. A segmental lesion will block the ascending afferent stimulus, abolishing the reflex. Pin pricking the skin in a caudal to cranial direction will identify the first level at which the reflex can be elicited. This segment

Table 4−6. SIGNS OF LESIONS IN THE SPINAL CORD

Site of Lesion	Sign
Cd1–Cd5	LMN—tail
S1–S3	UMN—tail
Pelvic plexus	LMN—anal sphincter, bladder
Pudendal nerve	
L4–S2	UMN—tail
Lumbosacral plexus	LMN—hind limbs
	UMN or LMN—bladder, sphincters
T3–L3	UMN—hind limbs, bladder, sphincter
	LMN—segmental spinal muscles
C6–T2	UMN—hind limbs, bladder
Brachial plexus	LMN—forelimbs
C1–C6 or brain	UMN—all four limbs, bladder

is normal, and the lesion will be one segment caudal to this level. The superficial pain pathways must be blocked in order to abolish the reflex. Normally, the panniculus reflex is most apparent in the thoracolumbar (saddle) area. A minimal response is obtained from a stimulus in the sacral or caudal regions, and no response is obtained from a cervical stimulus. Cervical pain is assessed by manipulation of the neck and deep palpation of the vertebrae. Although it may be difficult to define the location of the pain precisely, it usually is possible to determine whether it is in the rostral, middle, or caudal cervical segments by performing palpation carefully and gently.

Hypesthesia (decreased sensation) or anesthesia (no sensation) also are useful localizing signs. Single nerve root lesions usually will not produce a clinically detectable area of decreased sensation because of the overlapping pattern of cutaneous innervation (see Fig. 4–6). Multiple nerve roots may be involved in some lesions, especially in the area of the cauda equina. Lesions of the spinal cord may result in decreased perception of pain caudal to the lesion. The determination of the level of decreased sensation was discussed previously, and the prognostic implications of the loss of sensation will be discussed later. The motor examination localizes the lesion to one of six regions of the spinal cord or to the brain (Table 4–6). A carefully performed sensory exam-

Table 4−7. SIGNS OF LESIONS IN THE BRAIN

	Mental Status	Posture	Movement	Postural Reactions	Cranial Nerves
Cerebral cortex	Abnormal behavior, depression, seizures	Normal	Gait normal to slight hemiparesis (contralateral)	Deficits (contralateral)	Normal (vision may be impaired—contralateral)
Diencephalon (thalamus and hypothalamus)	Abnormal behavior, depression (Endocrine and autonomic)	Normal	Gait normal to hemiparesis or tetraparesis	Deficits (contralateral)	C.N. II
Brain stem (midbrain, medulla)	Depression, stupor, coma	Normal turning, falling	Hemiparesis to tetraparesis, ataxia	Deficits (ipsi- or contralateral)	C.N. III–C.N. XII
Vestibular, (central medulla)	Depression	Head tilt, falling	Hemiparesis, (usually ipsilateral), ataxia	Deficits (ipsi- or contralateral)	C.N. VIII, may also affect C.N. V and C.N. VII, nystagmus
Vestibular, peripheral (labyrinth)	Normal	Head tilt	Normal to ataxia	Normal, although may be awkward	C.N. VIII, sometimes C.N. VII or Horner's syndrome, nystagmus
Cerebellum	Normal	Normal	Tremors, dysmetria, ataxia	Normal to dysmetria	Normal, may be menace reaction deficit or nystagmus

ination will localize the lesion to within *three segments of the spinal cord* or to a peripheral nerve.

Localization in the Brain

If the lesion has been localized to the brain, the next step is to determine what part of the brain is involved. Localization to one of five regions of the brain or to the peripheral vestibular apparatus (labyrinth) is made on the basis of clinical signs (Table 4–7 and Fig. 4–8).

BRAIN STEM

Lesions of the brain stem (midbrain to medulla oblongata) will produce UMN signs in all four limbs (tetraparesis) or in the fore- and hind limbs on one side (hemiparesis). Abnormal posture, especially of the head and the neck, may be seen. Cranial nerve signs (C.N. III to C.N. XII) are present in brain stem lesions of significant size and provide good localizing signs (LMN or sensory) (Fig. 4–9). The evaluation of cranial nerves is outlined in Table 4–8 (see also Chapters 3, 12, and 13).

Cranial nerve signs are ipsilateral to the lesion, whereas motor signs may be ipsilateral or contralateral, depending on the level and the pathways involved. The animal's mental status may be altered, especially in lesions of the midbrain and the pons, which disrupt the reticular activating system. Signs vary from depression to coma (see Chapter 14).

DIENCEPHALON

Diencephalic lesions (thalamus, hypothalamus) may produce UMN signs in all four limbs (tetraparesis) or in the thoracic and pelvic limbs of one side (hemiparesis), depending on the extent of the lesion. The gait is not severely affected, but postural reaction deficits are obvious. C.N. II (optic) may be affected in diencephalic lesions. Space-occupying lesions (e.g.,

tumors, abscesses) of the diencephalon also may affect C.N. III, C.N. IV, and C.N. VI (see Table 4–8). Cranial nerve signs are *ipsilateral* to the lesion, whereas motor signs are *contralateral* to the lesion. The most characteristic signs of diencephalic lesions are related to abnormal function of the hypothalamus and its connections with the pituitary gland. The hypothalamus is the control center for the autonomic nervous system and most of the endocrine system.

All sensory pathways of the body, with the exception of olfaction, relay in the diencephalon en route to the cerebral cortex. Clinical signs of lesions in these systems usually are not localizing. A generalized hyperesthesia has been described as a result of an abnormality in the relay nuclei of the pain pathways. Large lesions in the diencephalon may produce alterations in the level of consciousness (stupor, coma) because of interference with the reticular activating system (see Chapter 14).

VESTIBULAR SYSTEM

Vestibular signs may be the result of central (brain stem) or peripheral (labyrinth) disease. It is important to differentiate central disease from peripheral disease because of the differences in treatment and prognosis. Signs of vestibular disease include falling, rolling, tilting of the head, circling, nystagmus, positional strabismus (deviation of one eye in certain positions of the head), and an asymmetric ataxia (Figs. 4–10 and 4–11).

Peripheral lesions involve the labyrinth in the petrosal bone. Middle ear lesions (bulla ossea) usually produce a head tilt with no other signs. Horizontal or rotatory nystagmus may be seen occasionally. Inner ear disease, which actually involves the receptors and the vestibular nerve, usually produces one or more of the signs listed earlier in addition to the head tilt. In either case, the head tilt is ipsilateral to the lesion. A Horner's sign (miosis, ptosis, enophthalmos) of the ipsilateral eye may be present with either middle or inner ear disease, because the sympathetic nerves pass through the middle ear in proximity to the petrosal bone. C.N. VII (facial) may be affected in inner ear disease as it courses through the petrosal bone, in contact with the vestibulocochlear nerve (C.N. VIII). The primary characteristics of peripheral vestibular disease are an asymmetric ataxia without deficits in postural reactions and a horizontal, or rotatory, nystagmus that does not change direction with different head positions. The quick phase of

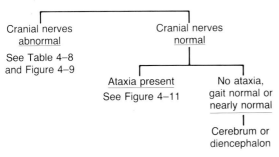

Figure 4–8. Evidence of brain lesion from Figure 4–7.

Text continued on page 75

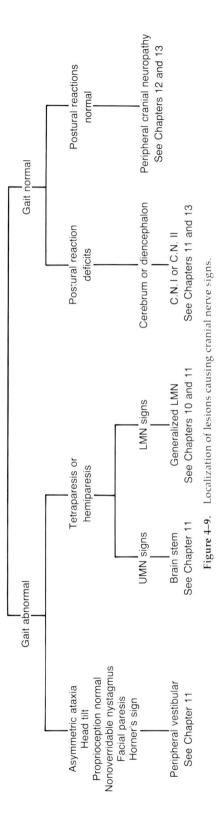

Figure 4–9. Localization of lesions causing cranial nerve signs.

Table 4–8. CRANIAL NERVES

Number and Name	Origin or Termination in Brain	Course	Function	Test	Normal Response	Abnormal Response	Occurrence
C.N. I—Olfactory	Pyriform cortex	Nasal mucosa, cribriform plate, olfactory bulbs, olfactory tract, olfactory stria, pyriform cortex	Sense of smell	Smelling of nonirritating volatile substances (alcohol, food)	Behavioral reaction: aversion or interest	No reaction	Rare: nasal tumors and infections (evaluation difficult)
C.N. II—Optic	Lateral geniculate nucleus (vision), pretectal nucleus (pupillary reflex)	Retina, optic nerve, optic tract, lateral geniculate nucleus, optic radiation, visual cortex or optic tract, pretectal nucleus, parasympathetic nucleus of C.N. III, oculomotor nerve	Vision, pupillary light reflexes	Menace reaction, behavior, placing reaction, pupillary reflex, ophthalmoscope	Blinks, avoids obstacles and responds to visual cues, visual placing good, pupillary light reflexes present, retina normal	No blink, poor avoidance of obstacles, no visual placing, direct pupillary light reflex absent ipsilaterally, retina or optic disk may be abnormal	Optic neuritis, neoplasia, orbital trauma, orbital abscess
C.N. III—Oculomotor	Midbrain, tegmentum (level of rostral colliculus)	Nucleus ventral to mesencephalic aqueduct, exits ventral to midbrain between cerebral peduncles, courses through tentorial notch, runs in cavernous sinus with C.N. IV and C.N. VI, exits orbital fissure	Constriction of pupil; ciliary muscle for accommodation reaction of lens; extraocular muscles: dorsal, ventral, and medial rectus, ventral oblique	Pupillary size, pupillary light reflex, eye position, eye movements	Pupils symmetric, pupils constrict to light, eyes centered in palpebral fissure, eyes move in all directions	Mydriasis, ipsilateral, no direct pupil response, ventrolateral strabismus, no movement except laterally (C.N. VI).	Orbital lesions, tentorial herniation
C.N. IV—Trochlear	Midbrain, tegmentum (level of caudal colliculus)	Nucleus ventral to mesencephalic aqueduct, exits dorsal to tectum, caudal to caudal colliculus, contralateral to origin, courses along ridge of petrosal bone, follows course of C.N. III	Dorsal oblique muscle, rotates dorsal portion of eye medioventrally	Eye position, eye movements	Eye centered in palpebral fissure, eyes move in all directions	Normal, rotation may be detected in animal with elliptical pupil or by position of vessels ophthalmoscopically	Rare—difficult to evaluate

Cranial Nerve	Nucleus	Course	Function	Normal	Abnormal	Diseases
C.N. V—Trigeminal (ophthalmic nerve, maxillary nerve, mandibular nerve)	*Motor nucleus:* pons. *Sensory nucleus:* pons, medulla, C1 spinal cord segment	*Motor:* Pons, exit at cerebellopontine angle, trigeminal canal of petrosal bone, oval foramen, mandibular nerve. *Sensory:* Same except trigeminal ganglion in trigeminal canal; ophthalmic, maxillary, and mandibular nerves	*Motor:* ability to close mouth, jaw tone. *Sensory:* palpebral reflex, pin prick or pinch of face, touch of nasal mucosa	Closed mouth, good jaw tone; no atrophy of temporal or masseter muscles; palpebral reflex present; behavioral response to noxious stimulus	Jaw hangs open (bilateral), poor jaw tone, atrophy, loss of palpebral reflex or behavioral response to noxious stimulus—check all three branches	Idiopathic mandibular paralysis, trigeminal neuritis, cerebellopontine angle tumors, trauma
C.N. VI—Abducent	Medulla (rostral and dorsal)	Medulla, lateral to pyramid, courses ventral to brain stem to join C.N. III and C.N. IV	Lateral rectus muscle, lateral movement of eye (abduct)	Eye position, eye movement	Eye centered in palpebral fissure, eye moves laterally	Medial strabismus, lack of lateral movement of eye	Orbital trauma, orbital abscess, brain stem tumors
C.N. VII—Facial	Medulla (rostral and ventrolateral)	*Motor:* Axons leave nucleus, loop around abducens nucleus, and exit ventrolateral medulla ventral to C.N. VIII to internal acoustic meatus, facial canal in petrosal bone, and stylomastoid foramen to muscles of face. *Taste:* Solitary nucleus and tract, medulla follows course of trigeminal nerve	Muscles of facial expression and taste, rostral two thirds of tongue	Facial symmetry, palpebral reflex, ear movements. *Taste:* atropine to rostral two thirds of tongue with cotton swabs	Face symmetric; normal movements of lips, ears, eyelids; palpebral reflex present; ears move in response to stimulation. *Taste:* aversive reaction immediately	Asymmetry of face, ptosis, lip drops, deviation of nasal philtrum, palpebral reflex absent (check C.N. V), ears do not move, no reaction until mouth is closed and material touches caudal portion of tongue	Idiopathic facial paralysis, inner ear infections, cerebellopontine angle tumors
C.N. VIII—Vestibulocochlear	Vestibular nuclei—medulla, cochlear nuclei—medulla	Inner ear, petrosal bone, internal acoustic meatus, Cerebellomedullary angle, medulla	Equilibrium, hearing	*Vestibular:* Posture and gait, eye movements, rotatory and caloric tests. *Hearing:* Startle response, electrophysiology (EEG alerting, brain stem-evoked response)	*Vestibular:* Normal posture and gait, oculocephalic responses normal, brief postrotatory nystagmus and caloric-induced nystagmus. *Hearing:* Startled reaction to handclap, evoked response present	*Vestibular:* Head tilt, head twist, circling, spontaneous nystagmus, prolonged or absent postrotatory nystagmus, abnormal or absent caloric response. *Hearing:* Poor startle reaction, no evoked response	Otitis media and otitis interna, encephalitis, cerebellopontine angle tumors, idiopathic vestibular disease (cats, old dogs)

Table continued on following page

Table 4–8. CRANIAL NERVES (Continued)

Number and Name	Origin or Termination in Brain	Course	Function	Test	Normal Response	Abnormal Response	Occurrence
C.N. IX—Glossopharyngeal	Medulla (caudal)	Sensory: solitary tract and nucleus Motor: parasympathetic, ambiguus nucleus, exit together along lateral surface of medulla, exit through jugular foramen	Sensory and motor to pharynx and palate, parasympathetic to zygomatic and parotid salivary glands (in C.N. V); sensory: carotid body and sinus	Gag reflex	Swallowing	Poor gag reflex, dysphagia	Rare
C.N. X—Vagus	Medulla (caudal)	Same as C.N. IX	Sensory and motor to pharynx and larynx, thoracic and abdominal viscera	Gag reflex, laryngeal reflex, oculocardiac reflex	Swallowing, coughing, bradycardia	Poor gag reflex, dysphagia, no reaction	Rare
C.N. XI—Accessory	Medulla (caudal) and cervical spinal cord	Ambiguus nucleus of medulla and cervical gray matter, axons run rostrally from cervical cord to join cranial roots, exit jugular foramen	Trapezius and parts of sternocephalicus and brachiocephalicus muscles	Palpate for atrophy of muscles	Normal muscles	Atrophied muscles	Rare
C.N. XII—Hypoglossal	Medulla (caudal)	Axons exit medulla lateral to pyramid, hypoglossal canal to tongue	Movements of tongue	Protrusion of tongue (wet nose), retraction of tongue	Tongue protrudes symmetrically and can lick in both directions, strong withdrawal of tongue	Tongue deviates to side of lesion, atrophy, weak withdrawal	Brain stem tumors, trauma

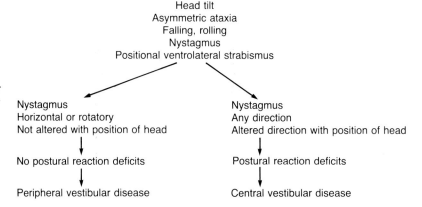

Figure 4–10. Algorithm for differentiation of central and peripheral vestibular diseases.

the nystagmus will be away from the side of the lesion (see Fig. 4–10).

Any signs of brain stem disease in association with vestibular signs indicate that central involvement is present. The most frequent differentiating feature is a deficit in postural reaction. Peripheral vestibular disease does not cause paresis or loss of proprioception, whereas central disease frequently does. Postural reactions must be evaluated critically, because an animal with peripheral vestibular disease has deficits in equilibrium, which make the performance of tests such as hopping awkward. An evaluation of proprioceptive positioning is an excellent method for discrimination. Alterations in mental status or deficits in C.N. V and C.N. VI also are indicative of central disease (see Fig. 4–10).

Lesions near the caudal cerebellar peduncle may produce what has been called a paradoxical vestibular syndrome. The signs are usually similar to those of central vestibular disease except that the direction of the head tilt is contralateral to the side of the lesion.[7]

Bilateral vestibular disease, which is usually peripheral, produces a more symmetric ataxia. The head often jerks from side to side. There is no nystagmus, and vestibular eye movements are usually absent.[8]

CEREBELLUM

Cerebellar lesions may be unilateral or bilateral, depending on the etiology. Characteristic signs include ataxia, a wide-based stance, dysmetria, and an intention tremor with little weakness. An involvement of the head differentiates cerebellar lesions from spinal tract lesions, which may produce similar signs in the limbs. For example, dysmetria usually is recognized as a severe head drop when the head is elevated and suddenly released. The animal

may stick its nose too far into its water dish when drinking or may even hit the edge of the dish. Intention tremors are uncoordinated movements that become much worse as the animal initiates an activity such as eating or drinking (see Fig. 4–11).[8]

Nystagmus may occur in cerebellar disease, but it is usually more of a tremor of the globe than the slow-quick (jerk) movements associated with vestibular disease. Cerebellar nystagmus is most pronounced as the animal shifts its gaze and fixates on a new field (an intention tremor).

Lesions of the anterior lobe of the cerebellum may produce increased extensor tone and opisthotonos, especially in acute lesions such as trauma. These signs are most pronounced when combined with brain stem lesions at the level of the midbrain or the pons.

Lesions of the flocculonodular lobes of the cerebellum produce signs similar to vestibular disease, including a loss of equilibrium, nystagmus, and a tendency to fall (see Chapter 11).

Diffuse cerebellar lesions may cause the menace reaction to be absent even if vision is normal.

CEREBRAL CORTEX

Cortical lesions usually will produce alterations in behavior or mental status, seizures, loss of vision with intact pupils, and a mild hemiparesis with deficits in postural reactions. Only one or two of these signs may be present, because the cerebrum is a relatively large structure with well-localized functional areas. Signs are generally contralateral to the lesion.

Behavioral changes usually reflect a lesion of the limbic system or the frontal lobe of the cortex. Frontal lobe lesions often cause a disinhibition that results in *excessive pacing of the an-*

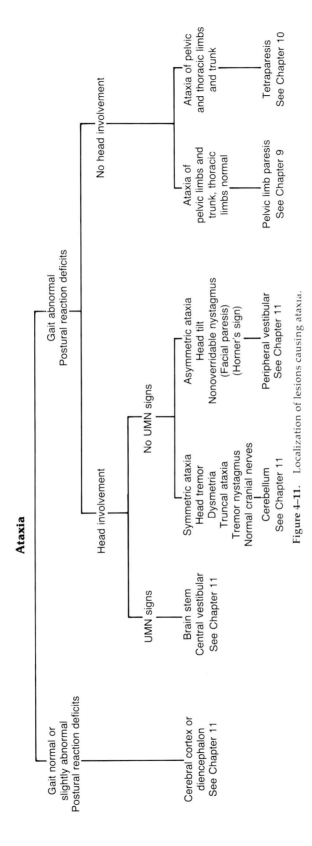

Figure 4–11. Localization of lesions causing ataxia.

imal. Compulsive pacing may continue until the animal walks into a corner and stands with its head pressed against the obstruction (see Chapter 16).

Depression, stupor, and coma represent decreasing levels of consciousness caused by a separation of the cerebral cortex from the reticular activating system of the brain stem. Severe depression usually is caused by brain stem lesions (see Chapter 14). Conscious visual perception requires intact visual pathways to the occipital lobes of the cerebral cortex. Occipital cortical lesions will cause blindness with intact pupillary reflexes (see Chapter 12).

The sensorimotor cortex is important for voluntary motor activity but is not necessary for relatively normal gait and posture. Animals with lesions in this area can stand, walk, and run with minimal deficits. The animal's ability for fine discrimination is lost, however, and it is unable to avoid obstacles smoothly or to perform fine maneuvers such as walking on the steps of a ladder. Markedly abnormal postural reactions are found.

Localization to one of the five regions of the brain is usually adequate for a clinical diagnosis. Cranial nerve signs provide positive evidence for precise localization within the brain stem.

Clinical signs referable to several parts of the nervous system indicate diffuse or multifocal disease, such as infection, metabolic disorder, or malignant neoplasia (see Chapter 17).

CASE HISTORIES

You now should be able to localize the lesion in the cases presented in Chapters 2 and 3. The signalment and pertinent neurologic abnormalities will be repeated. Make your assessment before reading ours.

Case History 4A

Signalment

West Highland white terrier, female, 6 years old.

History

Found down in back yard 4 days ago. Some voluntary movements in left thoracic and pelvic limbs. No change since onset. No pain observed. Appetite and eliminations normal. (See Case History 2A, Chapter 2.)

Physical Examination

Nothing significant found.

Neurologic Examination *

(See Case History 3A, Chapter 3.)
A. Observation
   1. Mental status: Alert.
   2. Posture: Recumbent; falls to right when placed on feet.
   3. Gait: None.
B. Palpation
   No abnormalities.

C. Postural Reactions

Left	Reactions	Right
	Proprioceptive positioning	
+1	PL	0
+2	TL	0
NE	Wheelbarrowing	NE
+1	Hopping, PL	0
+2	Hopping, TL	0
NE	Extensor postural thrust	NE
NE	Hemistand-hemiwalk	NE
NE	Tonic neck	NE
	Placing, tactile	
+1	PL	0
+2	TL	0
	Placing, visual	
+1	PL	0
+2	TL	0

---

*Key: 0 = absent, +1 = decreased, +2 = normal, +3 = exaggerated, +4 = very exaggerated or clonus, PL = pelvic limb, TL = thoracic limb, NE = not evaluated.

D. Spinal Reflexes

Left	Reflex / Spinal Segment	Right
+2	Quadriceps / L4–L6	+3
+2	Extensor carpi radialis / C7–T1	+2
NE	Triceps / C7–T1	NE
+2	Flexion, PL / L5–S1	+2
+2	Flexion, TL / C6–T1	+1
0	Crossed extensor	0
+2	Perineal / S1–S2	+2

E. Cranial Nerves

Left	Nerve + Function	Right
+2	C.N. II vision menace	+2
	C.N. II + C.N. III pupil size	
	Stim. left eye	
	Stim. right eye	
	C.N. II fundus	
	C.N. III, C.N. IV, C.N. VI Strabismus	
	Nystagmus	
	C.N. V sensation	
	C.N. V mastication	
	C.N. VII facial muscles	
	Palpebral	
	C.N. IX, C.N. X swallowing	
	C.N. XII tongue	

F. Sensation: Location
   Hyperesthesia _____ None _____
   Superficial pain Decreased in right thoracic limb
   Deep pain Decreased in right thoracic limb

Complete sections G and H before reviewing Case Summary.

G. Assessment (Anatomic diagnosis and estimation of prognosis)

H. Plan (Diagnostic)
   Rule-outs   Procedure
   1.
   2.
   3.
   4.

Case History 4B

Signalment

German shepherd, female, 7 years old.

History

Hip dysplasia since 1 year of age. Stumbling on pelvic limbs started 6 months ago and progressed slowly. Dog cannot go up steps, falls even with good footing. No evidence of pain. (See Case History 2B, Chapter 2.)

Physical Examination

Nothing significant found.

Neurologic Examination *

(See Case History 3B, Chapter 3.)
A. Observation
  1. Mental status: Alert.
  2. Posture: Difficulty getting up. Wide-based stance.
  3. Gait: Truncal ataxia, stumbles, crosses legs, knuckles toes of pelvic limbs.
B. Palpation
  Normal.

C. Postural Reactions

Left	Reactions	Right
	Proprioceptive positioning PL	
0	PL	0
+2	TL	+2
NE	Wheelbarrowing	NE
+1	Hopping, PL	+1
+2	Hopping, TL	+2
NE	Extensor postural thrust	NE
	Hemistand-hemiwalk	
	Tonic neck	
	Placing, tactile PL	
	TL	
	Placing, visual PL	
	TL	

D. Spinal Reflexes

Left	Reflex Spinal Segment	Right
+3	Quadriceps	+2
+2	Extensor carpi radialis C7–T1	+2
NE	Triceps C7–T1	NE
+2	Flexion, PL L5–S1	+2
+2	Flexion, TL C6–T1	+2
0	Crossed extensor	0
+2	Perineal S1–S2	+2

E. Cranial Nerves

Left	Nerve + Function	Right
+2	C.N. II vision menace	+2
	C.N. II + C.N. III pupil size	
	Stim. left eye	
	Stim. right eye	
	C.N. II fundus	
	C.N. III, C.N. IV, C.N. VI Strabismus	
	Nystagmus	
	C.N. V sensation	
	C.N. V mastication	
	C.N. VII facial muscles	
	Palpebral	
	C.N. IX, C.N. X swallowing	
	C.N. XII tongue	

F. Sensation: Location
  Hyperesthesia _____ No _____
  Superficial pain _____ +2 _____
  Deep pain _____ +2 _____
Complete sections G and H before reviewing Case Summary.
G. Assessment (Anatomic diagnosis and estimation of prognosis)

H. Plan (Diagnostic)
  Rule-outs   Procedure
  1.
  2.
  3.
  4.

*Key: 0 = absent, +1 = decreased, +2 = normal, +3 = exaggerated, +4 = very exaggerated or clonus, PL = pelvic limb, TL = thoracic limb, NE = not evaluated.

Case History 4C

Signalment

Feline, domestic short hair, female, 3 months old.

History

Clumsy since birth. One of four in litter: one born dead, other two normal. Peculiar prancing gait. Trembles at times. Seems to be able to get around better now. (See Case History 2C, Chapter 2.)

Physical Examination

Normal.

Neurologic Examination *

(See Case History 3C, Chapter 3.)
A. Observation
  1. Mental status: Alert.
  2. Posture: Slight wide-based stance. Tremor of head that disappears at rest.
  3. Gait: Ataxia, dysmetria of all four limbs.
B. Palpation
  Normal.

C. Postural Reactions

Left	Reactions	Right
	Proprioceptive positioning	
+2	PL	+2
+2	TL	+2
NE	Wheelbarrowing	NE
+3	Hopping, PL	+3
+3	Hopping, TL	+3
NE	Extensor postural thrust	NE
	Hemistand-hemiwalk	
	Tonic neck	
	Placing, tactile PL	
	TL	
	Placing, visual PL	
↓	TL	↓

*Key: 0 = absent, +1 = decreased, +2 = normal, +3 = exaggerated, +4 = very exaggerated or clonus, PL = pelvic limb, TL = thoracic limb, NE = not evaluated.

D. Spinal Reflexes

Left	Reflex Spinal Segment	Right
	Quadriceps	
NE	L4–L6	NE
↓	Extensor carpi radialis C7–T1	↓
↓	Triceps C7–T1	↓
+2	Flexion, PL L5–S1	+2
+2	Flexion, TL C6–T1	+2
0	Crossed extensor	0
+2	Perineal S1–S2	+2

E. Cranial Nerves

Left	Nerve + Function	Right
	C.N. II vision	
0	menace	0
+2	C.N. II + C.N. III pupil size	+2
↓	Stim. left eye	↓
↓	Stim. right eye	↓
↓	C.N. II fundus	↓
Pendular	C.N. III, C.N. IV, C.N. VI Strabismus	Pendular
+2	Nystagmus	+2
	C.N. V sensation	
	C.N. V mastication	
	C.N. VII facial muscles	
	Palpebral	
	C.N. IX, C.N. X swallowing	
↓	C.N. XII tongue	↓

F. Sensation: Location
  Hyperesthesia _____ No _____
  Superficial pain _____ +2 _____
  Deep pain _____ +2 _____

Complete sections G and H before reviewing Case Summary.
G. Assessment (Anatomic diagnosis and estimation of prognosis)

H. Plan (Diagnostic)
  Rule-outs   Procedure
  1.
  2.
  3.
  4.

Case History 4D

Signalment

Feline, Siamese, male, 2 years old.

History

Uveitis in right eye for 2 months. Lame in right thoracic limb. Head trembles when cat eats. Depressed last 2 days. (See Case History 2D, Chapter 2.)

Physical Examination

Anterior uveitis in right eye.

Neurologic Examination *

(See Case History 3D, Chapter 3.)
A. Observation
   1. Mental status: Depressed.
   2. Posture: Tremor of head that disappears at rest.
   3. Gait: Knuckles left thoracic limb.
B. Palpation
   Atrophy of triceps and muscles distal to elbow, left thoracic limb.

C. Postural Reactions

Left	Reactions	Right
	Proprioceptive positioning	
0	PL	+2
0	TL	+2
NE	Wheelbarrowing	NE
0	Hopping, PL	+2
+1	Hopping, TL	+2
0	Extensor postural thrust	+2
NE	Hemistand-hemiwalk	NE
	Tonic neck	
	Placing, tactile PL	
	TL	
	Placing, visual PL	
	TL	

*Key: 0 = absent, +1 = decreased, +2 = normal, +3 = exaggerated, +4 = very exaggerated or clonus, PL = pelvic limb, TL = thoracic limb, NE = not evaluated.

D. Spinal Reflexes

Left	Reflex Spinal Segment	Right
+3	Quadriceps L4−L6	+2
0	Extensor carpi radialis C7−T1	+2
NE	Triceps C7−T1	NE
+2	Flexion, PL L5−S1	+2
0	Flexion, TL C6−T1	+2
0	Crossed extensor	0
+2	Perineal S1−S2	+2

E. Cranial Nerves

Left	Nerve + Function	Right
+2	C.N. II vision menace	+2
Miosis	C.N. II + C.N. III pupil size	+2
+2	Stim. left eye	
	Stim. right eye	
	C.N. II fundus	
	C.N. III, C.N. IV, C.N. VI Strabismus	
	Nystagmus	
	C.N. V sensation	
	C.N. V mastication	
	C.N. VII facial muscles	
	Palpebral	
	C.N. IX, C.N. X swallowing	
	C.N. XII tongue	

F. Sensation: Location

Hyperesthesia	No
Superficial pain	+2
Deep pain	+2

Complete sections G and H before reviewing Case Summary.

G. Assessment (Anatomic diagnosis and estimation of prognosis)

H. Plan (Diagnostic)
   Rule-outs   Procedure
   1.
   2.
   3.
   4.

Case History 4E

Signalment

Yorkshire terrier, male, 8 months old.

History

Always small and thin. Episodes of abnormal behavior recently. Paces, is restless, and resents being held. These episodes have lasted for 2 to 3 hours, occasionally for a whole day, and have occurred every day for the last 3 weeks. (See Case History 2E, Chapter 2.)

Physical Examination

Thin.

Neurologic Examination *

A. Observation
 1. Mental status: Normal. Alert. Depressed during day.
 2. Posture: Normal.
 3. Gait: Paces. Sometimes bumps into table.
B. Palpation

C. Postural Reactions

Left	Reactions	Right
	Proprioceptive positioning PL	
+1		+1
+1	TL	+1
+1	Wheelbarrowing	+1
+1	Hopping, PL	+1
+1	Hopping, TL	+1
+1	Extensor postural thrust	+1
NE	Hemistand-hemiwalk	NE
NE	Tonic neck	NE
+1	Placing, tactile PL	+1
+1	TL	+1
+1	Placing, visual PL	+1
+1	TL	+1

*Key: 0 = absent, +1 = decreased, +2 = normal, +3 = exaggerated, +4 = very exaggerated or clonus, PL = pelvic limb, TL = thoracic limb, NE = not evaluated.

D. Spinal Reflexes

Left	Reflex Spinal Segment	Right
+2	Quadriceps L4–L6	+2
	Extensor carpi radialis C7–T1	
	Triceps C7–T1	
	Flexion, PL L5–S1	
	Flexion, TL C6–T1	
	Crossed extensor	
	Perineal S1–S2	

E. Cranial Nerves

Left	Nerve + Function	Right
+2	C.N. II vision menace	+2
	C.N. II + C.N. III pupil size	
	Stim. left eye	
	Stim. right eye	
	C.N. II fundus	
	C.N. III, C.N. IV, C.N. VI Strabismus	
	Nystagmus	
	C.N. V sensation	
	C.N. V mastication	
	C.N. VII facial muscles	
	Palpebral	
	C.N. IX, C.N. X swallowing	
	C.N. XII tongue	

F. Sensation: Location
 Hyperesthesia _____ No _____
 Superficial pain _____ +2 _____
 Deep pain _____ +2 _____
Complete sections G and H before reviewing Case Summary.
G. Assessment (Anatomic diagnosis and estimation of prognosis)

H. Plan (Diagnostic)
 Rule-outs   Procedure
 1.
 2.
 3.
 4.

The following abbreviated cases are presented to give you additional practice in localizing lesions. Use Table 4–5 or 4–8 or Figure 4–9 if necessary. The result of the neurologic examination is all that you need in order to localize the lesion.

Case History 4F

Signalment

Dachshund, male, 2 years old.

History

Physical Examination

Neurologic Examination *

A. Observation
   1. Mental status: Normal.
   2. Posture: Cannot stand.
   3. Gait: Moves thoracic limbs but not pelvic limbs.
B. Palpation
   Normal.

C. Postural Reactions

Left	Reactions	Right
	Proprioceptive positioning PL	
0		0
+2	TL	+2
+2	Wheelbarrowing	+2
0	Hopping, PL	0
+2	Hopping, TL	+2
0	Extensor postural thrust	0
NE	Hemistand-hemiwalk	NE
NE	Tonic neck	NE
	Placing, tactile PL	
0		0
+2	TL	+2
	Placing, visual PL	
0		0
+2	TL	+2

*Key: 0 = absent, +1 = decreased, +2 = normal, +3 = exaggerated, +4 = very exaggerated or clonus, PL = pelvic limb, TL = thoracic limb, NE = not evaluated.

D. Spinal Reflexes

Left	Reflex Spinal Segment	Right
0	Quadriceps L4–L6	0
+2	Extensor carpi radialis C7–T1	+2
+2	Triceps C7–T1	+2
0	Flexion, PL L5–S1	0
+2	Flexion, TL C6–T1	+2
0	Crossed extensor	0
0	Perineal S1–S2	0

E. Cranial Nerves

Left	Nerve + Function	Right
+2	C.N. II vision menace	+2
	C.N. II + C.N. III pupil size	
	Stim. left eye	
	Stim. right eye	
	C.N. II fundus	
	C.N. III, C.N. IV, C.N. VI Strabismus	
	Nystagmus	
	C.N. V sensation	
	C.N. V mastication	
	C.N. VII facial muscles	
	Palpebral	
	C.N. IX, C.N. X swallowing	
	C.N. XII tongue	

F. Sensation: Location
   Hyperesthesia _____ No _____
   Superficial pain _____ NE _____
   Deep pain _____ NE _____

Complete sections G and H before reviewing Case Summary.

G. Assessment (Anatomic diagnosis and estimation of prognosis)

H. Plan (Diagnostic)
   Rule-outs   Procedure
   1.
   2.
   3.
   4.

Case History 4G

Signalment

Feline, domestic, male, 6 years old.

History

Physical Examination

Neurologic Examination *

A. Observation
   1. Mental status: Normal.
   2. Posture: Recumbent.
   3. Gait: The cat has slight voluntary movements of limbs but cannot walk.

B. Palpation
   Normal.

C. Postural Reactions

Left	Reactions	Right
	Proprioceptive positioning	
0	PL	0
0	TL	0
0	Wheelbarrowing	0
0	Hopping, PL	0
0	Hopping, TL	0
0	Extensor postural thrust	0
0	Hemistand-hemiwalk	0
0	Tonic neck	0
	Placing, tactile	
0	PL	0
0	TL	0
	Placing, visual	
0	PL	0
0	TL	0

D. Spinal Reflexes

Left	Reflex / Spinal Segment	Right
	Quadriceps	
+3	L4−L6	+3
	Extensor carpi radialis	
+2	C7−T1	+2
	Triceps	
+2	C7−T1	+2
	Flexion, PL	
+2	L5−S1	+2
	Flexion, TL	
+2	C6−T1	+2
0	Crossed extensor	0
	Perineal	
+2	S1−S2	+2

E. Cranial Nerves

Left	Nerve + Function	Right
	C.N. II vision	
+2	menace	+2
	C.N. II + C.N. III pupil size	
	Stim. left eye	
	Stim. right eye	
	C.N. II fundus	
	C.N. III, C.N. IV, C.N. VI Strabismus	
	Nystagmus	
	C.N. V sensation	
	C.N. V mastication	
	C.N. VII facial muscles	
	Palpebral	
	C.N. IX, C.N. X swallowing	
	C.N. XII tongue	

F. Sensation: Location
   Hyperesthesia _____ No _____
   Superficial pain _____ +2 _____
   Deep pain _____ +2 _____

Complete sections G and H before reviewing Case Summary.

G. Assessment (Anatomic diagnosis and estimation of prognosis)

H. Plan (Diagnostic)
   Rule-outs   Procedure
   1.
   2.
   3.
   4.

---

*Key: 0 = absent, +1 = decreased, +2 = normal, +3 = exaggerated, +4 = very exaggerated or clonus, PL = pelvic limb, TL = thoracic limb, NE = not evaluated.

Case History 4H

Signalment

Quarter horse, male, 2 years old.

History

Physical Examination

Neurologic Examination *

A. Observation
   1. Mental status: Alert.
   2. Posture: Normal.
   3. Gait: Knuckles pelvic limbs, sways trunk. Difficulty in backing: will fall.

B. Palpation
   Normal.

C. Postural Reactions

Left	Reactions	Right
	Proprioceptive positioning PL	
+1		+1
+2	TL	+2
NE	Wheelbarrowing	NE
+1	Hopping, PL	+1
+2	Hopping, TL	+2
NE	Extensor postural thrust	NE
NE	Hemistand-hemiwalk	NE
NE	Tonic neck	NE
0	Placing, tactile PL	0
+2	TL	+2
NE	Placing, visual PL	NE
NE	TL	NE

D. Spinal Reflexes

Left	Reflex Spinal Segment	Right
+3	Quadriceps L4−L6	+3
+2	Extensor carpi radialis C7−T1	+2
NE	Triceps C7−T1	NE
+2	Flexion, PL L5−S1	+2
+2	Flexion, TL C6−T1	+2
0	Crossed extensor	0
+2	Perineal S1−S2	+2

E. Cranial Nerves

Left	Nerve + Function	Right
+2	C.N. II vision menace	+2
	C.N. II + C.N. III pupil size	
	Stim. left eye	
	Stim. right eye	
	C.N. II fundus	
	C.N. III, C.N. IV, C.N. VI Strabismus	
	Nystagmus	
	C.N. V sensation	
	C.N. V mastication	
	C.N. VII facial muscles	
	Palpebral	
	C.N. IX, C.N. X swallowing	
	C.N. XII tongue	

F. Sensation: Location

Hyperesthesia	No
Superficial pain	+2
Deep pain	+2

Complete sections G and H before reviewing Case Summary.

G. Assessment (Anatomic diagnosis and estimation of prognosis)

H. Plan (Diagnostic)
   Rule-outs   Procedure
   1.
   2.
   3.
   4.

---

*Key: 0 = absent, +1 = decreased, +2 = normal, +3 = exaggerated, +4 = very exaggerated or clonus, PL = pelvic limb, TL = thoracic limb, NE = not evaluated.

Case History 4I

Signalment

Cocker spaniel, female, 8 years old.

History

Physical Examination

Neurologic Examination *

A. Observation
1. Mental status: Normal.
2. Posture: Head tilt to right.
3. Gait: Tends to circle to the right. Disoriented when picked up for assessment of postural reactions.

B. Palpation
Normal.

C. Postural Reactions

Left	Reactions	Right
	Proprioceptive positioning PL	
+2		+2
+2	TL	+2
NE	Wheelbarrowing	NE
+2	Hopping, PL	+2
+2	Hopping, TL	+2
+2	Extensor postural thrust	+2
NE	Hemistand-hemiwalk	NE
NE	Tonic neck	NE
	Placing, tactile PL	
+2		+2
+2	TL	+2
	Placing, visual PL	
+2		+2
+2	TL	+2

D. Spinal Reflexes

Left	Reflex Spinal Segment	Right
	Quadriceps	
+2	L4−L6	+2
	Extensor carpi radialis C7−T1	
	Triceps C7−T1	
	Flexion, PL L5−S1	
	Flexion, TL C6−T1	
	Crossed extensor	
	Perineal S1−S2	

E. Cranial Nerves

Left	Nerve + Function	Right
	C.N. II vision	
+2	menace	0
+2	C.N. II + C.N. III pupil size	+2
+2	Stim. left eye	+2
+2	Stim. right eye	+2
+2	C.N. II fundus	+2
No	C.N. III, C.N. IV, C.N. VI Strabismus	No
Fast Left	Nystagmus	Horizontal
+2	C.N. V sensation	+2
+2	C.N. V mastication	+2
+2	C.N. VII facial muscles	Drooping
+2	Palpebral	0
+2	C.N. IX, C.N. X swallowing	+2
+2	C.N. XII tongue	+2

F. Sensation: Location
Hyperesthesia _____ No _____
Superficial pain _____ +2 _____
Deep pain _____ +2 _____

Complete sections G and H before reviewing Case Summary.

G. Assessment (Anatomic diagnosis and estimation of prognosis)

H. Plan (Diagnostic)
Rule-outs   Procedure
1.
2.
3.
4.

*Key: 0 = absent, +1 = decreased, +2 = normal, +3 = exaggerated, +4 = very exaggerated or clonus, PL = pelvic limb, TL = thoracic limb, NE = not evaluated.

Case History 4J

ignalment

Bovine, Jersey, female, 6 months old.

listory

hysical Examination

leurologic Examination *

A. Observation
  1. Mental status: Coma.
  2. Posture: Recumbent; increased extensor tone in all four limbs.
  3. Gait: None.

B. Palpation

C. Postural Reactions

Left	Reactions	Right
	Proprioceptive positioning PL	
0		0
	TL	
	Wheelbarrowing	
	Hopping, PL	
	Hopping, TL	
	Extensor postural thrust	
	Hemistand-hemiwalk	
	Tonic neck	
	Placing, tactile PL	
	TL	
	Placing, visual PL	
	TL	

D. Spinal Reflexes

Left	Reflex Spinal Segment	Right
	Quadriceps	
+3	L4−L6	+3
	Extensor carpi radialis	
+3	C7−T1	+3
	Triceps	
NE	C7−T1	NE
Slow; extensor hypertonus	Flexion, PL L5−S1	Slow; extensor hypertonus
Slow; extensor hypertonus	Flexion, TL C6−T1	Slow; extensor hypertonus
0	Crossed extensor	0
	Perineal	
+2	S1−S2	+2

E. Cranial Nerves

Left	Nerve + Function	Right
	C.N. II vision	
0	menace	0
Midposition	C.N. II + C.N. III pupil size	Midposition
0	Stim. left eye	0
0	Stim. right eye	0
+2	C.N. II fundus	+2
No eye movements	C.N. III, C.N. IV, C.N. VI Strabismus	No eye movements
0	Nystagmus	0
0	C.N. V sensation	0
+2	C.N. V mastication	+2
+2	C.N. VII facial muscles	+2
+2	Palpebral	+2
+1	C.N. IX, C.N. X swallowing	+1
+2	C.N. XII tongue	+2

F. Sensation: Location
   Hyperesthesia _____ No _____
   Superficial pain ___ Not conscious ___
   Deep pain _____ Not conscious _____

Complete sections G and H before reviewing Case Summary.

G. Assessment (Anatomic diagnosis and estimation of prognosis)

H. Plan (Diagnostic)
   Rule-outs   Procedure
   1.
   2.
   3.
   4.

*Key: 0 = absent, +1 = decreased, +2 = normal, +3 = exaggerated, +4 = very exaggerated or clonus, PL = pelvic limb, TL = thoracic limb, NE = not evaluated.

ASSESSMENT 4A

Postural reactions are abnormal in both limbs on the right side and, possibly, slow in the left pelvic limb. This finding is not characteristic of peripheral nerve lesions, which ordinarily are restricted to one limb or to all four limbs (generalized polyneuropathy). Since both pelvic and thoracic limbs are affected, the lesion must be rostral to T2. The right pelvic limb has an exaggerated quadriceps reflex, a UMN sign. Would the interpretation be different if the reflex were normal? No—it would not matter. Reflexes may be normal *or* exaggerated with UMN disease. The weak or absent myotatic reflexes in the thoracic limbs should not be considered diagnostic. They frequently are difficult to elicit. If there were a good response on one side and none on the other, you might be more confident in diagnosing an abnormality. The weak flexion reflex in the right thoracic limb is abnormal, however. This finding is a sign of sensory or motor deficit at the segmental level—an LMN sign. From this observation, you should assess the lesion to be between C6 and T2 on the right side.

The sensory examination confirms the assessment of a decrease in sensation in the right thoracic limb. Can the lesion be in the peripheral nerves of the brachial plexus? Not unless there is more than one lesion—remember the abnormalities of the right pelvic limb. One lesion in the C6–T2 spinal cord segments could account for both thoracic and pelvic limb abnormalities. A gray matter lesion affecting sensory and motor neurons to the brachial plexus and a white matter lesion affecting the proprioceptive and UMN pathways to the pelvic limb account for all the signs. Why is pain sensation still present in the pelvic limbs? The pain pathways are bilateral, and this lesion is unilateral. If the lesion were bilateral, both pelvic limbs would have severe postural reaction deficits. The slow initiation of hopping in the left pelvic limb may be caused by a partial loss of the proprioceptive pathways to that side. This hypothesis cannot be substantiated by proprioceptive positioning tests. Is the spinal cord lesion the only lesion? The animal's mental status and cranial nerves are normal, and there are no other signs that cannot be explained by one lesion. Always assume that there is one lesion unless there is evidence to the contrary.

Localization: spinal cord, C6–T2, right side.

Rule-outs (see Chapter 2):
1. vascular lesion,
2. trauma, and
3. inflammation (low probability).

The plan for a definitive diagnosis will be discussed at the end of Chapter 6.

ASSESSMENT 4B

Pelvic limb ataxia and paresis suggest a lesion caudal to T2. The postural reactions and the spinal reflexes confirm that the thoracic limbs are not affected. The spinal reflexes are normal or exaggerated in the pelvic limbs, indicating that the lesion is rostral to L4. Therefore, the lesion should be between T3 and L3. The sensory examination does not provide any definitive evidence for a more specific localization. The animal's

mental status and the reactions of the cranial nerves and the thoracic limbs do not suggest that there is more than one lesion.

Localization: spinal cord, T3–L3, symmetric.

Rule-outs (see Chapter 2):
1. degenerative disease,
2. neoplasia, and
3. inflammation.

The plan for a definitive diagnosis will be discussed at the end of Chapter 6.

ASSESSMENT 4C

Ataxia, dysmetria, and tremor are signs of cerebellar disease. Paresis is not associated with cerebellar disease, so it is important to be sure that there is no loss of voluntary movements. Brain stem or spinal cord disease may mimic some of the signs of cerebellar dysfunction. In this case, the head is affected, and there is a head tremor, an absent menace reaction, and pendular nystagmus, indicating brain disease. There is neither paresis nor proprioceptive deficits, although the postural reactions are not normal. The abnormality of the postural reactions is also a sign of ataxia and dysmetria. The absence of the menace reaction with an intact palpebral reflex (C.N. V and C.N. VII) and good vision is indicative of cerebellar disease. The nystagmus, which does not have a fast and slow component, is similar in origin to the intention tremor of the head. All of the signs are compatible with cerebellar disease, and there are no signs that cannot be explained by the presence of this lesion.

Localization: cerebellum.

Rule-outs (see Chapter 2):
1. anomaly and
2. trauma.

The plan for a definitive diagnosis will be discussed at the end of Chapter 6.

ASSESSMENT 4D

The animal's mental status and head tremor immediately should signal brain disease. Depression can be caused by a lesion in almost any part of the brain except the cerebellum, or it could be merely a manifestation of a generalized illness. The head tremor suggests cerebellar involvement. If the depression is caused by a brain lesion, there is more than one lesion. The postural reactions indicate a left hemiparesis. Hemiparesis is caused by brain disease more often than spinal cord disease. Because we are thorough, we assess the spinal reflexes even though it looks as if the cat has brain disease, and we find that they are absent in the left thoracic limb. This situation cannot be caused by brain disease! Absent reflexes with intact sensation are not an indication of peripheral nerve disease (with the exception of polyneuropathies), so the lesion must be in the ventral roots or the spinal cord gray matter. The pelvic limb has an upper motor neuron paresis, indicating that the spinal cord is involved. Where is the lesion? We have signs localizing it to the left C6–T2 spinal cord, the cerebellum, and, possibly, other brain structures (depression). In addition, there is an inflammatory lesion of the eye.

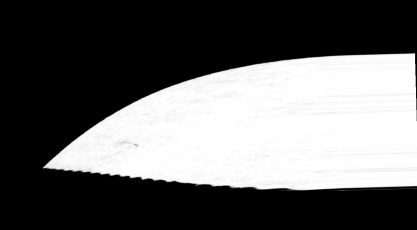

Therefore, the problem is a multifocal or a systemic disease. The signs cannot be explained by one lesion.

Localization: multifocal or systemic disease, left C6–T2 spinal cord, cerebellum; cerebrum or brain stem).

Rule-outs (see Chapter 2):
1. inflammation,
2. neoplasia, and
3. degenerative disease.

The plan for a definitive diagnosis will be discussed at the end of Chapter 6.

ASSESSMENT 4E

The primary abnormality is in the animal's mental status. The dog's mood fluctuates between depression and agitation. He does not always make appropriate responses. The slowness of the postural reactions must be interpreted cautiously in view of the dog's mental status. Severely depressed animals may not be cooperative when postural reaction tests are performed. Compulsive walking is usually a sign of prefrontal cerebral cortex disease. In severe forms of the disease, the animal will walk until it bumps into a corner and will stand pressing its head against the wall. The dog's neurologic signs suggest cerebral disease.

Localization: cerebrum.
Rule-outs (see Chapter 2):
1. metabolic disease and
2. toxic disease.

ASSESSMENT 4F

Normal thoracic limbs, LMN signs in the pelvic limbs.
Localization: L4–S3.

ASSESSMENT 4G

UMN signs in all four limbs, normal brain.
Localization: C1–C5.

ASSESSMENT 4H

Normal thoracic limbs, UMN signs in the pelvic limbs.
Localization: T3–L3.

ASSESSMENT 4I

The head tilt and the nystagmus indicate an abnormality of the vestibular system. The lack of paresis or proprioceptive deficits and the horizontal nystagmus that does not change are characteristic of peripheral vestibular lesions.

The lip and palpebral reflexes indicate involvement of the facial nerve (C.N. VII). C.N. VII and C.N. VIII are both affected in the labyrinth.

ASSESSMENT 4J

The animal's coma, decerebrate posture, tetraparesis, and cranial nerve signs indicate involvement of the brain stem. The menace reaction is absent because of the coma and the disconnection of the cortex from C.N. VII.

The pupils indicate a loss of both sympathetic and parasympathetic input and involvement of the midbrain. The eye movements indicate involvement of the core brain stem (medial longitudinal fasciculus). The lesion is in the midbrain (see Chapter 13).

A localization to the brain stem is adequate for the formulation of a clinical diagnosis.

REFERENCES

1. Weed, L. L.: Medical Records, Medical Education and Patient Care. Cleveland, Press of Case Western Reserve University, 1969.
2. Oliver, J. E., Jr.: Localization of lesions in the nervous system. *In* Hoerlein, B. F. Canine Neurology: Diagnosis and Treatment, 3rd ed. Philadelphia, W. B. Saunders Co., 1978.
3. Illingworth, R. D., and Molina-Negro, P.: Spontaneous and electrically-evoked activity in the anterolateral column of the spinal cord in dogs. J. Neurosurg. 40:58–64, 1974.
4. Breazile, J. E., and Kitchell, R. L.: A study of fiber systems within the spinal cord of the domestic pig that subserve pain. J. Comp. Neurol. 133:373–382, 1968.
5. Kennard, M.A.: The course of ascending fibers in the spinal cord of the cat essential to the recognition of painful stimuli. J. Comp. Neurol. 100:511–524, 1954.
6. Tarlov, I. M.: Spinal Cord Compression: Mechanism of Paralysis and Treatment. Springfield, IL, Charles C Thomas, 1957.
7. Holliday, T. A.: Clinical signs of acute and chronic experimental lesions of the cerebellum. Vet. Sci. Comm. 3:259–278, 1979/1980.
8. deLahunta, A.: Veterinary Neuroanatomy and Clinical Neurology. Philadelphia, W. B. Saunders Co., 1977.

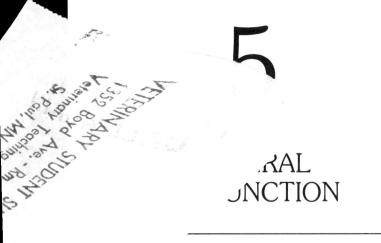

5

...RAL
...JNCTION

antagonist to the parasympathetic (cholinergic) system. This simplistic theory, which separates the autonomic system from the somatic system, does not explain well-defined somatovisceral and viscerosomatic reflexes.

Problems associated with micturition are common in neurologic disorders. Other visceral dysfunctions traditionally have been the concern of cardiologists or internists and are discussed in books on cardiology and internal medicine. This chapter reviews the anatomy, the physiology, and the clinical syndromes of micturition.

Abnormal visceral function may reflect a pathologic change in the nervous system; however, the importance of nervous control of the viscera is often overlooked.

The classical view of the autonomic nervous system as one with discrete boundaries is giving way to a concept of a more integrated system with no limits. For example, the classical theory was that the autonomic system controlled functions that the individual could not modify voluntarily. It has been proved, however, that one can regulate blood pressure, heart rate, micturition, and many other autonomic activities. In the classical view, the sympathetic (adrenergic) system functions as an

ANATOMY AND PHYSIOLOGY OF MICTURITION

Micturition is the reaction that ultimately will occur if a bladder is gradually distended, leading to the coordinated expulsion of its contents.[1] The micturition reflex is a complex integration of parasympathetic, sympathetic, and somatic pathways extending from the sacral segments of the spinal cord to the cerebral cortex. The components of the micturition reflex will be discussed in functional groups before a complete description of the micturition reflex is presented.

The Detrusor Reflex

The primary component of micturition is the detrusor (the muscle of the urinary bladder)

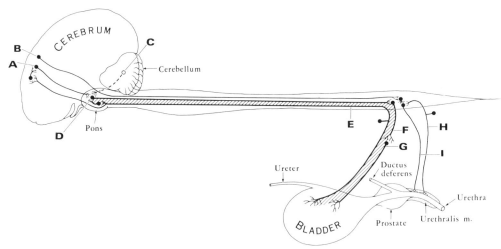

Figure 5–1. Anatomic organization of micturition. *A.* Cortical neurons for voluntary control of micturition. *B.* Cortical neurons for voluntary control of sphincters. *C.* Cerebellar neurons that have an inhibitory influence on micturition. *D.* Pontine reticular neurons that are necessary for the detrusor reflex. *E.* Afferent (sensory) pathway for the detrusor reflex. *F.* Preganglionic pelvic (parasympathetic) neuron to the detrusor. *G.* Postganglionic pelvic (parasympathetic) neuron to the detrusor. *H.* Afferent (sensory) neuron from the urethral sphincter, pudendal nerve. *I.* Efferent (motor) neuron from the urethral sphincter, pudendal nerve. (From Oliver, J. E., Jr., and Osborne, C. A.: Neurogenic urinary incontinence. *In* Kirk, R. W., ed.: Current Veterinary Therapy VII. Philadelphia, W. B. Saunders Co., 1980, pp. 1122–1127. Used by permission.)

reflex. As the bladder fills with urine, there is a very slight increase in bladder pressure with each increase in volume, until the limit of elasticity of the smooth muscle is reached. The sensory nerve endings in the bladder wall are tension-recorders and are arranged in series with the muscle fibers.[2] As the bladder nears its capacity, these nerves begin to discharge. The sensory fibers from the bladder are located in the pelvic nerve and originate from the sacral segments of the spinal cord (Fig. 5–1).[3] The sensory discharge ascends in the spinal cord to the pontine reticular formation in the brain stem. Integration occurs at this level, eventually giving rise to a motor discharge down the spinal cord to the preganglionic parasympathetic neurons in the intermediate horn of the sacral segments. The preganglionic parasympathetic nerves are located in segments S1–S3 in the cat and the dog.[3,4] The preganglionic neurons discharge and activate postganglionic neurons, which are located in the pelvic ganglia, along the course of the pelvic nerves, and in the wall of the bladder. Some integration of activity apparently takes place in the ganglia. Ultimately, the postganglionic neurons synapse on detrusor muscle fibers and cause a contraction—the detrusor reflex (Fig. 5–2A).

Integration in the brain stem is necessary in order for the detrusor reflex to be coordinated and sustained long enough for bladder evacuation. Complete lesions of any portion of this pathway will abolish the detrusor reflex.

VOLUNTARY CONTROL OF THE DETRUSOR REFLEX

The sensory pathway to the brain stem that signals distention of the bladder also sends collaterals to the cerebral cortex (see Fig. 5–1). Integration at the cortical level allows voluntary initiation (e.g., in territorial marking) or inhibition (e.g., in house training) of micturition. The precise location of the control center of cerebral cortex is not clear. Stimulation and evoked-response studies indicate that several areas of the cortex influence the detrusor reflex.[5] Lesions of the cerebral cortex may cause a loss of voluntary control of micturition and may reduce the capacity of the bladder.[6] For example, animals with cerebral tumors may start voiding in the house for no apparent reason.

CEREBELLAR INHIBITION OF THE DETRUSOR REFLEX

The cerebellum can inhibit the detrusor reflex (see Fig. 5–1). Stimulation of the fastigial nucleus abolishes detrusor reflex contraction.[7]

Lesions of the cerebellum, such as cerebellar hypoplasia, may produce increased frequency of voiding with a reduced bladder capacity.[8]

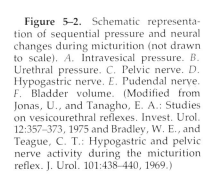

Figure 5–2. Schematic representation of sequential pressure and neural changes during micturition (not drawn to scale). *A.* Intravesical pressure. *B.* Urethral pressure. *C.* Pelvic nerve. *D.* Hypogastric nerve. *E.* Pudendal nerve. *F.* Bladder volume. (Modified from Jonas, U., and Tanagho, E. A.: Studies on vesicourethral reflexes. Invest. Urol. 12:357–373, 1975 and Bradley, W. E., and Teague, C. T.: Hypogastric and pelvic nerve activity during the micturition reflex. J. Urol. 101:438–440, 1969.)

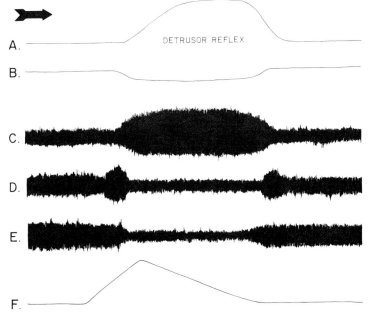

The Urethral Sphincter

The muscle surrounding the urethra contains muscle spindles that discharge in response to stretch, as do other skeletal muscles. Sensory discharges ascend in the pudendal nerves to the sacral segments. The pudendal urethral motor neurons are located in segments L7–S3 in the dog and the cat, although they are found primarily in S1 and S2 in both species.[4,9] Monosynaptic activation of the motor neurons is transmitted back down the pudendal nerve to the muscle (see Fig. 5–1). Afferent discharge through the pelvic nerves also activates the pudendal nerve. These pathways produce urethral contraction in response to a sudden stretch, maintaining continence during a cough, a sneeze, and so forth.

Voluntary control of the urethral sphincter is provided by cortical pathways to the sacral segments (see Fig. 5–1).

Lesions of the sacral segments or the pudendal nerve will cause a hypotonic paralysis of the sphincter. Cortical or spinal lesions may abolish voluntary control of the sphincter and may produce increased sphincter tone, which increases outflow resistance.[8] Typically, T3–L3 lesions of the spinal cord abolish the long-routed detrusor reflex and cause increased tone in the sphincter.

Sympathetic Innervation

The detrusor reflex is mediated through the parasympathetic nervous system (sacral). The skeletal muscle in the urethral sphincter is innervated by somatic nerves. Sympathetic nerves also are found in the pelvic plexus, the pelvic ganglia, and the urinary bladder, but their function is not clear.

The preganglionic sympathetic neurons to the bladder are located in the lumbar spinal cord (L2–L5 in the cat, L1–L4 in the dog).[3,4] The fibers course through the caudal mesenteric ganglion and the hypogastric nerve to the bladder and the pelvic plexus. Both alpha- and beta-adrenergic (sympathetic postganglionic) synapses have been found on neurons in the pelvic ganglia, in the bladder wall, and on the detrusor muscle, especially in the area of the trigone.[10]

Pharmacologic studies have demonstrated that alpha-adrenergic receptors are located primarily in the region of the trigone and the bladder neck and cause contraction of the smooth muscle.[11] Beta-adrenergic receptors are found in all parts of the bladder and cause relaxation of smooth muscle.[12] The presence of adrenergic synapses on cholinergic ganglion cells suggests that the sympathetic pathways also can modulate the activity of the parasympathetic pathway, but this effect has not been demonstrated in naturally occurring sympathetic firing.[13] Adrenergic innervation of the bladder neck and the trigone has been demonstrated to have major significance in the prevention of retrograde ejaculation.[14]

Lesions of the sympathetic pathways apparently do not have a significant effect on micturition; however, there has been an increasing acceptance of the theory that the sympathetic pathways play an important role in animals and in human beings with lesions of the parasympathetic pathways.[15] Patients with neurogenic bladder dysfunction complicated by a narrowing of the bladder neck or spasms of the urethra may be helped by alpha-adrenergic blockade.[16]

Sensory Pathways from the Bladder

Sensory fibers originating in the bladder run in both the pelvic and the hypogastric nerves. Stretch receptors in the bladder wall give rise to fibers that run through the pelvic nerve into the sacral spinal cord (S1–S3 in the cat and the dog) and ascend to the pontine reticular formation to initiate the detrusor reflex. Sensory fibers in the hypogastric nerve reach the spinal cord at the lumbar segments (L2–L5 in the cat, L1–L4 in the dog).[3,4] These fibers respond to overdistention of the bladder. Activation of these fibers is perceived as pain.[17] It is possible for a lesion of the lower lumbar or sacral spinal cord to abolish micturition, although the animal still will be able to perceive overdistention of the bladder as a painful sensation mediated through the hypogastric nerve.

Motor Innervation of the Detrusor Muscle

Each motor nerve in the bladder wall innervates many muscle cells, although not all muscle cells have direct innervation. The neuromuscular junction is characterized by a varicosity of the axon containing synaptic vesicles, a thinning of the Schwann cell layer, and a close apposition to specialized areas of the detrusor muscle fibers. Excitation of the innervated muscle cell (pacemaker cell) initiates a spread of excitation and contraction through adjacent cells by means of "tight junctions."[18] It also has been hypothesized that the spread of excitation occurs by diffusion of a neurotransmitter in the extracellular space to adjacent detrusor muscle fibers.

Disruption of tight junctions between muscle fibers may occur when the bladder is overdistended (e.g., in obstruction of the urethra). If tight junctions are disrupted, the wave of excitation cannot spread, and a flaccid bladder will result. Reconnection of the junction will occur in 1 to 2 weeks if the distention is relieved early enough. If the bladder remains distended too long or if infection is present, fibrosis develops between the cells, preventing restoration of function.

Reflex Integration

The micturition reflex involves a coordinated and sustained contraction of the detrusor muscle and relaxation of the urethra. Pelvic nerve sensory neurons that produce the detrusor reflex also send collaterals to inhibitory interneurons in the sacral spinal cord.[19,20] The inhibitory interneurons synapse on the pudendal motor neurons, which are also in the sacral segments to reduce motor activity in the pudendal nerves and the periurethral striated muscle (see Fig. 5–2B and E). As the detrusor contracts, the urethra relaxes, allowing urine to pass. If the long pathways are intact, voluntary activation of the pudendal neurons by the corticospinal pathways can override this effect and block micturition. Lesions of the long tracts or at the segmental level may interfere with reflex integration. Detrusor contraction without urethral relaxation is called *reflex dyssynergia.*[21]

Reflex connections between the pelvic (parasympathetic) nerve afferents and the lumbar (sympathetic) motor neurons also have been demonstrated.[13,17,19,22] The effect seems to be similar to that observed in the pudendal (somatic) nerve, that is, as the pelvic motor neuron begins to fire to initiate a detrusor contraction, the hypogastric nerve becomes silent (see Fig. 5–2C and D). When the pelvic nerve stops firing as the bladder is emptied, the hypogastric nerve discharges once more. Whether the effect of the hypogastric nerve is on bladder storage, urethral contraction, both, or neither has not been firmly established. At present, it

appears that it has an effect on both but is not essential for either.

The Micturition Reflex

Urine is transported from the kidneys to the bladder through the ureters. Peristaltic waves move the urine into the bladder in spurts. Vesicoureteral reflux is prevented by the oblique course of the ureter through the bladder wall, resulting in the formation of a flap valve. The detrusor spirals around the ureter, assisting in the maintenance of the valve effect.

The bladder fills without a significant increase in pressure as the smooth muscle stretches (see Fig. 5–2A and F). The sympathetic (adrenergic) pathways may assist by inhibiting parasympathetic (cholinergic) neurons or by direct relaxation of smooth muscle. If the bladder fills beyond the normal elasticity of the smooth muscle, pressure increases linearly with the increase in volume.

In the intact animal, as the limits of stretch of the smooth muscle are approached, stretch receptors in the bladder wall are excited and send sensory discharges through the pelvic nerves to the sacral spinal cord. These discharges are relayed up the spinal cord to the reticular formation in the pons. The activation of neuronal pools in the pons results in a motor discharge down the spinal cord to the sacral segments. Preganglionic parasympathetic motor neurons in the intermediate horn of the sacral gray matter are activated. The motor discharge passes down the pelvic nerves to activate postganglionic neurons in the pelvic ganglia and in the wall of the bladder, which in turn activate the bladder smooth muscle (detrusor). The sustained discharge of neurons through these pathways produces a coordinated, sustained contraction of the detrusor muscle (see Fig. 5–2A and C).

The fibers of the detrusor spiral into the neck of the bladder and help to maintain continence in the relaxed state. As the fibers contract, the bladder neck is pulled open into a funnel shape. Simultaneously, sensory discharges from the pelvic nerves are relayed to the lumbar segments, inhibiting the output of the sympathetic pathway, and to the pudendal motor neurons in the ventral horn of the sacral segments, inhibiting the tonic output in the nerves to the skeletal sphincter (see Fig. 5–2C, D, and E).

The result is a coordinated contraction of the

bladder and a relaxation of the sphincter, which is maintained until voiding is complete (see Fig. 5–2A and B). Sustaining of the contraction also is enhanced by sensory fibers in the urethra, which respond to the flow of urine.[1]

When the bladder is empty, the sensory discharge in the pelvic nerve stops, resulting in a cessation of motor discharge in the pelvic nerve and a return of activity in the sympathetic and pudendal nerves. The bladder relaxes, and the sphincter closes.

DISORDERS OF MICTURITION

The principal neurogenic disorders of micturition are inappropriate voiding; inadequate voiding with an overflow of urine; increased frequency, reduced capacity, or both; or incomplete voiding when normal voiding reactions are interrupted by abrupt contractions of the urethral sphincter.[8,23]

Clinical Signs (Tables 5–1 and 5–2)

Detrusor Areflexia with Sphincter Hypertonus. The most frequently recognized disorder of micturition is a loss of the detrusor reflex with increased tone in the urethral sphincter. Lesions from the pontine reticular formation to the L7 spinal cord segments may cause these complications. The most common cause is compression of the spinal cord, such as a herniated disk, which disrupts the long pathways that are responsible for the detrusor reflex and the upper motor neuron (UMN) pathways to the skeletal muscle of the urethral sphincter. The animal is unable to void, the bladder becomes greatly distended, and it is difficult or impossible to express the bladder manually. The perineal reflex is intact.

Detrusor Areflexia with Normal Sphincter Tone. Lesions of the spinal cord or the brain stem may produce detrusor areflexia without producing increased tone in the urethral sphincter. Traumatic injuries of the pelvis may damage the pelvic plexus without damaging the pudendal nerve. The animal is unable to void, but manual expression can be accomplished. Female dogs have a short skeletal sphincter so that even with UMN lesions, sphincter tone may not be excessive. Perineal reflexes are intact.

Detrusor Areflexia with Sphincter Areflexia. Lesions of the sacral spinal cord or the nerve roots, such as fractures of the L6 or L7 vertebrae, cause a loss of the detrusor and urethral sphincter reflexes. The bladder is easily expressed and may leak urine continuously. Perineal reflexes are diminished or absent.

Detrusor Areflexia from Overdistention. Loss of excitation-contraction coupling in the detrusor muscle may occur as a result of severe overdistention of the bladder. Manual expression of the bladder may be difficult, because the sphincter is normal. The animal may empty the bladder partially by abdominal contraction. Attempts to void indicate that sensory pathways are intact and suggests a primary detrusor muscle abnormality. The most frequent cause is obstruction of the outflow tract (e.g., calculi or feline urologic syndrome).

Detrusor Hyperreflexia. Frequent voiding of small quantities of urine, often without warning, may be caused by partial lesions of the long pathways or of the cerebellum. Inflammation of the bladder (cystitis) may produce similar signs. There is little or no residual urine, the capacity of the bladder is reduced, and perineal reflexes are intact.

Reflex Dyssynergia. Normal initiation of voiding is followed by interruption of the stream through an involuntary contraction of the urethral sphincter. The stream of urine is normal at first. It is followed by short spurts and then by a complete cessation of the flow. Frequently, the animal continues to strain with no success. Reflex dyssynergia is seen primarily in male dogs. The pathogenesis is not certain but is presumed to be the result of a partial UMN lesion, causing a loss of the normal inhibition of the pudendal nerves during the detrusor reflex. The detrusor reflex is present, and the perineal reflex is often hyperactive.

Normal Detrusor Reflex with Decreased Sphincter Tone. Loss of normal urethral resistance with a normal detrusor reflex causes leaking of urine when voiding is delayed. The animal can empty the bladder, but as soon as a small amount of urine accumulates, leakage occurs. The leakage may be related to an abdominal press (barking, coughing) or may occur during complete rest. The most frequent cause is the lack of sex hormones in a neutered animal. Estrogen-responsive incontinence has been well documented in the ovariectomized bitch.[24] We have seen a similar syndrome in neutered male dogs. Both cases are responsive to hormone replacement therapy. A similar clinical picture may be seen in some animals that are not responsive to hormone therapy. The lesion may be a structural abnormality of the urethra, a loss of pudendal innervation, or

Table 5–1. EFFECT OF LESIONS OF THE NEUROMUSCULAR SYSTEM*

Location of Lesion	Normal Function	Bladder					Sphincter			
		Voluntary Control	Sustained Detrusor Reflex	Tone	Volume	Residual Urine	Voluntary Control	Reflexes (Perineal Bulboureth.)	Tone	Synergy with Detrusor
Cerebral cortex to brain stem	Voluntary control to detrusor and sphincter	Absent	Normal	Normal	May be greater or smaller than normal	None	Absent	Normal to hyperreflexic	Normal to increased	Normal
Cerebellum	Modulation (inhibition) of detrusor reflex	Normal, but increased frequency	Possible hyperreflexia	Normal	Small	None	Normal	Normal	Normal	Normal
Brain stem (pons) to sacral spinal cord	Sustained detrusor reflex	Absent	Lost early; small unsynchronized contractions late	Atonic early; possibly increased late	Large	Large	Absent	Normal to hyperreflexic	Normal to increased	Absent
Partial lesions (reflex dyssynergia)	Sustained detrusor reflex	May be present	May be present	Normal to atonic	Large	Small to large	May be normal	Normal	Normal to increased	Absent
Sacral spinal cord or roots	LMN to detrusor and sphincter	Absent	Absent	Atonic	Large	Large	Absent	Absent	Flaccid	Absent
Disruption of tight junctions of detrusor	Spread of excitation in detrusor	Absent	Absent	Atonic	Large	Large	Normal	Normal	Normal	Normal (cannot evaluate, however)

*From Oliver, J. E., Jr., and Osborne, C. A.: Neurogenic urinary incontinence. In Kirk, R. W.: Current Veterinary Therapy VI. Philadelphia, W. B. Saunders Co., 1977. Used by permission.

Table 5-2. SIGNS OF ABNORMAL MICTURITION

Problem	Voiding	Attempts to Void	Expression of Bladder	Residual Urine	Perineal Reflex	Probable Lesion
Detrusor areflexia, sphincter hypertonus	Absent	No	Difficult	Large amount	Present	Brain stem to L7, spinal cord
Detrusor areflexia, normal sphincter tone	Absent	No	Possible, some resistance	Large amount	Present	Brain stem to L7 spinal cord
Detrusor areflexia, sphincter areflexia	Absent	No	Easy, often leaks	Large to moderate amount	Absent	Sacral spinal cord or nerve roots
Detrusor areflexia (overdistention)	Absent	Yes	Possible, some resistance	Large amount	Present	Detrusor muscle
Detrusor hyperreflexia	Frequent, small quantity	Yes	Possible, some resistance	None	Present	Brain stem to L7, partial or cerebellum; rule out inflammation of bladder
Reflex dyssynergia	Frequent, spurting, unsustained	Yes	Difficult	Small to large amount	Present, may be exaggerated	Brain stem to L7, partial
Normal detrusor reflex, incompetent sphincter	Normal, but with leakage of urine with stress or full bladder	Yes	Easy	None	May or may not be present	Pudendal nerves, sympathetic nerves, estrogen deficiency

a loss of sympathetic innervation to the urethra.

Diagnosis

The minimum data base recommended for the evaluation of an animal with a problem associated with micturition is presented in Table 5–3. The minimum data base is designed to reveal any additional problems as well as to provide the information necessary to make a diagnosis and to formulate a prognosis. Figure 5–3 outlines the process of establishing a diagnosis. Specific steps in the process will be discussed in the following sections.[23]

HISTORY

In addition to the usual items in a history, the examiner should obtain some specific information pertinent to micturition.

Past History. The clinician should determine the animal's pattern of micturition habits from as early an age as possible (see Chapter 16). Age at house training, frequency of micturition at various ages, and changes in habits may provide insights into the onset of a problem prior to the owner's recognition of its significance.

Signs of abnormality in the nervous system or the urinary tract or previous trauma are important. Previous operative procedures, especially neurologic, abdominal, or pelvic surgery (e.g., ovariohysterectomy), should be analyzed in relation to the onset of the problem.

History of the Problem. Information regarding the onset and the chronologic course of the problem will allow the examiner to construct a sign-time graph, which is useful for determining the etiology of the disease (see Chapter 2).

Voluntary control of micturition is often best established by the owner's perceptions, which are supplemented and confirmed by direct observation of the animal in natural surroundings (e.g., outside on the grass). If the animal can volitionally initiate voiding, the *detrusor reflex* probably is present. Voluntary control also implies that micturition can be withheld for a reasonable length of time (house training) and can be interrupted if necessary. Interruption of micturition is difficult to evaluate. A dog that is lead-trained can be interrupted by a pull on the lead and a command to "come." Individual interpretation of interruption is quite subjective.

Reflex dyssynergia usually will appear as a normal initiation of voiding followed by a narrowing of the stream and a sudden interruption of the flow. The animal often will persist in straining and may continue voiding in brief spurts. Dyssynergia must be differentiated from partial obstruction (e.g., urethral calculi), which usually is recognized by catheterization and urethral contrast radiography.

Various types of incontinence may be described by the owner. Precipitate voiding (detrusor hyperreflexia), in which the animal voids suddenly in inappropriate places without apparent warning, is characteristic of cerebellar lesions and some partial spinal cord or brain stem lesions (see Table 5–2). Differentiation between precipitate voiding and loss of normal voluntary control, as in cortical lesions or behavioral changes, may be difficult on the basis of the history alone.

Dribbling of urine may result from loss of urethral resistance or overflow from an areflexic bladder (see Table 5–2).

PHYSICAL EXAMINATION

Observation of the animal may confirm the characteristics of micturition as described in the history. The differences in the various abnormalities of micturition may be very subtle, so it is critical that the problem described by the owner be verified by the examiner.

The presence of a *detrusor reflex* can be assumed if voiding is sustained (see Fig. 5–3). However, bladder contractions with incomplete voiding are common in neurologic disorders. Such contractions are not the result of

Table 5–3. MINIMUM DATA BASE FOR DIAGNOSIS OF DISORDERS OF MICTURITION*

History
Physical examination
    Includes: observation of voiding and measurement of residual urine
Neurologic examination
    Includes: sphincter reflexes
Clinical pathology
    Includes: CBC, urinalysis, BUN or creatinine determinations
Radiologic examination
    Includes: survey of abdomen and pelvis contrast cystography and urethrography intravenous pyelogram

*Modified from Oliver, J. E., Jr., and Osborne, C. A.: Neurogenic urinary incontinence. In Kirk, R. W.: Current Veterinary Therapy VI. Philadelphia, W. B. Saunders Co., 1977.

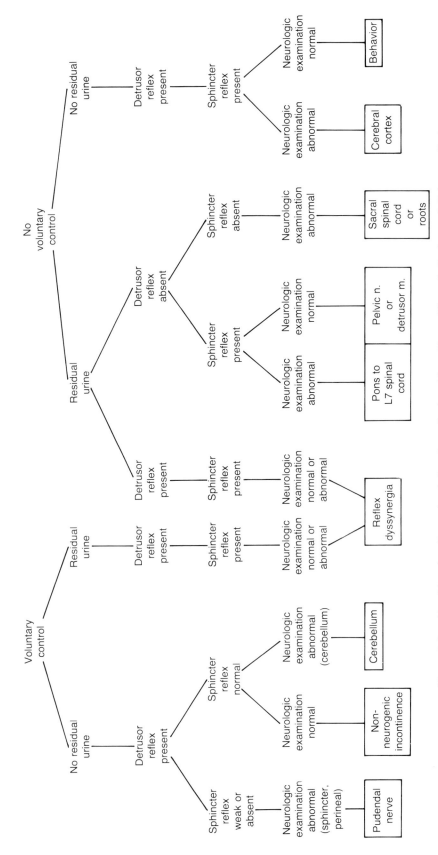

Figure 5–3. Algorithm for diagnosis of disorders of micturition. (From Oliver, J. E., Jr., and Osborne, C. A.: Neurogenic urinary incontinence. *In* Kirk, R. W., ed.: Current Veterinary Therapy VII. Philadelphia, W. B. Saunders Co., 1980, pp. 1122–1127. Used by permission.)

a true detrusor reflex. Therefore, the *residual urine* must be measured in every animal with a problem associated with micturition. After the animal has voided, preferably outside in natural surroundings, the bladder is catheterized and the residual urine is measured. Residual urine should be less than 10 per cent of the normal volume. Most animals have less than 10 ml.

Except for urethral flaps (which are rare), obstructions in the urethra can be detected when a catheter is passed. A flap can be demonstrated only by excretory urethrography.[25]

Palpation of the bladder before and after voiding provides some information regarding bladder tone. The tone of the detrusor muscle is intrinsic and is not directly related to innervation; however, a normal bladder contracts to accommodate the volume of urine present. An overdistended bladder with rupture of the tight junctions does not contract. A chronically infected bladder is often small and has thickened, fibrotic walls. A small contracted bladder with infection may not be the primary problem, since bladder infection is a common sequela to urine retention from neurogenic disorders. Some of the non-neurogenic causes of incontinence, such as tumors or calculi, may be identified by palpation.

Manual expression of the bladder provides some information regarding urethral sphincter tone. Normally, expression of the bladder is more difficult in the male than in the female. Urethral sphincter tone is decreased in lesions of the sacral spinal cord, the sacral roots, or the pudendal nerve (lower motor neuron) and is increased in lesions between the L7 spinal cord segment and the brain stem (see Table 5–2). The sacral spinal cord segments lie within the body of the fifth lumbar vertebra, so lesions of the vertebrae from L5–L6 caudally can affect the sacral roots.

NEUROLOGIC EXAMINATION

The complete neurologic examination has been described in Chapter 3. Reflexes related to the sacral spinal cord segments are especially important in neurogenic bladder dysfunction.

The anal and urethral sphincters are innervated by the pudendal nerve, primarily from sacral segments 1 and 2, but occasionally with fibers from S3. Anal sphincter function is easy to observe or to palpate, whereas the urethral sphincter is evaluated best by electrodiagnostic procedures.

The tone of the anal sphincter can be observed, or the sphincter can be palpated with a gloved digit. Two sacral reflexes also can be evaluated. The *bulbocavernosus reflex* is a sharp contraction of the sphincter in response to a squeeze of the bulb of the penis or the clitoris. The *perineal reflex* is a contraction of the sphincter in response to a pinch or pin prick of the perineal region. The perineal reflex also is used to test sensory distribution in the perineal region. Unilateral lesions are detected in this manner.

Lesions of the sacral spinal cord, the sacral roots, or the pudendal nerves will abolish these reflexes, and the anal sphincter will be atonic.

The history, the physical examination, and the neurologic examination provide sufficient data to differentiate neurogenic from non-neurogenic bladder disorders and to localize the lesion in the nervous system if a neurogenic disorder is present (see Tables 5–1 and 5–2). Additional data are necessary for the formulation of an etiologic diagnosis and a prognosis.

CLINICAL PATHOLOGY

The minimum data base includes a complete blood count (CBC), a urinalysis, and a determination of blood urea nitrogen (BUN) or creatinine values. Each is essential for the formulation of a prognosis of urinary tract dysfunction and may assist in the diagnosis of non-neurogenic problems of micturition.[23–25]

All animals with neurogenic bladder disorders are likely to have urinary tract infections. Constant surveillance and appropriate treatment, when indicated, are imperative if a favorable outcome is to be expected. Ureteral reflux is also a frequent complication of neurogenic bladder dysfunction. Reflux of infected urine may lead to pyelonephritis, uremia, and death.[26]

RADIOLOGIC EXAMINATION

Radiography is important for the identification of non-neurogenic problems, for the evaluation of the extent of urinary tract disease, which may be a complication of neurogenic disorders, and for the assessment of the primary neurologic problem.

Contrast cystourethrography performed during voiding has not been evaluated adequately in animals but could provide considerable information about the functional morphology of the lower urinary tract.[26]

ELECTROPHYSIOLOGIC EXAMINATION

Electrophysiologic tests have not been included in the minimum data base because they currently are not widely available. In some

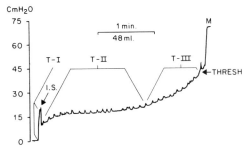

Figure 5–4. Cystometrogram of a dog showing segments of the tonus limb. *T-I* = Resting pressure. *T-II* = Bladder filling pressure change (smooth muscle elasticity). *T-III* = Bladder filling pressure change after the capacity is reached. Scale indicates time and volume. *Thresh* = Threshold of the detrusor reflex. *M* = Maximal contraction. *I.S.* = Initial spike, an artifact. (From Oliver, J. E., Jr., and Young, W. O.: Air cystometry in dogs under xylazine-induced restraint. Am. J. Vet. Res. 34:1433–1435, 1973. Used by permission.)

cases, however, electrophysiologic tests are necessary in order to make a definitive diagnosis.

The cystometrogram (CMG) measures intravesical pressure during a detrusor reflex (Fig. 5–4).[27,28] A sustained detrusor reflex is difficult to document clinically in most cases. Additionally, the CMG provides data on the threshold volume and pressure, the capacity, the ability of the bladder to fill at a normal pressure (a measure of elasticity of the bladder wall), and the presence of uninhibited bladder contractions (a sign of denervation). Normal data from the CMG of the dog are presented in Table 5–4.

Electromyography (EMG) of the skeletal muscles of the anal and urethral sphincters and other muscles in the pelvic diaphragm provides direct evidence of the status of innervation. The perineal or bulbocavernosus reflex also can be tested while a recording is being taken directly from these muscles in cases in which clinical evaluation is equivocal.

An EMG recording that is taken from the anal sphincter while the urethra or the bladder is being stimulated with a catheter electrode is termed *electromyelography* (EMyG).[29] Urethral stimulation evokes a response similar to the bulbocavernosus reflex. Stimulation of the bladder wall evokes a comparable response, except that the sensory pathway is in the pelvic nerves. An EMyG from bladder stimulation provides evidence of the integrity of the pelvic nerves. The main advantages of the electrical tests are: (1) the response is objective, (2) the response can be measured accurately, and (3) latencies are recorded that provide information about partial denervation. The urethral pressure profile measures the pressure along the length of the urethra.[30] The maximum urethral closure pressure and the functional profile length are the most important parameters (Fig. 5–5). Normal values are listed in Table 5–5.

Averaged evoked responses can be recorded from the scalp (cortex) or the spinal cord from stimulation of the bladder or the urethra (see the section on the somatosensory-evoked response in Chapter 6). The cortical-evoked response (CER) is a method of evaluating the sensory pathways.

Data from all of the tests are useful for establishing the location of the abnormality that is causing the problem. Table 5–6 summarizes the data provided by each test.

The final diagnosis should include (1) the location of the lesion in the nervous system, (2) the etiology of the lesion, (3) the functional central nervous system (CNS) deficit, and (4) the functional deficit related to micturition.

Table 5–4. NORMAL VALUES FOR CYSTOMETROGRAMS (CMG) OF DOGS USING XYLAZINE FOR RESTRAINT *

Measurement	Mean ± S.D. Values of CMG (N=41)†
Tonus Limb I	9.7 ± 4.3
Tonus Limb II	12.6 ± 12.2
Threshold Pressure	24.4 ± 10.0
Threshold Pressure Minus Tonus Limb I	14.4 ± 8.7
Threshold Volume	206.6 ± 184.4
Maximal Contraction Pressure	77.6 ± 33.8

*From Oliver, J. E., Jr., and Young, W. O.: Air cystometry in dogs under xylazine-induced restraint Am. J. Vet. Res. 34:1433–1435, 1973. Used by permission.

†N = number of CMG. All values are given in centimeters of water except for threshold volume, which is given in milliliters of air. (See Fig. 5–4.)

Table 5–5. NORMAL VALUES FOR URETHRAL PRESSURE PROFILES OF DOGS USING XYLAZINE FOR RESTRAINT *†

	Maximal Urethral Pressure (mm Hg)	Maximal Urethral Closure Pressure (mm Hg)	Functional Profile Length (cm)
Female dogs	27.1 ± 12.5	23.9 ± 11.8	7.2 ± 1.9
Male dogs	32.7 ± 4.1	28.3 ± 4.0	28.3 ± 3.9

*Modified from Rosin, A., Rosin, E., and Oliver, J. E., Jr.: Canine urethral pressure profile. Am. J. Vet. Res. 41:1113–1116, 1980.

†All values are mean ± standard deviation.

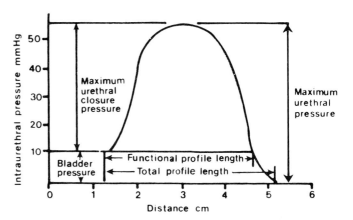

Figure 5–5. Schematic representation of the urethral closure pressure profile. (From Rosin, A., Rosin, E., and Oliver, J. E., Jr.: Canine urethral pressure profile. Am. J. Vet. Res. 41:1113–1116, 1980. Used by permission.)

Treatment

The management of a case is dependent on the final diagnosis. The treatment of primary CNS disease is described throughout this text. Functional deficits of micturition secondary to CNS disease may be temporary or permanent, depending on the reversibility of the CNS lesion and the maintenance of the integrity of the urinary system. If the bladder is severely infected and secondary fibrosis of the bladder wall occurs, normal function cannot be restored, even if the CNS lesion is corrected. The management of the urinary tract based on the functional disorder of micturition will be presented in this section.

Detrusor Areflexia with Sphincter Hypertonus. Lesions from the pons to the L7 spinal cord segments may abolish the detrusor reflex and may produce an UMN-type sphincter characterized by hyperreflexia and increased tone (see Table 5–2). The animal is unable to void, and it is difficult if not impossible to express the bladder manually.

The primary consideration in all neurogenic bladder disorders is to evacuate the bladder completely at least three times daily. When tone in the urethra is exaggerated, manual expression is not only ineffective but also dangerous. Aseptic catheterization is required. Indwelling catheters are associated with a high risk of infection, and their use should be avoided. One exception is in cases of detrusor areflexia from overdistention (see later).

Urethral tone may be reduced pharmacologically, making management easier. Phenoxybenzamine, an alpha-adrenergic blocking agent, sometimes is effective at doses of 10 mg per day. The dosage is increased every fourth day to a maximum of 30 mg. Hypotension is

Table 5 – 6. ELECTROPHYSIOLOGIC TESTS OF MICTURITION

	Detrusor Reflex	Detrusor Tone	Urethral Reflex	Urethral Tone	Pelvic Nerve	Pudendal Nerve	Sacral Spinal Cord	Spinal Cord and Brain
Cystometrogram	+	+			+		+	+
Urethral electromyogram			+			+	+	
Urethral pressure profile				+				
Electromyelogram of bladder					+	+	+	
Electromyelogram of urethra						+	+	
Cortical-evoked response of bladder					+		+	+
Cortical-evoked response of urethra						+	+	+

+ = test evaluates this function or this anatomic component

the most common side effect. Bethanechol is a cholinergic agent that stimulates bladder contraction. It should not be used when urethral resistance is increased, except in combination with an adrenergic blocking agent.[31]

Urinalysis is performed weekly or any time that the urine appears abnormal. At the first sign of infection, urine is obtained for quantitative culture and sensitivity tests.[25] Appropriate antibiotic therapy should be continued until urinalysis verifies correction of the problem. Animals receiving anti-inflammatory drugs such as corticosteroids are at increased risk for urinary tract infection. In addition, corticosteroids can suppress the inflammatory response to infection. Asymptomatic infection may go undetected unless urine is cultured repeatedly for micro-organisms.

If catheterization is necessary for prolonged periods (over 1 week), prophylactic antibacterial agents, such as methenamine, may be indicated. These products do not replace an aseptic catheterization technique.

If the detrusor reflex returns with good voiding of urine, the bladder is catheterized periodically to ensure that there is no residual urine. Voiding is often incomplete in the early stages, and residual urine in quantities of 10 to 20 ml or more can result in a urinary tract infection.

Bethanechol, a cholinergic agent, can be used to stimulate bladder contraction. We have not found it effective if the bladder is areflexic, however. If bladder contractions are present but are inadequate for good voiding, bethanechol in doses of 2.5 to 10 mg given subcutaneously tid may be beneficial. Side effects include increased motility of the gastrointestinal tract. Oral doses of up to 50 mg also may be effective. The combination of bethanechol and phenoxybenzamine may be necessary in order to reduce urethral resistance.[16]

Detrusor Areflexia with Normal Sphincter Tone. Some lesions of the spinal cord and the brain stem may abolish the detrusor reflex without producing hypertonus of the urethral sphincter. The bladder can be expressed manually in many of these cases. The urethra of the female dog is short, and the examiner will encounter less resistance with bitches than with male dogs. Manual expression may be effective even in face of sphincter hypertonus. Manual expression, if adequate, is less likely to produce infection when compared with repeated catheterization.

Other aspects of management are the same as those described earlier.

Detrusor Areflexia with Sphincter Areflexia. Lesions of the sacral spinal cord or the roots will produce a lower motor neuron deficit of both the bladder and the sphincter. The management of the bladder is the same as that described previously.

An additional management problem is created by the constant leakage of urine through the incompetent sphincter. Frequent evacuation of the bladder reduces the problem but does not eliminate it. Continual soiling of the skin with urine quickly leads to irritation and formation of decubital ulcers. Frequent hydrotherapy and protective emollients are useful adjuncts.

The problem of long-term management of the patient with paralysis of the sphincter has not been solved. Surgical reconstruction of the bladder neck and the urethra is sometimes successful in humans but has had no significant trials in animals. Timm and others have developed prosthetic devices that offer promise of a solution.[32] The cost of these devices probably will limit their applicability in veterinary medicine.

Detrusor Areflexia from Overdistention. Severe overdistention of the bladder can produce a separation of the tight junctions between the detrusor muscle fibers, which prevents excitation-contraction coupling. The neural elements may be normal.

The bladder must be treated early if an irreversible deficit is to be avoided. Complete evacuation of the bladder must be accomplished and maintained for 1 to 2 weeks. Manual expression is not recommended because of the increased stress on the detrusor muscle. Intermittent aseptic catheterization can be performed at least tid but preferably qid. An indwelling catheter for the first 5 to 7 days followed by intermittent catheterization, if needed, is the procedure of choice. This is one of the few instances in which an indwelling catheter is recommended. Function should return in 1 to 2 weeks if the treatment is successful. Bethanechol may be of benefit, especially if partial contractions are present.

Antibiotics or urinary antiseptics are administered throughout the treatment period. Frequent urinalysis, with cultures when indicated, is mandatory. Infection in the overdistended bladder leads to fibrosis, and adequate function will not be restored in this case.

Detrusor Hyperreflexia. Frequent voiding of small volumes of urine, often without much warning and with little or no residual urine, is characteristic of detrusor hyperreflexia. Partial long tract lesions or abnormalities of the cerebellum may produce these signs. The condition is not usually detrimental to the patient, but it may be an early sign of a progressive disease of the nervous system. Additionally, it is socially unacceptable in the house pet. The condition must be differentiated from the small, contracted, irritable bladder associated with chronic cystitis.

Anticholinergic medication may be of benefit. Propantheline (Pro-Banthine) is used in dosages of from 7.5 to 30 mg tid or qid. The lowest dose should be tried first and should be increased in small increments until a response is obtained. Overdosage may result in urinary retention in addition to the other side effects characteristic of this group of drugs.[31]

Reflex Dyssynergia. Initiation of a detrusor reflex with voiding followed by an uncontrolled reflex contraction of the urethral sphincter is termed reflex dyssynergia. Partial lesions of the long tracts are presumed to be responsible, although the condition has been seen in a dog with a cauda equina lesion.

The problem may be related to uninhibited reflexes of the external urethral sphincter (skeletal muscle) or to increased tonus in the smooth muscle related to adrenergic innervation.[33] Limited reports in human beings and in dogs have not yet provided a definitive therapeutic regimen. Skeletal muscle reflexes may be reduced with diazepam (Valium) or baclofen, a new drug that has not been tested clinically in animals. Sympathetic (adrenergic) activity can be reduced with an alpha-blocking agent such as phenoxybenzamine (Dibenzyline, 10-mg capsules). The dosage must be determined by trial, starting with 10 mg per day and increasing every fourth day if indicated. The major side effect of alpha-blocking agents is hypotension.

Normal Detrusor Reflex with Decreased Sphincter Tone. If hormone therapy is ineffective in an animal with normal voiding but leakage, an alpha-adrenergic stimulating drug, such as phenylpropanolamine, may be effective. The dosage is 12.5 to 50 mg tid, orally. Side effects include restlessness and irritability.

The management of neurogenic bladder disorders is critical for the ultimate prognosis of both reversible and irreversible CNS disorders. A study of chronically paralyzed people revealed that 75 per cent die of renal failure secondary to neurogenic bladder dysfunction.[34]

CASE HISTORIES

In the cases in this section, you should concentrate on the problem related to micturition, even though it may be only a part of the total deficit. Using Table 5—2, decide the location of the lesion that causes the problem.

Case History 5A

Signalment. Dachshund, male, 5 years old.
History. The dog became paralyzed in the pelvic limbs last night. The dog was alone in a fenced-in back yard when the owners found him.
Physical Examination. The bladder is large and easily palpated. It cannot be expressed, even with considerable pressure.
Neurologic Examination. The dog is alert and drags himself around the examination room. The thoracic limbs are normal. There are no voluntary movements of the pelvic limbs. The postural reactions are normal in the thoracic limbs and absent in the pelvic limbs. The spinal reflexes are normal in the thoracic limbs. The quadriceps reflex is exaggerated (+3) bilaterally, and the flexion reflexes are strong in the pelvic limbs. The perineal and bulbocavernosus reflexes are present. The anal sphincter has good tone. Hyperesthesia is evident on palpation of the T13—L2 area. The panniculus reflex is absent caudal to L1. Deep pain sensation is present in the pelvic limbs.

Case History 5B

Signalment. Pekingese, female, 6 years old.
History. The dog suddenly became paralyzed in the pelvic limbs while playing with the children of the owners. When first seen by the referring veterinarian 4 hours later, the dog had complete pelvic limb paralysis, increased tone in the pelvic limbs, exaggerated quadriceps reflexes, and no sensation caudal to L4. The dog was referred to you.
Physical Examination. The dog is presented 12 hours after the onset of paralysis. Urine has leaked during the trip to the clinic, and the dog is obviously in pain. The bladder is large and easily expressed on palpation.
Neurologic Examination. The dog is alert and anxious. The thoracic limbs are normal. The postural reactions and the spinal reflexes are absent in the pelvic limbs. The perineal reflex is absent, and the anal sphincter is dilated. There is no sensation caudal to T13.

Case History 5C

Signalment. Chihuahua, male, 3 years old.
History. The dog has had generalized seizures at least three times in the last 2 weeks. The previous medical history is noncontributory. Questioning about other changes reveals that the dog has started urinating in the house within the past 3 months, although before this

problem he had not urinated in the house since he was a puppy. The dog has not been on medication.

Physical Examination. The skull is dome-shaped, and the fontanelle is 1.5 cm in diameter. The bladder is empty.

Neurologic Examination. The postural reactions are judged to be a bit slow, but the rest of the examination is normal.

ASSESSMENT 5A

The neurologic examination indicates a UMN paralysis of the pelvic limbs. The sensory examination localizes the lesion to T13–L2. The bladder problem can be characterized as detrusor areflexia with sphincter hypertonia, which is typical of a lesion rostral to L7. Cystometry confirms the detrusor areflexia. Management of the bladder should include intermittent aseptic catheterization (at least tid). The dog has a herniated intervertebral disk, which is decompressed by hemilaminectomy. Seven days after surgery, voluntary movements of the pelvic limbs are seen, and voiding begins with minimal pressure of the abdomen. Voiding returns to normal in 10 days.

ASSESSMENT 5B

The dog has lower motor neuron paralysis of the pelvic limbs and the sphincters. This finding indicates a lesion from L4 through S3. The loss of sensation has progressed from L4 to T13 in 8 hours, indicating a progressive lesion. There is detrusor areflexia and sphincter areflexia, which is consistent with a lesion of the sacral segments of the spinal cord. The dog has a herniated disk with hemorrhagic myelomalacia (*see* Chapter 9). The prognosis is so poor that no other tests are performed. Cystometry would confirm the detrusor areflexia. The urethral pressure profile would be expected to have pressures below normal. Electromyography would demonstrate no voluntary or reflex activity, but fibrillation potentials would not be present this early. If management were attempted, manual evacuation of the bladder probably would be effective.

ASSESSMENT 5C

The seizures indicate abnormality of the cerebrum or diencephalon or a metabolic problem. The change in urinary habits also could be either cerebral or metabolic (polyuria). A laboratory evaluation is indicated in order to rule out metabolic diseases. The evaluation was performed, and all tests were normal.

Rule-outs:
1. hydrocephalus,
2. encephalitis,
3. tumor (unlikely), and
4. idiopathic epilepsy.

The cystometrogram was normal and showed adequate capacity and a good detrusor reflex. An electro-encephalogram showed high-voltage slow waves in all leads. This finding is typical of hydrocephalus. A ven-

tricular tap confirmed the diagnosis. The dog was treated with corticosteroids, and complete remission of the signs resulted. (See Chapter 14 for a discussion of hydrocephalus.) The voiding behavior was related to cerebral dysfunction.

REFERENCES

1. Barrington, F. J. F.: The nervous mechanism of micturition. Q. J. Exp. Physiol. 8:33–71, 1914.
2. Iggo, A.: Tension receptors in the stomach and the urinary bladder. J. Physiol. 128:593–607, 1955.
3. Oliver, J. E., Jr., Bradley, W. E., and Fletcher, T. F.: Spinal cord representation of the micturition reflex. J. Comp. Neurol. 137:329–346, 1969.
4. Purinton, P. T., and Oliver, J. E., Jr.: Spinal cord origin of innervation to the bladder and urethra of the dog. Exp. Neurol. 65:422–434, 1979.
5. Gjone, R., and Setekleiv, J.: Excitatory and inhibitory bladder responses to stimulation of the cerebral cortex in the cat. Acta Physiol. Scand. 59:337–348, 1963.
6. Langworthy, O. R., and Hesser, F. H.: An experimental study of micturition released from cerebral control. Am. J. Physiol. 115:694–700, 1936.
7. Bradley, W. E., and Teague, C. T.: Cerebellar influence on the micturition reflex. Exp. Neurol. 23:399–411, 1969.
8. Oliver, J. E., Jr., and Selcer, R. R.: Neurogenic causes of abnormal micturition in the dog and cat. Vet. Clin. North Am. 4:517–524, 1974.
9. Oliver, J. E., Jr., Bradley, W. E., and Fletcher, T. F.: Spinal cord distribution of the somatic innervation of the external urethral sphincter in the cat. J. Neurol. Sci. 10:11–23, 1970.
10. Hamberger, B., and Norberg, K. A.: Adrenergic synaptic terminals and nerve cells in bladder ganglia of the cat. Int. J. Neuropharmacol. 4:41–45, 1965.
11. Nergardh, A., and Boreus, L. O.: Autonomic receptor function in the lower urinary tract of man and cat. Scand. J. Urol. Nephrol. 6:32–36, 1972.
12. Gregg, R. A., Boyarsky, S., and Labay, P.: Blocking of beta adrenergic receptors in the urinary bladder using sotalol. South. Med. J. 62:1366–1373, 1969.
13. DeGroat, W. C., and Saum, W. R.: Sympathetic inhibition of the urinary bladder and of pelvic ganglionic transmission in the cat. J. Physiol. 214:297–314, 1972.
14. Gennser, G., Owman, C., Owman, T., and Wehlin, L.: Significance of adrenergic innervation of the bladder outlet during ejaculation. Lancet 1:154, 1969.
15. Sundin, T., and Dahlstrom, A.: The sympathetic innervation of the urinary bladder and urethra in the normal state and after parasympathetic denervation at the spinal root level. Scand. J. Urol. Nephrol. 7:131–149, 1973.
16. Applebaum, S. M.: Pharmacologic agents in micturitional disorders. Urology 16:555–568, 1980.
17. DeGroat, W. C.: Nervous control of the urinary bladder of the cat. Brain Res. 87:201–211, 1975.
18. Bradley, W. E., and Timm, G. W.: Physiology of micturition. Vet. Clin. North Amer. 4:487–500, 1974.
19. Bradley, W. E., and Teague, C. T.: Spinal cord organization of micturition reflex afferents. Exp. Neurol. 22:504–516, 1968.
20. Bradley, W. E., and Teague, C. T.: Electrophysiology of pelvic and pudendal nerves in the cat. Exp. Neurol. 35:378–393, 1972.
21. Jonas, U., and Tanagho, E. A.: Studies on vesicourethral reflexes. Invest. Urol. 12:357–373, 1975.

22. Bradley, W. E., and Teague, C. T.: Hypogastric and pelvic nerve activity during the micturition reflex. J. Urol. 101:438–440, 1969.
23. Oliver, J. E., Jr., and Osborne, C. A.: Neurogenic urinary incontinence. *In* Kirk, R. W., ed., Current Veterinary Therapy VI. Philadelphia, W. B. Saunders Co., 1977.
24. Osborne, C. A., and Oliver, J. E., Jr.: Non-neurogenic urinary incontinence. *In* Kirk, R. W., ed., Current Veterinary Therapy VI. Philadelphia, W. B. Saunders Co., 1977.
25. Osborne, C. A., Low, D. G., and Finco, D. R.: Canine and Feline Urology. Philadelphia, W. B. Saunders Co., 1972.
26. Bors, E., and Comarr, A. E.: Neurological Urology, Baltimore, University Park Press, 1971.
27. Oliver, J. E., Jr., and Young, W. O.: Evaluation of pharmacologic agents for restraint in cystometry in the dog and cat. Am. J. Vet. Res. 34:665–668, 1973.
28. Oliver, J. E., Jr., and Young, W. O.: Air cystometry in dogs under xylazine-induced restraint. Am. J. Vet. Res. 34:1433–1435, 1973.
29. Bradley, W. E., Timm, G. W., Rockswold, G. L., and Scott, F. B.: Detrusor and urethral electromyelography. J. Urol. 114:891–894, 1975.
30. Rosin, A., Rosin, E., and Oliver, J. E., Jr.: Canine urethral pressure profile. Am. J. Vet. Res. 41:1113–1116, 1980.
31. Rosin, A. H., and Ross, L.: Diagnosis and pharmacological management of disorders of urinary continence in the dog. Comp. Cont. Ed. Pract. Vet. 3:601–612, 1981.
32. Timm, G. W.: Electromechanical restoration of voiding. Vet. Clin. North Amer. 4:525–533, 1974.
33. Krane, R. J., and Olsson, C. A.: Phenoxybenzamine in neurogenic bladder dysfunction. II. Clinical consideration. J. Urol. 110:653–656, 1973.
34. Tribe, C. R.: Renal Failure in Paraplegia. London, Pitman Medical Publishing Co., 1969.

6

CHAPTER

CONFIRMING A DIAGNOSIS

After the history has been taken and the physical and neurologic examinations have been completed, a list of problems is made. For each problem, the examiner makes a list of most likely diseases to be ruled out by appropriate diagnostic tests. Chapters 2 through 5 have provided the information necessary for identifying the problem and making an anatomic diagnosis. Chapters 8 through 17 will elaborate on each problem in terms of arriving at a differential diagnosis through appropriate diagnostic tests. This chapter discusses the tests that are available; indicates the feasibility of performing them; suggests references for further reading on techniques and interpretation; and outlines the indications, the contraindications, and the limitations of the tests.

Table 6-1. MINIMUM DATA BASE: NEUROLOGIC PROBLEM

History (see Chapter 2)
Physical examination
Neurologic examination (see Chapter 3)
Clinical laboratory profile
  Complete blood count
    At least: Packed cell volume
            Hemoglobin level
            White blood count and differential
  Urinalysis
  Chemistry profile
    Recommended: Serum urea nitrogen level (BUN)
              Serum alanine transaminase level (SGPT)
              Alkaline phosphatase level
              Calcium level
              Blood glucose level (with animal fasting at least 24 hours)
              Total serum protein level
              Albumin level

CLINICAL LABORATORY STUDIES

Hematology, Blood Chemistry Analysis, and Urinalysis

AVAILABILITY

All clinical practices should have the facilities to perform routine hematology, chemistry analysis, and urinalysis.

INDICATIONS

A minimum data base is established for all sick animals in order for common diseases to be ruled out and information about the general status of the animal to be accessible. In addition to the history, the physical examination, and the neurologic examination, it is recommended that a laboratory profile be developed (Table 6-1). The studies that are performed may vary, depending on the availability of automated chemistry profiles, the experience of the examiner in the practice, or the influence of economic considerations. The function of the major organ systems should be evaluated. Glucose and calcium levels always are included in the assessment of patients presenting with seizures. The primary indications are summarized in Table 6-2.

Cerebrospinal Fluid (CSF) Analysis

AVAILABILITY

CSF analysis can be performed in any practice.

CSF is collected routinely by cisternal puncture. The examiner should perform the procedure often enough to maintain confidence. Lumbar puncture is more difficult in dogs but can be performed at the lumbosacral interspace in cats and in large animals. Lumbar CSF is more likely to provide positive information in cases of spinal cord disease.

CSF is collected with the animal under general anesthesia in order to avoid movements during the placement of the needle. The skin is clipped and prepared for an aseptic procedure. The needle (a 22G, 1½-inch disposable spinal needle with a stylet for most small animals; a 20G, 2½-inch needle for most large animals) should be handled with sterile gloves. The landmarks for the midline are the occipital protuberance and the spine of the axis (C2) (Fig. 6-1). The needle is inserted on the midline near the cranial border of the wings of the atlas (C1). A slight loss of resistance is felt as the needle penetrates the subarachnoid space. The stylet is withdrawn, and fluid is removed

Table 6–2. CLINICAL LABORATORY PROFILE

Test	Indications	Probable Usefulness	Contraindications	Availability
Hematology	Inflammation	Moderate to high	None	Practice
	Neoplastic disease	Low		
	Toxic disease	Low		
Blood chemistry analysis	Metabolic disease	High	None	Practice
Urinalysis	Metabolic disease	Moderate	None	Practice
Cerebrospinal fluid analysis	Degenerative disease	Moderate	Increased	Practice
	Demyelinating disease	Low	intracranial	
	Neoplastic disease	Moderate	pressure	
	Inflammation	High		
	Trauma	Moderate		
	Toxic disease	Low		

from the hub of the needle as it flows. The syringe is not attached to the needle, because aspiration is likely to cause hemorrhage. The techniques for lumbar puncture are described in several texts.[1–3]

Total and differential white blood cell (WBC) counts are the most important parts of a CSF analysis. Unless a preservative is added, cell counts must be determined within 30 minutes of collection, because WBCs deteriorate rapidly. Techniques for using a preservative and a filtration method of obtaining cell counts have been described by Roszel.[4] Not all laboratories are prepared to use this method.

Cell counts are performed on fresh specimens with a hemacytometer. One chamber of the hemacytometer is filled with CSF, and cells within all nine squares are counted. The number of cells counted is multiplied by 1.1 to give the total count per cu mm. WBCs can be differentiated from red blood cells (RBCs) because they are larger, more granular, and more refractile, especially with reduced illumination. The CSF can be diluted with a crystal violet–acetic acid fluid to lyse RBCs and to stain WBCs. The CSF is drawn into a pipette (1.0 ml) with 0.1 ml of the diluting fluid. The count is determined as just described, but the total count is multiplied by 1.2 to give the number of cells per cu mm. Subtracting this number from a total count on undiluted fluid gives the number of RBCs per cu mm.

The remaining CSF is centrifuged. The supernate is used for protein determination, and the sediment is smeared and stained for a differential WBC count. The addition of a few drops of canine serum to the sediment improves the quality of the cells in the smear. Any stain used for blood is acceptable.

The examiner should observe the appearance of the CSF. Hemorrhage caused by the puncture produces a red tinge to the fluid that decreases as the flow continues. Centrifugation should leave a clear, colorless fluid. A yellowish tinge to the CSF is called xanthochromia and is caused by free bilirubin. Previous subarachnoid hemorrhage is the usual cause, although prolonged icterus can produce xanthochromia. Turbidity is caused by an increase in the cell content of the fluid. Usually, more than 500 cells per cu mm are required to produce turbidity. Shaking the sample will produce foam if the protein content is markedly elevated. Fibrin clots may be seen if the elevated protein includes fibrinogen.

Measurement of CSF protein is necessary for a complete examination. Simple qualitative studies such as the Pandy test are adequate, although quantitative methods are preferred. The Pandy test can be performed in the practice.[1] Quantitative analysis also can be done in the practice, or the sample can be sent to a reference laboratory.

Other chemical values, including glucose levels, creatine phosphokinase (CPK) levels, and lactic dehydrogenase (LDH) levels, may be determined. Quantities necessary for these tests are difficult to obtain from small animals, and the usefulness of the studies has not been demonstrated clearly. CSF glucose levels may be decreased in bacterial infections, but the increase in cells and protein is more significant. Increased CPK concentrations occur when nervous tissue is destroyed, but the increase usually parallels the increase in protein values. LDH concentrations have been reported to increase in central nervous system (CNS) lymphosarcoma.

A strong clinical suspicion of bacterial infection, an increase in WBCs, or the presence of neutrophils is an indication for CSF culture and sensitivity testing. Fluid should be obtained in two sterile syringes, one for laboratory analysis and one for culture.

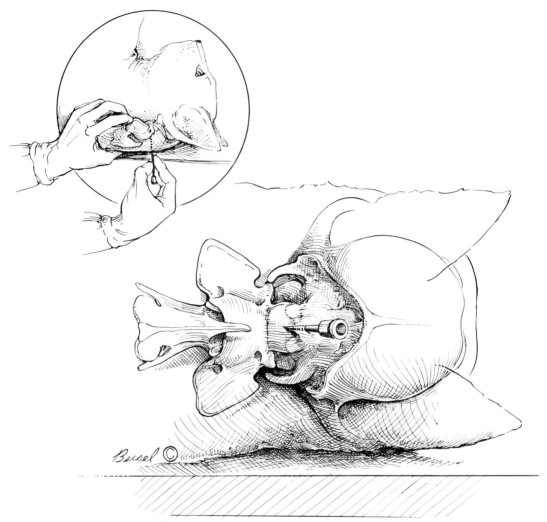

Figure 6–1. Landmarks for cerebrospinal fluid collection. (From Greene, C. E., and Oliver, J. E., Jr.: Neurologic examination. *In* Ettinger, S. J.: Textbook of Veterinary Internal Medicine, 2nd ed., Philadelphia, W. B. Saunders Co., 1982. Used by permission.)

CSF pressure may be a useful measurement in some situations. It is technically difficult to perform and frequently results in hemorrhage that can contaminate the CSF if the clinician is inexperienced.

INDICATIONS

CSF analysis is the best test for the diagnosis of CNS inflammatory disease. Increased WBC counts and increased protein are expected with active inflammatory diseases. The WBCs are predominantly polymorphonuclear leukocytes in bacterial diseases and predominantly lymphocytes in viral diseases. Fungal and protozoal diseases may cause mixed populations of leukocytes (Table 6–3).

Any disease that causes degeneration of nervous tissue without inflammation will cause an increase in CSF protein with little or no increase in cells. Primary degenerative or demyelinating diseases, neoplasia, or any compression of the CNS may produce this change (Table 6–3).

Free blood or xanthochromia may be seen following subarachnoid hemorrhage. Hemorrhage may be caused by trauma, primary vascular disease, or secondary vascular lesions from inflammation or neoplasia.

CONTRAINDICATIONS

The animal should be anesthetized when CSF is collected; therefore, if anesthesia is contraindicated, CSF should not be obtained.

CSF should not be collected if increased in-

Table 6-3. CEREBROSPINAL FLUID*

Disease	Appearance	Pressure (mm H$_2$O)	White Blood Cells/cu mm	Cell Type	Protein (mg/dl)	Other
Normal dog	Clear	<170	<5	Mononuclear	<25	Glucose: 60% to 70% of blood glucose
Normal cat	Clear	<100	<5	Mononuclear	<25	
Normal horse	Clear	<400	<5	Mononuclear	<70	
Normal cow	Clear	<200	<5	Mononuclear	<40	
Inflammatory						
I. Meningitis						
Bacterial	Turbid	Slight increase	Increased, usually >100	Mostly neutrophils	Increased, usually >100	Glucose decreased
Viral	Clear	Slight increase	Increased, usually <100	Mostly mononuclear	Increased	Fluorescent antibody for distemper
Feline infectious peritonitis	Clear to turbid	Increased	Increased, usually >100	Mixed, mostly mononuclear	Increased, usually >100	
Fungal	Turbid	Increased	Increased, usually >100	Mixed	Increased, usually >100	Organisms may be seen, especially *Cryptococcus*
Protozoal	Clear	Increased	Increased, usually >100	Mononuclear, sometimes neutrophils	Increased, usually >100	
Parasitic	Clear to xanthochromic		Increased, variable	Mixed, sometimes eosinophils	Increased, usually >100	
II. Encephalitis—usually similar to above except cell count and protein are lower if meninges are not involved.						
Degenerative, including compression	Clear	Normal	Normal to slight increase, usually <15	Mononuclear	Increased, usually <100	
Neoplastic	Clear	Increased	Normal to slight increase, usually <10	Mononuclear	Increased, usually <100	Tumor cells, e.g., lymphosarcoma, metastatic tumors, or ependymoma, rarely are seen. Usually *contraindicated* in suspected brain tumors. Not very useful for diagnosis and dangerous if intracranial pressure is elevated.
Traumatic	Xanthochromic	Increased	Normal to increased	RBCs, WBCs	Increased, variable	Usually *contraindicated.* Not needed for diagnosis and dangerous if intracranial pressure is elevated.

*Modified from Hoerlein, B. F.: Canine Neurology: Diagnosis and Treatment, 3rd ed. Philadelphia, W. B. Saunders Co., 1978; Kornegay, J. N.: Cerebrospinal fluid collection, examination, and interpretation in dogs and cats. Comp. Cont. Ed. Pract. Vet. 3:85–92, 1981; and deLahunta, A.: Veterinary Neuroanatomy and Clinical Neurology. Philadelphia, W. B. Saunders Co., 1977.

tracranial pressure is suspected. Removal of CSF from a cisternal or a lumbar puncture causes a pressure shift that pushes the cerebrum or the cerebellum in a caudal direction. Herniation of the cerebellum causes death of the animal from compression of the medullary respiratory centers. The slight increase in pressure associated with inflammatory disease is not sufficient to cause a problem. Increased pressure from brain tumors or intracranial trauma can cause herniation. The information obtained from the CSF analysis may not be worth the risk to the animal in these cases.

RADIOGRAPHY

Radiography is the most frequently used and the most useful diagnostic tool in neurology (Table 6–4).

AVAILABILITY

Most veterinary practices have a radiographic capability that is adequate for the formulation of a neurologic diagnosis in small animals. Meticulous technique is essential for the detection of the subtle changes that are often the key to a diagnosis.[1,5] Positioning of the animal, correct exposure, and proper development are all imperative. Beyond these parameters, the only limitation is the interpretive skill of the veterinarian. Interpretive skill is developed through practice. An approach to the interpretation of radiographs is outlined in Table 6–5.

Contrast procedures, especially myelography, are within the capabilities of most practices. As is the case with most procedures, however, they must be performed often enough to enable the veterinarian to be confident of both the technique and the interpretation. Table 6–4 indicates all contrast procedures available in specialty practice. Arteriography requires rapid-sequence film exposure, which necessitates equipment that

Table 6–4. RADIOGRAPHY

Test	Indications	Possible Usefulness	Contraindications	Availability
Spinal radiography	Degenerative disease (vertebral)	High	Anesthesia usually required	Practice
	Anomaly	High		
	Neoplasia	Moderate		
	Inflammatory disease (vertebral)	High		
	Trauma	High		
Myelography	Degenerative disease	High	Anesthesia required	Specialty practice
	Anomaly	High	Not done if active inflammation is present.	
	Neoplasia	High		
	Inflammatory disease	Low		
	Trauma	High	Spinal tap not done if intracranial pressure is increased	
Epidurography (primarily for evaluation of caudal lumbar and sacral area)	Degenerative disease	Variable	Anesthesia required	Specialty practice
	Anomaly	Variable		
	Neoplasia	High		
	Inflammatory disease	Variable		
	Trauma	Low		
Vertebral sinus venography	Same as those for epidurography			
Skull radiography	Anomaly	High	Anesthesia required	Practice
	Neoplasia	Low		
	Inflammatory disease (especially otitis interna)	Low (except in cases of otitis)		
	Trauma	High		
Ventriculography	Anomaly (hydrocephalus)	High	Anesthesia required	Specialty practice
	Neoplasia	Low		
Cavernous sinus venography	Neoplasia (floor of skull)	Moderate	Anesthesia required	Specialty practice
Cerebral arteriography	Neoplasia	High	Anesthesia required	Specialty practice, institutions
Radioisotope scans	Neoplasia	Moderate	Anesthesia required	Institutions
Computerized axial tomography	Degenerative disease	Moderate	Anesthesia required; procedure is expensive	Institutions (few)
	Anomaly	High		
	Neoplasia	High		
	Trauma	High		

Table 6–5. SYSTEMATIC APPROACH TO THE INTERPRETATION OF RADIOGRAPHS

1. Scan the entire radiograph for quality of exposure, positioning, and presence of artifacts or motion. Recognize the limitations imposed by these factors.
2. Scan the structures on the radiograph that are not of primary interest, such as soft tissue, abdomen, chest, and so forth.
3. Systematically evaluate the area of primary interest.

Spine

a. Scan the entire vertebral column for contour: ventral surface of vertebral bodies, floor of spinal canal, lamina, articulations, spinous processes. See Table 6–6: Displacement and Proliferation.
b. Scan the entire vertebral column for changes in bone density, such as lytic or proliferative changes. See Table 6–6: Lysis and Proliferation.
c. Scan the spinal canal for changes in density, especially at the intervertebral foramina and the disk space.
d. Compare the size of adjacent intervertebral disk spaces, intervertebral foramina, and the joint space of facets. Narrowing of one or more of these spaces is suggestive of disk herniation.
e. Stand back and scan the spine again. Sometimes, changes in contour or spacing are more apparent from a distance.

Skull

a. Ventrodorsal and frontal (anteroposterior) views are especially useful because the two sides can be compared.
b. Scan the periphery of the calvarium for asymmetry, cracks, deviations, or abnormal shape. See Table 6–6: Proliferation, Lysis, and Abnormal Shape.
c. Compare the nasal passages, the frontal sinuses, and the bulla of the middle ear for similarity in density.
d. Survey the calvarium for changes in density (proliferative or lytic), normal digital impressions, presence of open suture lines or fontanelles, or linear fractures.
e. Evaluate the structures inside the calvarium—osseous tentorium cerebelli, foramina, petrous temporal bone.

included in the discussion of each disease (see Chapters 8 through 17).

Contrast procedures are used to confirm a suspected lesion that cannot be identified definitively on survey radiographs or to identify the extent or the location of the lesion more precisely.

Myelography (radiographs following the injection of contrast material into the subarachnoid space) is the most frequently used contrast procedure.[1,5,6] Masses that occupy space in the spinal canal (tumors, abscesses, disks, and so forth) cause alterations in the contrast column. The epidural, intradural-extramedullary, or intramedullary location can be deter-

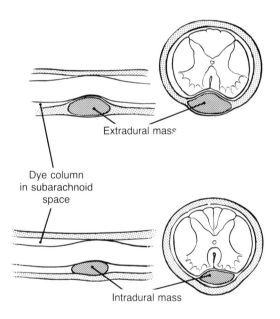

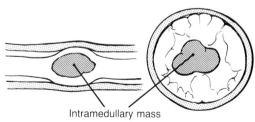

Figure 6–2. Effect of a mass lesion on a myelogram. *Top:* An extradural mass causes thinning or complete obliteration of the dye column. *Middle:* An intradural-extramedullary mass deviates the spinal cord and obstructs the dye column. The cranial and the caudal borders of the mass may have a cup-shaped outline of contrast material. *Bottom:* An intramedullary mass expands the spinal cord, causing thinning or obliteration of the dye column on all sides.

is usually available in institutional settings. Radioisotope brain scans and computerized axial tomography are available only in larger clinics and hospitals.

INDICATIONS

Nervous tissue has essentially the same radiographic density as other soft tissues. Radiographs of the head and the spinal column detect changes in the skull and the vertebrae. Lesions of nervous tissue, such as hemorrhage, tumor, or degeneration, are not detected, except in rare cases with calcification of the lesion. The most common radiographic changes and their causes are listed in Table 6–6. Examples of radiographic changes associated with specific disease processes are

Table 6–6. RADIOGRAPHIC FINDINGS AND INTERPRETATION

Radiographic Change	Possible Causes	Radiographic Change	Possible Causes
	Vertebrae		space, foramen, and facet space)
Proliferation	*Degenerative:* Spondylosis, dural ossification (linear density in spinal canal)		*Anomalous:* Hemivertebrae, agenesis of dens (atlantoaxial luxation)
	Neoplastic: Primary or metastatic vertebral tumor		*Neoplastic:* Pathologic fractures
	Nutritional: Ankylosing spondylosis, hypervitaminosis A		*Nutritional:* Pathologic fractures
			Inflammatory: Pathologic fractures
			Traumatic: Fractures, luxations
	Inflammatory: Osteomyelitis involving disk space, diskospondylitis (osteomyelitis usually is proliferative and lytic)		**Skull**
		Proliferation	*Degenerative:* Hypertrophic osteopathy of the mandible and skull (possibly inflammatory)
	Traumatic: Healing fracture		*Neoplastic:* Primary or metastatic tumor
Lysis	*Neoplastic:* Primary or metastatic vertebral tumor, widening of spinal canal (spinal cord tumor), widening of intervertebral foramen (nerve root tumor)		*Inflammatory:* Osteomyelitis, otitis media and otitis interna
		Lysis	*Anomalous:* Loss of digital markings, open fontanelles or suture lines, loss of osseous tentorium (may be caused by chronic hydrocephalus)
	Nutritional: Generalized loss of density, hypocalcemia, hyperparathyroidism		*Neoplastic:* Primary or metastatic tumor
	Inflammatory: Osteomyelitis involving disk space, diskospondylitis (osteomyelitis usually is proliferative and lytic)		*Nutritional:* Generalized loss of density, hypocalcemia, hyperparathyroidism
			Inflammatory: Osteomyelitis, otitis media and otitis interna
Abnormal shape of vertebrae	*Degenerative:* Cervical instability	Abnormal shape	*Anomalous:* Hydrocephalus, rarely otocephaly, hydranencephaly, and other cranial malformations
	Anomalous: Hemivertebrae, spina bifida, fused vertebrae		
	Traumatic: Compression fractures		*Traumatic:* Fractures
Displacement	*Degenerative:* Cervical spondylopathy (Wobbler syndrome), lumbosacral spondylopathy, intervertebral disk herniation (narrowing of inter-	Alterations in shape of foramina	*Anomalous:* Occipital dysplasia, hydrocephalus
			Neoplastic: Tumor of a cranial nerve

mined by the type of distortion occurring in the contrast column (Fig. 6–2).[6] Focal degenerative changes in the spinal cord are recognized as a narrowing of the cord with a widening of the contrast column. Severe malacia may allow the contrast media to pool in the cord substance (Fig. 6–3).

Epidurography (radiographs following the injection of contrast material into the epidural space of the spinal canal) with the use of water-soluble contrast agents is receiving renewed attention.[1,7] The toxic effects of the procedure are minimized with the use of this medium, and the technique is simple. It is indicated primarily for the evaluation of the lumbosacral region, where the subarachnoid space is very small or is not present. Although the technique is easy, considerable experience with normal variations is required for proper interpretation of the results.

Vertebral sinus venography requires filling the venous sinuses on the floor of the spinal canal with contrast material. Injection into the body of a caudal vertebra is used most frequently in veterinary medicine, although introduction of a catheter through the femoral vein to a lumbar vein is used in human beings.[8,9] The results of this procedure are no better than those of epidurography, and the technique is more difficult.

Ventriculography is the delineation of the cerebral ventricular system following the injection of air or a positive contrast agent (Fig. 6–4).[1,10] Ventriculography is the procedure of choice for the diagnosis of hydrocephalus. Masses in the cranial vault can be detected by shifts in the ventricular system. Precise localization is better accomplished with arteriography, however.

Cavernous sinus venography is a relatively easy procedure, requiring injection of contrast material into the angularis oculi vein on the face.[11] The medium flows through the orbit into the cavernous sinuses on the floor of the

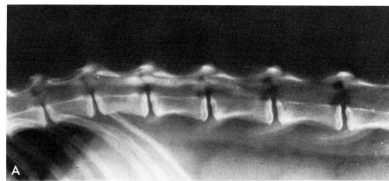

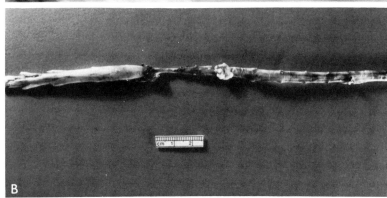

Figure 6–3. *A.* Myelogram of a cat with malacia of the spinal cord caused by infarction. Note the contrast media pooled in the area of the malacia. *B.* Spinal cord showing the area of the malacia.

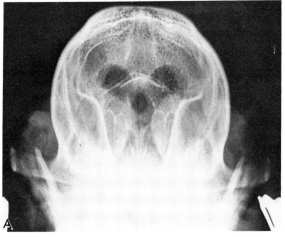

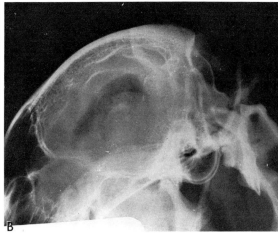

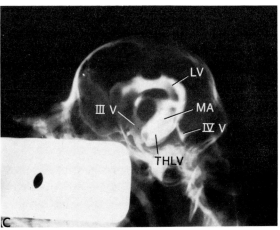

Figure 6–4. Frontal (*A*) and lateral (*B*) views of a pneumoventriculogram of a normal dog. The lateral ventricles are filled with air. A portion of the third ventricle can be seen in the lateral view. *C.* Positive contrast ventriculogram. *LV* = Lateral ventricle. *III V* = Third ventricle. *MA* = Mesencephalic aqueduct. *IV V* = Fourth ventricle. *THLV* = Temporal horn of lateral ventricle.

113

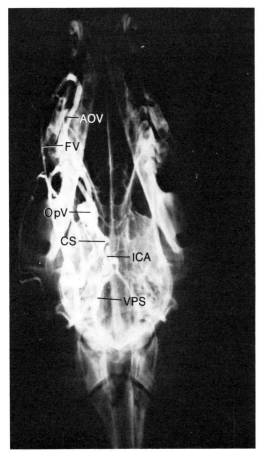

Figure 6–5. Cavernous sinus venogram of a normal dog. *AOV* = Angularis oculi vein. *FV* = Facial vein. *Op V* = Ophthalmic vein. *CS* = Cavernous sinus. *ICA* = Internal carotid artery (negative image inside CS). *VPS* = Ventral petrosal sinus.

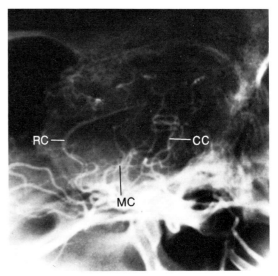

Figure 6–6. Cerebral arteriogram of a normal dog. *RC* = Rostral cerebral artery. *MC* = Middle cerebral artery. *CC* = Caudal cerebral artery.

cranial vault (Fig. 6–5). Compression or occlusion of the sinus from masses in the area of the pituitary gland can be demonstrated.

Cerebral arteriography is performed by injecting contrast material into the internal carotid or vertebral arteries.[1,12-14] In the dog, the internal carotid artery provides more consistent filling of the cerebral circulation rostral to the caudal cerebral artery, whereas the vertebral artery provides more consistent filling of the caudal portions of the intracranial circulation (Fig. 6–6). The internal carotid artery usually is cannulated by direct exposure. Using fluoroscopic control, the medium is injected into the vertebral artery following catheterization of the artery by way of the femoral artery. Arteriography requires rapid exposure of sequential films. Arteriography is the procedure of choice for the diagnosis of brain tumors. The interpretation of cerebral arteriograms requires a knowledge of the anatomy of the normal cerebral circulation.[15,16] Radioisotope imaging and computerized axial tomography are excellent alternatives, but they are available at only a few institutions.[17,18]

CONTRAINDICATIONS

Anesthesia is required for good-quality radiographs of the nervous system. Many patients with CNS disease are poor risks for anesthesia. The veterinarian must make a decision by weighing the risks of the procedure against the risk of doing nothing. For example, spinal fractures usually require early decompression if spinal cord function is to be preserved. These patients may be in shock and may have several other injuries. The question of risk versus benefit must be resolved on an individual basis.

Increased intracranial pressure is a contraindication for a spinal puncture; hence, myelography cannot be performed in such cases. Because contrast media are irritating, myelography is not done in the face of subarachnoid inflammation. When the puncture is made for a myelogram, a cell count of the CSF is determined. If the count indicates active inflammation, the myelogram is not performed unless it is considered essential for treatment (e.g., when there is strong suspicion of an abscess).

ELECTROPHYSIOLOGY

AVAILABILITY

Equipment for electrophysiologic techniques is expensive and requires training and experience for valid interpretation. These factors generally limit its availability to specialty practices and institutional settings. Electroencephalography and electromyography are the most widely used techniques and are available in a number of specialty practices. The other techniques are in varying stages of development for clinical application and are available primarily at research institutions (Table 6–7).

INDICATIONS

Electroencephalography (EEG), the graphic recording of the electrical activity of the brain, is useful for the evaluation of cerebral disease.[19] As with most diagnostic tools, the EEG often does not provide a specific diagnosis, but it supports the determination of a category of disease. The EEG varies with the level of consciousness: Low voltage and fast activity are seen in the alert animal, and higher voltage and slower activity occur during drowsiness and sleep. Drugs such as sedatives, tranquilizers, and anesthetics produce higher voltage and slower activity (similar to sleep patterns). The EEG usually can indicate that cerebral disease is present and whether it is focal or diffuse, acute or chronic, and inflammatory or degenerative.[19,20]

The following general principles of EEG changes have been listed by Klemm and Hall: [21] (1) Low voltage, fast activity (LVFA) and spikes (very fast activity) indicate irritation from any cause (usually inflammatory disease). (2) High voltage, slow activity (HVSA) suggests neuronal death or compression. (3) Neither change is diagnostic of a disease; rather, it reflects the kind of process occurring (e.g., inflammation or degeneration). (4) Focal EEG abnormality indicates a focal cortical lesion. (5) Generalized EEG abnormality indicates diffuse cortical disease *or* a subcortical abnormality that alters the activity of the majority of the cerebral cortex. (6) The EEG can change with time, suggesting the progression or resolution of the disease process. Table 6–8 outlines the more common EEG changes in various diseases.

Table 6–7. ELECTROPHYSIOLOGY

Test	Indications	Probable Usefulness	Contraindications	Availability
Electroencephalography	Degenerative disease	Moderate	None	Specialty practice
	Anomaly	High		
	Metabolic disease	Moderate		
	Neoplasia	Moderate		
	Inflammatory disease	High		
	Trauma	Low		
	Toxic disease	Moderate		
Electromyography, nerve conduction, and nerve stimulation	Lower motor neuron diseases	High	None	Specialty practice
	Peripheral neuropathies	High		
	Myopathies	High		
Electroretinography	Retinal disease	High	None	Specialty practice
Evoked response (cortical, brain stem, and spinal)	Localization of lesions in pathways	Insufficient data in most areas	None	Primarily institutions
Visual-evoked response		Low at present		
Auditory-evoked response	Test of hearing, location of brain stem lesions	High		
Somatosensory-evoked response		Questionable at present		
Echoencephalography	Midline shifts of cerebrum	Low	None	Institutions (few)
Urodynamics (cystometrogram, urethral pressure, sphincter reflexes)	Neurogenic bladder disorders	Moderate	None	Institutions (few)
Tympanometry	Otitis media, otitis interna, hearing disorders	Moderate, early development	None	Institutions (few)

Table 6–8. ELECTROENCEPHALOGRAPHIC CHANGES IN DISEASE

	EEG Findings	Pathology	Diseases*
Generalized	Low voltage, fast activity (LVFA)	Irritation of neurons	Metabolic, neoplastic (subcortical—unusual), *inflammatory, toxic*
	High voltage, slow activity (HVSA)	Neuronal death or depression of neurons	*Degenerative, anomalous (hydrocephalus)*, neoplastic (subcortical), inflammatory (late stages), traumatic (brain stem, cerebral edema)
	Mixed LVFA and HVSA	Both irritation and destruction of neurons	*Toxic* (heavy metals), *anomalous* (hydrocephalus), *inflammatory*
Focal	LVFA	Localized irritation of neurons	Epilepsy (cortical focus), *neoplastic* (cortical), inflammatory (focal cortical), traumatic (cortical)
	HVSA	Localized death or depression of neurons	Degenerative, neoplastic (cortical), traumatic

Italics indicate diseases that are most likely with each abnormal pattern on the EEG.

Electromyography (EMG) (the measurement of the electrical activity of muscle) and measurement of nerve conduction velocity (NCV) are performed on the same equipment, usually during the same examination. EMG and NCV are the best diagnostic tools for the evaluation of neuropathies and myopathies.[22,23] The information provided by these procedures regarding the location and the extent of the abnormality may support an etiologic diagnosis.

The EMG examination includes the evaluation of the electrical activity of the muscle at the following times: (1) during insertion or movement of the electrode (insertion activity), (2) when the muscle is resting (resting activity), (3) during muscle contraction (voluntary or reflex), and (4) in response to electrical stimulation of the motor nerve (also called electrodiagnostic testing [EDT]). Mechanical distortion of the muscle membrane by the needle electrode causes the membrane to depolarize, producing a brief burst of electrical activity (i.e., insertion activity). Resting muscle is electrically silent.

Loss of nerve supply to a muscle causes an increase in the excitability of the muscle membrane. Insertion activity is greatly prolonged. Small, abnormal potentials (called *fibrillation potentials* and *positive sharp waves*) are produced spontaneously while the muscle is at rest. Contraction of the muscle voluntarily by

activation of a reflex or by direct stimulation of a nerve usually is reduced because of denervation (Table 6–9).

Myopathies may have EMG changes similar to those of neuropathies, except that muscle activation is possible and may even be hyperactive (Table 6–9).

Localization to a spinal cord segment, a spinal nerve root, or a peripheral nerve is determined on the basis of the distribution of abnormal findings (Table 6–10).

Electroretinography (ERG) is the electrical recording of the retinal response to light. Simple strip chart recorders can be used, but a cathode ray oscilloscope is necessary in order to obtain better results. Signal-averaging computers provide even better resolution.[24] The ERG is helpful for differentiating retinal blindness from central blindness.

The *visual-evoked response* (VER) is the cortical electrical activity that occurs in response to a light stimulus administered to the eye. A signal-averaging computer is required in order to record this response. The response provides an objective evaluation of central visual pathways. At present, the VER appears to be masked completely by the ERG in the dog, even with recording electrodes placed over the occipital poles of the cerebrum (scalp recording).[25] Successful recording of wave forms not related to the ERG has been reported.[26] With some modification of the technique, including

Table 6-9. ELECTROMYOGRAPHIC CHANGES IN DISEASES

Parameter	Normal	Neuropathy	Myopathy
Insertion activity	Brief burst of activity	Prolonged activity	Prolonged activity
Resting activity	Silent	Many fibs and + waves*	Few fibs and + waves*
Muscle contraction	Interference pattern	Decreased	Normal to increased
Stimulation of nerve	Large, usually triphasic response	Reduced or normal amplitude, increased duration and number of phases (absent if nerve is not functional)	Decreased amplitude and duration, increased number of phases

*fibs = fibrillation potentials; + waves = positive sharp waves

the use of an alternating grid-pattern stimulus, a useful clinical tool may be developed.

The *brain stem auditory-evoked response* (BAER) is the recording of brain stem potentials in response to a click stimulus in the ear canal. A signal-averaging computer is necessary in order to record this response.[27,28] Hearing can be evaluated rapidly and accurately with this system. Partial hearing losses require pure tone stimuli, which present more difficult technical problems. Brain stem function also can be evaluated. The recording consists of a series of waves that represent electrical activity at successive levels of the brain stem. A lesion at one level of the brain stem will block the responses at that level and at all succeeding levels. The BAER is used to evaluate hearing and the level of brain stem lesions and to confirm a diagnosis of complete loss of brain stem function when brain death has occurred.

Table 6-10. EXAMPLE OF LOCALIZATION OF LOWER MOTOR NEURON LESION WITH ELECTROMYOGRAPHY

Lesion	
L7 cord segment	Partial denervation of muscles innervated by sciatic nerve with preservation of some normal activity in each muscle; usually bilateral
L7 nerve root	Same as cord segment, except usually unilateral
Cauda equina at lumbosacral junction (L7, sacral and caudal nerves)	Partial denervation of muscles innervated by sciatic nerve (L7 and S1), denervation of anal sphincter and urinary bladder (S1–S3) and tail (Cd1–Cd5); usually bilateral
Sciatic nerve	Denervation of muscles innervated by sciatic nerve; unilateral

Other tests for hearing include monitoring of the EEG and of respiration with presentation of an auditory stimulus. An alerting response is recorded on the EEG, and panting is interrupted briefly.[19] These methods are moderately reliable but do not indicate the location of the abnormality.

Impedance audiometry (IA) is a method of assessing the integrity of the middle ear system. IA measures the compliance of the tympanic membrane at rest, with changes in pressure, and in response to auditory stimuli. Middle ear effusion, occlusion of the auditory (eustachian) tube, conduction alterations in the ossicles, retrocochlear hearing loss, and facial motor nerve function (through the stapedial reflex) can be identified through IA.[29]

The *somatosensory-evoked response* (SER) is the recording of spinal cord, brain stem, or cortical potentials in response to a stimulus administered to a peripheral nerve.[30-32] A signal-averaging computer is required. The SER is used to determine the functional capacity of sensory pathways, for example, in a paraplegic animal with questionable sensory function on neurologic examination. Adequate information is not yet available to determine the clinical value of this test. The fastest potentials recorded are those of the faster pathways (e.g., the dorsal columns). More trials are required before it can be determined whether the slower-conducting pain pathways can be evaluated in clinical patients.[32]

Echoencephalography uses pulsed ultrasound (1 to 2 megahertz) to record the location of tissue interfaces. Midline structures of the brain can be determined in relation to the bony calvarium.[33] Shifts of the midline structures caused by masses in the cranial vault (tumor, hemorrhage) can be detected.[34] The technique is noninvasive, requires minimal patient co-operation, and appears to be reliable, although there have been limited trials in veterinary medicine.

Urodynamics includes cystometrograms (CMG), urethral pressure profiles (UPP), and electrophysiologic testing of bladder and sphincter reflexes (see Chapter 5 for details).

CONTRAINDICATIONS

There are no significant contraindications to any of the electrophysiologic tests. Anesthesia or tranquilization may be necessary for some procedures, especially if the animal is uncooperative.

BIOPSY

AVAILABILITY

A biopsy of neural or muscular tissue can be performed by any veterinary surgeon; however, the difficulties in obtaining good diagnostic samples generally limit the use of this procedure to specialty practices and institutions. Histopathologic evaluation requires a trained pathologist. A ventricular tap can be performed by any veterinarian with training (Table 6-11).

INDICATIONS

A biopsy of the brain is used to confirm a diagnosis of a diffuse encephalopathy, such as viral inflammation or storage disease.[35] Samples of the cerebral cortex or the cerebellum can be obtained. Many of these diseases cannot be diagnosed antemortem in any other way. Because of the invasive nature of the procedure, it is not generally recommended; however, it is very useful for establishing a diagnosis in a potential animal model of a genetic disease or for when the owner of the animal wants a definitive diagnosis of a potentially untreatable disease. Minimal deficits in neurologic function are produced by removal of small samples of the cerebral or cerebellar cortex.

A biopsy of the spinal cord is not feasible because of the severe deficits produced by excising the tissue.

A biopsy of a peripheral nerve is indicated in peripheral neuropathies. Small sensory nerves usually are removed. Excision of a few fascicles of a mixed nerve is preferred if a motor neuropathy is suspected.[36]

A muscle biopsy usually is performed along with a peripheral nerve biopsy in order to differentiate neuropathies from myopathies. Tissues must be handled properly for satisfactory histopathologic evaluation. The nerve or muscle specimen must be maintained straight, without excess tension, during fixation. This positioning usually is attained by suspending the nerve with a weight on the end or by use of double clamps on the muscle.[36]

Ventricular puncture is indicated primarily for confirmation of hydrocephalus[1,37] rather than for procurement of CSF. The thickness of the cerebral cortex can be estimated by the depth of the needle in the site where CSF first is obtained. Questionable cases can be confirmed by pneumoventriculography. Animals with open fontanelles or suture lines can be tapped easily. If the skull is closed, the procedure is more difficult.[1,10]

CONTRAINDICATIONS

The invasive nature of these procedures must be weighed against the benefits of the information to be derived. A brain biopsy usually is reserved for animals with serious, usually untreatable, encephalopathies. The

Table 6-11. BIOPSY

Test	Indications	Probable Usefulness	Contraindications	Availability
Brain	Degenerative disease, demyelinating disease, inflammatory disease	High	Invasive	Specialty practice
Spinal cord			Destructive	
Peripheral nerve	Peripheral neuropathies	High	Must be selective	Practice
Muscle	Neuropathies, myopathies	High	Must be selective	Practice
Ventricular tap	Hydrocephalus; alternate source of cerebrospinal fluid if intracranial pressure is elevated	High	Invasive; excessive removal of fluid may cause subdural hematoma	Specialty practice

Table 6-12. SELECTION OF DIAGNOSTIC TESTS

Disease Category	Diagnostic Tests	
	Useful	*Usually Diagnostic*
Degenerative		
Brain	EEG, CSF	Biopsy
Spinal cord	Myelography, CSF	None
Vertebrae	CSF	Radiography, myelography
Demyelinating		
Brain	EEG, CSF	Biopsy
Spinal cord	Myelography, CSF	None
Peripheral nerve	EMG, EDT	Biopsy
Anomalous		
Brain	Examination	Radiography
Spinal cord	Radiography	Myelography
Vertebrae	Examination	Radiography
Metabolic	History	Clinical laboratory profile
Neoplastic		
Brain	EEG, radiography	Arteriography, scans
Spinal cord	CSF, radiography	Myelography
Peripheral nerve	EDT	Biopsy
Nutritional	History	Radiography
Inflammation	History, examination	CSF
Traumatic	History, examination	Radiography
Toxic	History	Clinical laboratory profile

brain biopsy has gained favor as a procedure for the diagnosis of certain human viral encephalitides, such as herpes encephalitis. The deficits produced by the biopsy are minimal. A spinal cord biopsy is contraindicated, because the procedure seriously compromises spinal cord function. Peripheral nerve and muscle biopsies are performed more commonly and do not produce serious deficits if care is exercised in the selection of the peripheral nerve. A ventricular tap not only is diagnostic but also may be therapeutic in an animal with increased intracranial pressure. Excessive removal of fluid can cause collapse of the cerebral cortex and subdural hematoma.

The most useful diagnostic tests for evaluating each category of disease are outlined in Table 6–12.

CASE HISTORIES

The case studies presented in Chapters 2, 3, and 4 involved the history (Chapter 2), which was used to develop a sign-time graph and a list of probable categories of disease (rule-outs); the neurologic examination (Chapter 3); and, from it, localization of the lesion (Chapter 4). At this point in each case, an anatomic diagnosis and a list of rule-outs have been established. The next step is to perform appropriate diagnostic tests to confirm or deny the possible causes of the problem and, in some cases, to pinpoint the location of the lesion. The signalment, the localization, and the list of rule-

outs will be repeated. Decide which diagnostic tests are appropriate in each case before reading the diagnostic plan.

Case History 6A

Signalment. Canine, West Highland white terrier, female, 6 years old.
Problems. Right hemiparesis, left pelvic limb slight paresis.
Localization. (see Chapter 4) Spinal cord, C6–T2, primarily the right side.
Rule-outs. (see Chapter 2)
1. vascular lesion,
2. trauma, and
3. inflammation.

Case History 6B

Signalment. Canine, German shepherd, female, 7 years old.
Problems. Pelvic limb ataxia and paresis.
Localization. (see Chapter 4) Spinal cord, T3–L3, symmetric.
Rule-outs. (see Chapter 2)
1. degenerative disease,
2. neoplasia, and
3. inflammation.

Case History 6C

Signalment. Feline, domestic short hair, female, 3 months old.

Problems. Ataxia and dysmetria, nystagmus, and menace deficit.

Localization. (see Chapter 4) Cerebellum.

Rule-outs. (see Chapter 2)

1. anomaly and
2. trauma.

Case History 6D

Signalment. Feline, Siamese, male, 2 years old.

Problems.

1. depression,
2. head tremor,
3. left hemiparesis, and
4. uveitis in left eye.

Localization. (see Chapter 4)

1. left C6–T2 spinal cord,
2. cerebellum, and
3. possibly cerebrum or brain stem.

Rule-outs. (see Chapter 2)

1. inflammation,
2. neoplasia, and
3. degenerative disease.

Case History 6E

Signalment. Canine, Yorkshire terrier, male, 8 months old.

Problems.

1. Mental status: episodic depression and agitation.
2. Compulsive walking with slight dysmetria and mild postural reaction deficits.

Localization. (see Chapter 4) Cerebrum diffuse.

Rule-outs. (see Chapter 2)

1. metabolic disease and
2. toxic disease.

Assessments

DIAGNOSTIC PLAN 6A

Radiographs: Rule out trauma (vertebral fracture or luxation).

Cerebrospinal fluid (CSF) analysis: Rule out inflammation. Possible evidence of hemorrhage.

Myelogram: Rule out compression from trauma. Check for possible swelling of the spinal cord, which may be seen with a vascular lesion.

Infarctions usually are diagnosed by exclusion, as in this case. The CSF may have a slight increase in protein and, more rarely, may be xanthochromic. See Chapter 9 for a discussion of spinal cord infarction.

DIAGNOSTIC PLAN 6B

Radiographs: Rule out vertebral inflammation (diskospondylitis) or vertebral neoplasia.

CSF analysis: Rule out inflammation.

Myelogram: Rule out degenerative disk disease and spinal cord tumor. Primary degenerative diseases of the spinal cord or the brain are diagnosed by exclusion, since the lesion is microscopic. Tumors and intervertebral disks also may cause these signs, so they must be ruled out. This dog had a protruding disk that was demonstrated on the myelogram and was corrected surgically. For a discussion of these diseases, see Chapter 9.

DIAGNOSTIC PLAN 6C

This kitten has been abnormal since birth—a congenital lesion. Trauma is a possible diagnosis if we consider the possibility of a birth injury. The problem has been present for at least 6 to 8 weeks (from the time of significant motor activity) and probably since birth (poor nursing). The lack of progression and the severity of the signs suggest a static lesion, which is not likely to be treatable. This syndrome is typical of cerebellar malformations associated with in utero infections of panleukopenia virus. Diagnostic tests other than a cerebellar biopsy are not likely to be rewarding. Sometimes, the client should be advised not to waste any more money on diagnostic procedures. The cat can live a reasonably normal life if she stays in the house. See Chapter 11 for a discussion of this syndrome.

DIAGNOSTIC PLAN 6D

Funduscopic examination: Characterize the eye lesion.

Hematology and chemistry analysis: Rule out systemic disease.

CSF analysis: Rule out inflammation and neoplasia.

Serum titers: Rule out feline infectious peritonitis and feline leukemia virus.

Radiographs and myelograms are taken if these tests are negative. Rule out neoplasia.

The funduscopic examination is an integral part of the neurologic examination. Inflammatory and neoplastic diseases of the nervous system often produce retinal lesions as well. Hematology and chemistry analyses should be performed for any animal with neurologic disease (see the section on the minimum data base in Chapter 4), but they are likely to provide positive evidence in this case. The chronic progressive history and the multifocal signs are most likely caused by an infectious agent or a metastatic neoplasia. Feline infectious peritonitis (FIP) and feline leukemia virus (FeLV) are the most likely causes of this syndrome. Specific immunologic tests for these diseases are available and should be used if the results are questionable. It is unlikely that radiographs are needed. This cat had an increased plasma protein (9.2), primarily in the globulin fraction (6.2). There was a granulomatous uveitis and retinitis on ophthalmoscopic examination. The CSF had a protein level of 400 mg/dl and 300 WBCs, which were 80 per cent neutrophils and 20 per cent lymphocytes. These findings are typical of FIP.

The FeLV test was positive, and the FIP titer was high. For a discussion of these diseases, see Chapter 17.

DIAGNOSTIC PLAN 6E

Consider the results of the minimum data base (MDB—see Chapter 4) before proceeding. The complaints on the history and the clinical findings are typical of hepatic encephalopathy. Any suggestion of liver disease on the MDB will indicate the need for specific tests. Levels of serum enzymes that indicate acute liver disease (SGPT, alkaline phosphatase) may be normal. Decreased values of serum urea nitrogen (BUN) and serum albumin are significant. Specific tests include sulfobromophthalein sodium excretion (BSP), blood ammonia levels, and the ammonia tolerance test. For a discussion of hepatic encephalopathy, see Chapter 17.

REFERENCES

1. Hoerlein, B. F.: Canine neurology: Diagnosis and Treatment, 3rd ed. Philadelphia, W. B. Saunders Co., 1978.
2. Kornegay, J. N.: Cerebrospinal fluid collection, examination, and interpretation in dogs and cats. Comp. Cont. Ed. Pract. Vet. 3:85–92, 1981.
3. deLahunta, A.: Veterinary Neuroanatomy and Clinical Neurology. Philadelphia, W. B. Saunders Co., 1977.
4. Roszel, J. F.: Membrane filtration of canine and feline cerebrospinal fluid for cytologic evaluation. JAVMA 160:720–725, 1972.
5. Ticer, J. W.: Radiographic Techniques in Small Animal Practice. Philadelphia, W. B. Saunders Co., 1975.
6. Suter, P. F., Morgan, J. P., Holliday, T. A., and O'Brien, T. R.: Myelography of the dog: Diagnosis of tumors of the spinal cord and vertebrae. JAVRS 12:29–44, 1971.
7. Klide, A. M., Steinberg, S. A., and Pond, M. J.: Epiduralograms in the dog: The uses and advantages of the diagnostic procedure. JAVRS 8:39–44, 1967.
8. McNeel, S. V., and Morgan, J. P.: Intraosseous vertebral venography: A technic for examination of the canine lumbosacral junction. JAVRS 19:168–175, 1978.
9. LePage, J. R.: Transfemoral ascending lumbar catheterization of the epidural veins. Radiology 111:337–339, 1974.
10. Oliver, J. E., Jr., and Conrad, C. R.: Cerebral ventriculography. In Ticer, J. W.: Radiographic Technique in Small Animal Practice. Philadelphia, W. B. Saunders Co., 1975.
11. Oliver, J. E., Jr.: Cranial sinus venography in the dog. JAVRS 10:66–71, 1969.
12. Conrad, C. R., and Oliver, J. E., Jr.: Cerebral arteriography. In Ticer, J. W.: Radiographic Technique in Small Animal Practice. Philadelphia, W. B. Saunders Co., 1975.
13. Dorn, A. S.: A standard technique for canine cerebral angiography. JAVMA 161:1669–1675, 1972.
14. Rising, J. L., and Lewis, R. E.: Femorovertebral cerebral angiography in the dog. Am. J. Vet. Res. 33:665–676, 1970.
15. Dorn, A. S.: Radiographic interpretation of the normal canine cerebral angiogram. JAAHA 11:478–483, 1975.
16. Dorn, A. S.: Radiographic interpretation of the abnormal canine cerebral angiogram. JAAHA 11:484–490, 1975.
17. Kallfelz, F. A., deLahunta, A., and Allhands, R. V.: Scintigraphic diagnosis of brain lesions in the dog and cat. JAVMA 172:589–597, 1978.
18. Fike, J. R., LeCouteur, R. A., Cann, C. E., and Pflug-felder, C. M.: Computerized tomography of brain tumors of the rostral and middle fossas in the dog. Am. J. Vet. Res. 42:275–281, 1981.
19. Redding, R. W.: Canine electroencephalography. In Hoerlein, B. F.: Canine Neurology: Diagnosis and Treatment, 3rd ed. Philadelphia, W. B. Saunders Co., 1978.
20. Klemm, W. R.: Animal Electroencephalography. New York, Academic Press, 1969.
21. Klemm, W. R., and Hall, C. L.: Current status and trends in veterinary electroencephalography. JAVMA 164:529, 1974.
22. Bowen, J. M.: Peripheral nerve electrodiagnostics, electromyography, and nerve conduction velocity. In Hoerlein, B. F.: Canine Neurology: Diagnosis and Treatment, 3rd ed. Philadelphia, W. B. Saunders Co., 1978.
23. Chrisman, C. L.: Diseases of peripheral nerves and muscles. In Ettinger, S. J.: Textbook of Veterinary Internal Medicine. Philadelphia, W. B. Saunders Co., 1975.
24. Coulter, D. B., and Martin, C. L.: Signal averaging of electroretinograms. Ga. Vet. 30:14–17, 1978.
25. Malnati, G. A., Marshall, A. E., and Coulter, D. B.: Electroretinographic components of the canine visual evoked response. Am. J. Vet. Res. 42:159–163, 1981.
26. Redding, R. W., and Ingram, J. T.: The visual evoked response of the dog. Proc. AVNA, Washington, D.C., 1980.
27. Morgan, J. L., Coulter, D. B., Marshall, A. E., and Goetsch, D. D.: Effects of neomycin on the wave form of auditory-evoked brain stem potentials in dogs. Am. J. Vet. Res. 41:1077–1081, 1980.
28. Marshall, A. E., Byars, T. D., Whitlock, R. H., and George, L. W.: Brainstem auditory evoked response in the diagnosis of inner ear injury in the horse. JAVMA 178:282–286, 1981.
29. Penrod, J. P., and Coulter, D. B.: The diagnostic uses of impedance audiometry in the dog. JAAHA 16:941–948, 1980.
30. Holliday, T. A.: Percutaneous recording of evoked spinal cord potentials of dogs. Am. J. Vet. Res. 40:326–333, 1979.
31. Parker, A. J.: Evoked cisterna cerebellomedullaris potentials in the clinically normal dog. Am. J. Vet. Res. 39:1811–1815, 1978.
32. Kornegay, J. N., Marshall, A. E., Purinton, P. T., and Oliver, J. E., Jr.: Somatosensory-evoked potential in clinically normal dogs. Am. J. Vet. Res. 42:70–73, 1981.
33. Smith, C. W., Marshall, A. E., and Knecht, C. D.: Use of A-mode echoencephalography in the dog. Am. J. Vet. Res. 33:2415–2421, 1972.
34. Smith, C. W., Marshall, A. E., and Knecht, C. D.: Detection of artificially produced intracranial midline shifts of the brain in the dog with A-mode echoencephalography. Am. J. Vet. Res. 33:2423–2427, 1972.
35. Swaim, S., Vandevelde, M., and Faircloth, J. C.: Evaluation of brain biopsy techniques in the dog. JAAHA 15:627–633, 1979.
36. Braund, K. G., Walker, T. L., and Vandevelde, M.: Fascicular nerve biopsy in the dog. Am. J. Vet. Res. 40:1025–1030, 1979.
37. Savell, C. M.: Cerebral ventricular tap: An aid to diagnosis and treatment of hydrocephalus in the dog. JAAHA 10:500–501, 1974.

7

CHAPTER

PRINCIPLES OF MEDICAL TREATMENT OF THE NERVOUS SYSTEM

MANAGEMENT OF CENTRAL NERVOUS SYSTEM INFECTIONS

Effective therapy for central nervous system (CNS) infections depends upon identification of the cause and selection of the appropriate antimicrobial agent. Identification is based upon cerebrospinal fluid (CSF) analysis and culture. Selection of the appropriate antimicrobial agent depends upon two principles: (1) The agent must be effective against the microbial target without severely injuring the patient, and (2) it must be delivered to and must penetrate the CNS. Unfortunately, anatomic and physiologic barriers to successful therapy for CNS infections appear when certain drugs are used. The combined effects of these obstacles create a functional blood-brain barrier.

The Blood-Brain Barrier

The combined functions of the CNS capillaries and the choroid plexus create a barrier to the movement of drugs from the capillary or pericapillary fluid into nervous tissue or cerebrospinal fluid. Discrepancies between serum and CNS drug concentrations occur because of two factors: the special anatomy of CNS capillaries and the secretory selectivity of the choroid plexus. In capillaries outside the CNS, drugs and other agents pass from the blood through clefts between endothelial cells and

through fenestrations in the capillary basement membrane. In the CNS, capillary endothelial cells are joined by tight junctions that seal the intercellular clefts. The capillary basement membrane has no fenestrations. In addition, glial cell foot processes surround the capillaries. In the CNS, a drug must penetrate an inner bimolecular lipid membrane, the endothelial cell cytoplasm, an outer lipid membrane, and a basement membrane and, finally, must traverse a tangle of glial foot processes. Penetration of the drug is largely a function of its endothelial membrane solubility. Membrane solubility is favored by (1) a low degree of ionization at the physiologic pH, (2) a low degree of plasma protein binding, and (3) a high degree of lipid solubility of the un-ionized drug.[1] Certain highly lipid-soluble drugs bind strongly to tissue sites in the brain, permitting high concentrations within nervous tissue.

Regulation of CSF solutes occurs at the choroid plexus. Plasma dialysate that filters through fenestrated capillaries is selectively secreted by choroid epithelial cells. Certain CSF constituents also are actively reabsorbed by the choroidal epithelial cell, which tends to clear these substances from the CSF and from nervous tissue. This active transport system for weak organic acids removes such drugs as penicillin and gentamycin. Inflammation may block this active transport system, allowing drug concentrations to increase. In addition, inflammation may increase the permeability of endothelial membranes to certain antibiotics, allowing these drugs to penetrate nervous tissue in cases of disease. In the normal animal, these antibiotics penetrate poorly.

Use of Antimicrobial Agents in Bacterial Infections

Antimicrobial agents are grouped by their capacity to achieve concentrations in CSF sufficient to inhibit micro-organisms throughout the period of therapy.[1] Table 7–1 lists these drugs relative to achievable concentrations in CSF. Antibiotics such as the aminoglycosides diffuse poorly, even in the presence of inflammation. Intrathecal administration may be required in order for adequate CSF concentrations to be achieved.

ANTIBIOTIC SYNERGISM AND ANTAGONISM

Much has been written concerning the antagonism and the synergism of antibiotic combinations. Synergistic combinations include penicillin G or ampicillin plus an ami-

Table 7–1. ACHIEVABLE CONCENTRATIONS OF ANTIBIOTICS IN CSF

High	Adequate in Meningitis	Inadequate
Chloramphenicol	Penicillin G*	Penicillin G benzathine
Sulfonamides	Ampicillin*	Cephalosporins‡
Trimethoprim	Methicillin*	Aminoglycosides
Metronidazole	Nafcillin*	Polymyxin B
Isoniazid	Carbenicillin*	Colistin
	Tetracycline	Novobiocin
	Minocycline†	Amphotericin B§
	Doxycycline†	Lincomycin
	Oleandomycin	Erythromycin‖
	Vancomycin‖	
	Bacitracin	
	Ristocetin	
	Flucytosine	

*High intravenous doses are needed to achieve the maximal effect.
†Lipid-soluble tetracyclines that achieve higher concentrations in CSF than do other tetracyclines.
‡May be effective early in bacterial meningitis; concentrations dramatically decrease with repair of the blood-brain barrier.
§May be effective in cryptococcal meningitis.
‖Penetration in the face of inflammation is unpredictable.

noglycoside, such as gentamycin, against the enterococcus and staphylococcus bacteria, carbenicillin and gentamycin against *Pseudomonas aeruginosa*, and amphotericin B and flucytosine against *Cryptococcus neoformans*. Synergistic activity in CNS infections may be compromised by the inability of one antibiotic to penetrate nervous tissue. Antagonism occurs between ampicillin and oxytetracycline and between penicillin and chloramphenicol. Unless there are clear-cut indications for their use, these combinations should be avoided. In situations in which it is deemed necessary to give penicillin with chloramphenicol, the penicillin should be given in high doses and should be started at least 24 hours before the administration of chloramphenicol.[1]

Bacterial Infections

BACTERIAL MENINGITIS

Primary bacterial meningitis, although common in human beings, is rare in dogs and cats. It occurs primarily in association with bacteremia or endocarditis or as a later finding in diskospondylitis. In the dog, organisms associated with canine bacterial meningitis include the *Pasteurella* species, *Pasteurella multocida*, and the *Staphylococcus* species (*S. aureus, S. epidermidis,* and *S. albus*).[2] *Staphylococcus aureus* is probably the most important. Gramnegative septicemia with *Salmonella, Esche-*

richia coli, Proteus, and *Pseudomonas* occasionally has been found to be associated with purulent meningoencephalomyelitis.[3]

Definitive treatment of bacterial meningitis is based upon isolation of the organism from the CSF and determination of its antibiotic sensitivity. In addition, the source of infection (i.e., endocarditis, bacteremia) should be identified and should be managed therapeutically. The initial therapy for bacterial meningitis is based upon the assumption that staphylococcal organisms are the cause. The antibiotics of choice are penicillin, ampicillin, or a penicillinase-resistant antibiotic, such as methicillin. We prefer to use penicillin G, 10,000 units per kg, every 4 to 6 hours or ampicillin, 5 mg per kg every 6 hours. The antibiotics are given intravenously for at least 7 days. Chloramphenicol, 10 mg per kg every 4 to 6 hours intravenously, also can be used as a substitute for penicillin; however, many strains of staphylococcal organism are resistant to this antibiotic.[2] Chloramphenicol probably should be used only when the organism has been determined to be sensitive to its action. Although the aminoglycoside antibiotics penetrate very poorly into nervous tissue, gentamycin commonly is combined with penicillin or ampicillin. The basis for this combination is the assumption that the source of infection is not the CNS. The drug is given intravenously or intramuscularly at a dosage of 2 mg per kg every 8 hours. Renal function must be monitored carefully, and treatment should not exceed 14 days. *Under no circumstances should gentamycin or any other aminoglycoside antibiotic be given as the sole antimicrobial agent in bacterial meningitis.* Antibiotic therapy should be modified if results of culture and sensitivity testing suggest that the initial therapy will not be effective.

After 7 to 14 days, intravenous therapy can be stopped and oral antibiotics begun. Antibiotics should be given for 4 to 6 weeks in order to prevent relapse. The prognosis for recovery is fair to good.

Gram-negative meningoencephalomyelitis presents some unusual problems in therapy, inasmuch as the effective antibiotics may not penetrate the CNS, even in the presence of inflammation. Empiric antibiotic therapy includes the concomitant administration of chloramphenicol and gentamycin parenterally. Intrathecal gentamycin, 5 to 10 mg per day, should be considered. A serious drawback to the intrathecal use of antibiotics in dogs or cats is the multiple anesthetic episodes required for its administration. If *Pseudomonas aeruginosa* is isolated, the optimal therapy is a combination of sodium carbenicillin and gentamycin. In systemic salmonellosis with CNS involvement, chloramphenicol is the initial drug of choice, unless it is contraindicated by sensitivity testing. Alternative regimens include trimethoprim-sulfa or ampicillin-gentamycin combinations. Cephalothin may be effective in vitro but penetrates the CNS very poorly. As for the aminoglycosides, cephalosporins should not be used as the sole antibiotic regimen in the treatment of bacterial meningitis. Other gram-negative infections should be treated according to culture and sensitivity results.

Occasionally, systemic infection extending to the nervous system occurs from *Brucella canis*. The best therapy for neurobrucellosis includes a combination of streptomycin and minocycline. Based on human data, streptomycin should be administered for 2 weeks by parenteral injection. Minocycline should be given orally for 4 weeks, in combination with the 2-week schedule for streptomycin. Occasionally, trimethoprim-sulfa combinations are effective.[1]

BACTERIAL BRAIN ABSCESS

An abscess of the brain usually results from extension of purulent otitis media and otitis interna or from rhinitis or sinusitis. It can occur in association with foreign body penetration or migration through the CNS. The causative agents are usually *Staphylococcus, Streptococcus,* or *Pasteurella* organisms. Successful treatment includes appropriate antibiotics and surgical drainage or removal of the abscess. Because of the organisms involved, penicillin, ampicillin, methicillin, and chloramphenicol are the antibiotics of choice. The treatment of bacterial brain abscess is difficult, the relapse rate is high, and the prognosis is very poor.

DISKOSPONDYLITIS

The most common cause of diskospondylitis is *Staphylococcus aureus;* and occasionally, *Brucella canis* organisms are the source.[4] The disease is associated with a high incidence of urinary tract infection and bacteremia. In staphylococcal diskospondylitis, various antibiotics may be effective. Ampicillin, cephalosporins, chloramphenicol, and gentamycin have been effective. Vertebral curettage in addition to antibiotic therapy for 4 to 6 weeks results in more predictable clinical resolution than does antibiotic therapy alone.[4]

In *Brucella canis* diskospondylitis, therapy is expensive and may not eradicate the infection effectively. Streptomycin-minocycline combinations are used. The dog should be neutered and should be isolated from other dogs. Human infection has occurred with this organism.

Mycotic Infections

The more common mycotic infections of the CNS are caused by *Cryptococcus neoformans, Blastomyces dermatitidis, Histoplasma capsulatum,* and *Coccidioides immitis.* A definitive diagnosis is made by isolation or identification of the organism in the CSF or other body secretions. Except for cryptococcal meningitis, each of these diseases is treated in nearly the same way as the others.

CRYPTOCOCCAL MENINGITIS

The mainstay of therapy for the deep mycotic agents is amphotericin B. This drug is poorly absorbed from the gastrointestinal tract and must be given intravenously for a full therapeutic effect. Amphotericin B diffuses very poorly into the CSF; however, it remains the drug of choice for many CNS mycotic infections. Several therapeutic regimens have been described. We have used a modified schedule. Fifty mg of amphotericin B is dissolved with 10 ml of sterile water. This solution is added to an amber multidose bottle containing 240 ml sterile 5 per cent dextrose in water. The initial dosage of this solution is 1.1 ml per kg (0.22 mg per kg). The solution is injected slowly, intravenously, over 3 to 5 minutes. Before each subsequent injection, a BUN analysis is performed in order to monitor renal toxicity. Treatment is stopped if the BUN level increases one and one half to two times over the pretreatment figure. Day 3, a second injection is given at a dosage of 1.65 ml per kg (0.33 mg per kg). Day 5, a third injection is given at a dosage of 2.2 ml per kg (0.4 mg per kg). Thereafter, injections are given three times a week at this dosage. Although a maximum of 12 injections is recommended, some animals may require additional therapy. Extended therapy is given provided that renal function remains stable. After reconstitution, amphotericin B remains active for 1 week. Solutions should be stored in dark, sterile containers in a refrigerator.

Amphotericin B is a very toxic antibiotic. Untoward effects include fever, vomiting, and phlebitis at the site of the injection. The drug is very irritating to tissues, and care must be exercised in order to avoid extravascular spillage. Serious side effects include acute hepatic failure and irreversible renal failure. Decreased renal function is expected in most patients given amphotericin B; however, critical monitoring of the animal allows the clinician to suspend therapy before renal failure becomes irreversible. Renal effects include a reversible decrease in glomerular filtration and concentrating ability of relatively short duration. A more prolonged decrease in renal blood flow occurs. These effects usually disappear when therapy is stopped and do not contraindicate retreatment.

Intrathecal amphotericin B may be helpful. Five ml of spinal fluid is removed and mixed with 10 to 20 mg of soluble hydrocortisone or methylprednisolone. The solution is instilled slowly intrathecally. After 5 to 10 minutes, 5 ml of spinal fluid is removed again, and a solution containing 0.1 to 0.5 mg of amphotericin B is added. The mixture is injected slowly intrathecally. The procedure is repeated two to three times per week until a total dosage of 10 to 15 mg has been given. Spinal arachnoiditis and cranial toxic neuropathy are major hazards, even if the clinician takes precautions.

Flucytosine, when combined with amphotericin B, acts synergestically in vitro against *Cryptococcus neoformans*. It achieves satisfactory concentrations in CSF. Studies on human beings indicate that 6 weeks of intravenous amphotericin B at 0.3 mg per kg daily combined with 150 mg per kg of flucytosine daily is at least equivalent to 10 weeks of therapy with amphotericin B at 0.4 mg per kg daily.[1] The rate of relapse is considerably lower with the combined therapy. Side effects include leukopenia, thrombocytopenia, vomiting, and diarrhea. Controlled studies with the combined therapy in dogs and cats are lacking; however, combined therapy should be used because it may remove the need for intrathecal injections.

COCCIDIOIDAL MENINGITIS

Coccidioides immitis is not susceptible to the synergistic activity of combined amphotericin B and flucytosine therapy. The levels of amphotericin B achieved in CSF following intravenous administration are usually below the levels needed to inhibit most coccidioidal strains. Intrathecal administration of amphotericin B is recommended for the management of coccidioidal meningitis.

Ketoconazole is an orally effective broad-spectrum antifungal agent. It may be effective against the following organisms: *Candida* species, *Coccidioides immitis, Paracoccidioides brasiliensis, Histoplasma capsulatum,* and *Cryptococcus neoformans.* The drug has not been evaluated thoroughly in dogs and cats; however, it may be active against several deep mycotic infections in these animals. Ketoconazole should not be used for CNS fungal infections, because it penetrates poorly into the CSF. For infections of other body systems, a dosage of 10 mg per kg per day is suggested.

HISTOPLASMA MENINGITIS

Histoplasma capsulatum is very sensitive to amphotericin B. Most cases can be treated intravenously. In vitro studies suggest that amphotericin B and rifampin work synergistically. The clinical use of this combination is under investigation.

BLASTOMYCES MENINGITIS

Systemic blastomycosis in dogs frequently is associated with CNS involvement. Dogs with eye lesions almost always have CNS involvement. The organism is quite susceptible to amphotericin B and is treated with the intravenous regimen. As in all CNS mycotic infections, the prognosis is poor and the treatment is expensive.

INTRACRANIAL CANDIDIASIS

This condition is very rare in dogs and cats. It is of some importance in immunosuppressed patients. The treatment consists of intravenous amphotericin B. The *Candida* species are susceptible to the synergestic activity of combined intravenous amphotericin B and oral flucytosine.

INTRACRANIAL ASPERGILLOSIS

This disease results from an extension of an infection in the nose or sinuses into the brain. Many isolates of the *Aspergillus* species are resistant to amphotericin B, 75 per cent are resistant to flucytosine, and most are resistant to rifampin. Combined amphotericin B and flucytosine or amphotericin B and rifampin work synergistically against many strains of the *Aspergillus* species. Combined chemotherapy should be used, because the disease can be very fulminant. Controlled studies in the dog and cat are lacking. The prognosis is very poor.

INTRACRANIAL SPOROTRICHOSIS

Intravenous amphotericin B is the treatment of choice. Iodide therapy usually is not effective and should be reserved for diseases that are confined to the skin and the regional lymphatics.

Actinomycetes Infections

TUBERCULOUS MENINGITIS

Although it is nearly nonexistent in dogs and cats, this disease occurs occasionally in primates. Most of the antituberculous drugs readily penetrate the CNS. A combination of isoniazid and ethambutol is suggested. Other effective drugs include rifampin, ethionamide, pyrazinamide, and cycloserine.

NOCARDIOSIS

The drugs of choice include triple sulfonamides or trimethoprim-sulfa combinations. The drugs should be given in high doses, and precautions should be taken to prevent nephrotoxicity. Alternate drugs for patients intolerant of sulfonamides include minocycline and cycloserine. In vitro synergism between ampicillin and erythromycin has been demonstrated; however, clinical trials in dogs and cats have not been reported.

ACTINOMYCOSIS

The drug of choice is penicillin G, given intravenously at 25,000 units per kg per day.[1] Therapy is continued with amoxicillin or minocycline.

Viral Infections

Viral infection of the CNS may fit into one of four categories: (1) viral invasions resulting in inflammation (viral meningitis, encephalitis, or poliomyelitis), (2) postinfectious, noninflammatory encephalopathic states, (3) postinfectious and postvaccinal inflammatory states (old dog encephalitis, perhaps polyradiculoneuritis, brachial plexus neuropathy), and (4) slow virus infections (scrapie, Aleutian mink disease). The important viral diseases affecting the CNS in dogs and cats include rabies and pseudorabies. In dogs, distemper and canine herpes virus are of great importance. In cats, feline infectious peritonitis virus and feline leukemia virus are the most important.

Viral diseases of all species will be described in Chapter 17.

RABIES AND PSEUDORABIES

There is no effective therapy for these diseases. Treatment should not be attempted because of public health risks.

CANINE DISTEMPER

No effective therapy is known. Reports of cures following massive vitamin C therapy, ether therapy, or intravenous administration of modified live virus vaccine are unsubstantiated. Therapy is largely symptomatic. Seizure therapy will be discussed in the sections dealing with this subject.

Chronic progressive forms of distemper encephalitis (old dog encephalitis) resemble subacute sclerosing panencephalitis of human beings. The human disease is caused by a measles-like paramyxovirus that is antigenically related to canine distemper virus. Although controlled studies are lacking, corticosteroid therapy may cause temporary improvement in animals with this disease. Complete remission is unlikely. Occasionally, corticosteroid therapy may hasten the clinical course. Inasmuch as the disease is progressive and fatal, corticosteroid therapy should be evaluated carefully.

HERPES ENCEPHALITIS

Although a herpes virus is known to cause encephalitis in neonatal dogs, its association with other forms of chronic or acute encephalitis in dogs and cats has not been proved. *Herpes simplex* encephalitis is well documented in man and can be confirmed only by a demonstration of the virus in brain tissue.

Adenine arabinoside may be effective in lowering overall mortality rates in human beings. In canine herpes infections, the mortality may be lowered by raising the environmental temperature of puppies to 90 to 95 degrees F.

FELINE INFECTIOUS PERITONITIS (FIP)

The noneffusive form of FIP can produce a severe pyogranulomatous meningitis and ependymitis. There is no definitive therapy. Corticosteroids in doses of 2 to 4 mg per kg per day may cause temporary improvement. Complete remissions are unlikely.

FELINE CNS LYMPHOSARCOMA

This viral-induced disease will be discussed with the treatment of other neoplastic conditions.

LARGE ANIMAL VIRAL DISEASES

Very little is known about specific treatment of viral diseases of large animals. Supportive treatment is indicated.

MANAGEMENT OF CNS EDEMA, COMPRESSION, AND PAIN

These problems frequently occur in association with each other. Edema and pain frequently result from compressive lesions. The consequences of CNS compression (traumatic or neoplastic) is edema that may cause neuronal death and myelin degeneration. Therapy is directed at removal of the compression and control of the resulting edema. Edema also may accompany several metabolic or biochemical diseases, such as heat stroke, status epilepticus, hypoglycemic coma, hyperosmolar diabetic coma, water intoxication, hepatic encephalopathy, or hydrocephalus.

There are two basic types of cerebral edema: vasogenic and cytotoxic. Vasogenic edema involves expansion of the extracellular fluid space (EFS) because of a breakdown in the blood-brain barrier (BBB). Cytotoxic edema involves an intracellular shift of water caused by damage to cell membranes. In most conditions, both types of edema play a role in the increase of CNS pressure.

Treatment Considerations

Clinical management of an animal with increased CNS pressure from compression or edema, or both, is directed at the particular mechanism responsible for the illness. In compressive disorders, decompression and stabilization are extremely important. In addition, medical therapy is administered to control any tissue swelling. Certain drugs or procedures are used to treat a variety of conditions resulting in CNS edema. Each of these drug groups will be discussed relative to its mechanism of action and indications.

CORTICOSTEROIDS

Of the various corticosteroids studied, dexamethasone appears to be the most successful in the treatment of CNS edema. The effectiveness of dexamethasone in human beings with brain tumors and related edema has been well established. Studies of dogs indicate that dexamethasone in dosages of 0.5 to 2.0 mg per kg per day will prevent the cerebral edema that results from the experimental implantation of psyllium seed into the cerebral cortex.[5] Thus, dexamethasone is clearly indicated in the management of primary and metastatic CNS neoplasia.

The benefits of this drug in animals with CNS trauma are more controversial. Studies of human beings suggest that high-dose dexamethasone therapy reduces mortality in patients with severe head injury.[6] Dosages of 1 to 2 mg per kg are used. These dosages of dexamethasone correlate well to the levels suggested for dogs and cats with CNS trauma or compression. Two mg per kg of dexamethasone is given intravenously; the dose is repeated in 4 to 6 hours. Thereafter, the drug is given intravenously or intramuscularly at 0.25 mg per kg every 8 to 12 hours.

It has been suggested that dexamethasone has several mechanisms of action: (1) restoration of the damaged blood-brain barrier, (2) inhibition of CSF formation, and (3) a direct effect on the pressure-volume function of brain elasticity. In addition, the anti-inflammatory effects of this drug are beneficial in the treatment of several diseases, including intervertebral disk disease and immune-mediated diseases. The drug is also beneficial in the medical management of hydrocephalus. The indications for dexamethasone therapy are summarized in Table 7–2.

Side effects should be expected with high-dose corticosteroid therapy. Polyuria, polydipsia, polyphagia, weight gain, and adrenocortical suppression are common side effects. Gastric bleeding and ulceration also occur, particularly when dogs are on dexamethasone for longer than 5 days at dosages exceeding 0.5

Table 7–2. INDICATIONS AND CONTRAINDICATIONS FOR DEXAMETHASONE (CORTICOSTEROID) THERAPY IN CNS DISEASE

Effective	Probably Effective	Contraindicated
CNS neoplasia	Heat stroke	Bacterial meningitis
Hydrocephalus	Status epilepticus	Viral
Immune polymyositis	CNS trauma	encephalomyelitis
Severe hypoglycemia	Head injury	Diskospondylitis
	Spinal cord compression	Hepatic
	(disk disease and so forth)*	encephalopathy
	Noneffusive FIP†	
	Lymphosarcoma†	
	Hypercalcemia	
	Hyperosmolar coma	

*Used with strict cage confinement in cases of disk disease.
†Beneficial effects are short-term.

to 1.0 mg per kg per day. Bloody vomiting and diarrhea are indications to stop therapy. Decreased resistance to infection and delayed wound healing also are encountered occasionally.

OSMOTIC AGENTS

Hyperosmolar solutions may reduce increased intracranial pressure and CNS swelling rapidly. Mannitol and urea establish an osmotic gradient between the brain and various intracranial compartments, resulting in a net loss of CNS water. Both urea and mannitol enter nervous tissue; however, mannitol enters at a much slower rate. As these agents are cleared from the systemic circulation, blood concentrations drop below the CNS concentrations, favoring the movement of water back into CNS tissue. This activity occurs within 6 hours for urea, but blood levels of mannitol are higher than brain levels for up to 24 hours. Thus, mannitol is associated with a lower risk of pressure rebound than is urea. Mannitol at doses of 1.0 to 1.5 gm per kg is the preferred agent. The drug is given intravenously over a 30-minute period. The dose should be repeated 4 hours later. Thereafter, it is hoped that sustained antiedema effects will be provided by concomitant dexamethasone therapy. Clinically, concern has arisen regarding the use of mannitol in the face of possible active brain hemorrhage. Inasmuch as the clinician cannot actually determine the presence of ongoing hemorrhage, it is best to administer the drug because of its ability to decrease CNS swelling acutely. Mannitol does increase capillary oozing at surgery; nevertheless, it is a desirable agent in the management and control of edema resulting from surgical trauma. Sustained mannitol therapy can produce dehydration and

hypovolemia. Mannitol should not be given to a patient that is hypovolemic. The drug is cleared by the kidneys.

Glycerol is an osmotic agent that can be given orally. It seldom is used in animals. Experimentally, dimethyl sulfoxide (DMSO) has reduced CNS swelling and pressure. When given intravenously, it may cause hemolysis and red blood cell crenation. This drug is not recommended until clinical trials have been completed. DMSO may be helpful in the management of intraoperative trauma when it can be applied directly to CNS tissue.

DIURETICS

Certain diuretics have direct inhibitory effects on CSF production. Furosemide and acetazolamide significantly reduce edema from cold-induced brain lesions in cats. When combined with dexamethasone, the antiedema effects are enhanced. Diuretics also may delay rebound cerebral edema when combined with mannitol or urea therapy. Furosemide-mannitol combined therapy should be considered in the initial management of raised intracranial pressure. Furosemide also is effective in the medical management of hydrocephalus. It usually is combined with dexamethasone for treatment of this disease.

HYPOCAPNIA

Controlled hyperventilation to relax the brain and the spinal cord is a routine procedure in neurosurgery. A decreased pCO_2 (hypocapnia) results in CNS vasoconstriction, which may reduce intracranial pressure. In general, a pCO_2 of 25 to 30 mm Hg is desirable. In addition to neurosurgery, hyperventilation can be used in patients that are comatose from head injuries.

ANALGESICS AND ANTI-INFLAMMATORY AGENTS

Many CNS diseases are associated with severe pain. Diseases affecting the meninges or the vertebral periosteum are likely to be very painful. At times, symptomatic control of this pain is desirable; however, complete suppression of pain may be contraindicated in diseases in which decreased patient activity is desirable (i.e., intravertebral disk disease). These drugs are not substitutes for a correction of the underlying cause of the pain.

NON-NARCOTIC ANALGESICS

In this group, aspirin, acetaminophen, and phenylbutazone are the most frequently used compounds. Because of its multiple effects (antipyretic, anti-inflammatory, and platelet-inhibiting), aspirin is often useful for reasons other than its analgesic action. Vomiting or bleeding from gastirc irritation or ulceration is common but can be minimized by administration of the drug with food or use of enteric-coated tablets. The dosage in dogs is 10 to 25 mg per kg q8h. Because cats metabolize aspirin at a slower rate, a dosage of 10 mg per kg q52h is recommended for this species. Acetaminophen can be used in dogs; however, because this drug produces hemolytic anemia in cats, it should not be used in this species. Meperidine hydrochloride (Demerol) and codeine, as compared with morphine, rarely produce excitement in cats. In dogs, the following dosages are recommended: morphine, 1 mg per kg prn; meperidine hydrochloride, 10 mg per kg prn; and codeine, 2 mg per kg q6h. In cats, the following dosages are recommended: Meperidine hydrochloride, 3 mg per kg prn and codeine, 0.5 to 1.0 mg per kg. Codeine frequently is combined with aspirin in the same tablet. Unfortunately, these products present problems when used in dogs or cats. When the appropriate amount of codeine is given, the aspirin concentration is excessive. Therefore, separate codeine and aspirin products are indicated to ensure that accurate doses are administered.

Pentazocine (Talwin) has been used in dogs; however, its analgesic effects are inferior to those of the other drugs previously described.

ANTIANXIETY AGENTS AND MUSCLE RELAXANTS

Phenothiazine tranquilizers and benzodiazepines sometimes are used to relax and quiet animals that are in pain. Phenothiazine compounds should not be used to relax animals

with head injuries or following intracranial surgery, because these agents lower the threshold for seizures. Diazepam is more effective, because it relieves anxiety, produces mild sedation, relaxes muscles, and suppresses seizure activity. It is available in tablets for oral use or in ampuls for parenteral injection. The oral dosage must be adjusted to fit the individual needs of the animal. Oral dosages of 2.5 to 10 mg every 6 to 8 hours usually are given. Parenterally, dosages of 2.5 to 5 mg every 4 to 6 hours are recommended. Higher doses sometimes are required to control seizures.

Phenobarbital is the drug of choice if long-term sedation is required in both dogs and cats. Five mg per kg every 24 hours is recommended. It is the drug of choice for initial seizure control in cats.

Methocarbamol (Robaxin) is a close chemical relative of mephenesin carbamate and is of some value in the treatment of acute muscle spasm and as adjunct therapy in the treatment of tetanus. A dosage of 250 to 500 mg tid is recommended.

MANAGEMENT OF CONVULSIVE DISORDERS AND NARCOLEPSY

The treatment of these disorders will be discussed in Chapter 15.

MANAGEMENT OF CNS NEOPLASIA

The medical management of CNS neoplasia is directed at decreasing nervous tissue edema with corticosteroids (dexamethasone) and, in some instances, specific chemotherapy. Dexamethasone in dosages of 10 to 15 mg per day usually is effective. After 5 to 7 days, the dosage can be decreased in many dogs to 2 to 4 mg per day.

The blood-brain barrier (BBB) presents a unique problem in CNS chemotherapy. The BBB is impermeable to many of the chemotherapeutic agents that currently are used. In certain tumors, the BBB is not intact at the center of the mass; however, the integrity of the BBB improves at the periphery of the neoplasm. Thus, only those agents that have a small molecular weight, a low degree of ionization, and lipid solubility will penetrate the BBB. The nitrosoureas (BCNU, CCNU, and methyl-CCNU) meet these requirements and have been used in the treatment of gliomas in human beings. In addition, methotrexate can be given intrathecally in the management of CNS lymphoma.

PHYSICAL THERAPY

Much has been said in this chapter regarding specific drug therapy in the management of CNS diseases. Physical rehabilitation is also very important for the return of neurologic function, however,. Physical therapy is often neglected in veterinary practice. It is time-consuming and labor-intensive and is often boring. Pet owners can be taught to help, and many do a better job than veterinarians.

Hydrotherapy

Exercises performed in water or whirlpools are very effective for relaxing contracted muscles and stimulating circulation in atrophied muscles. They also help to keep the patient clean. Paralyzed dogs should undergo hydrotherapy sessions twice a day. Muscles and legs should be exercised passively. Sodium hypochlorite is used as a disinfectant in bathtubs and whirlpools to help suppress wound infections.

Exercise

Exercise can be passive or active, depending upon the degree of neurologic dysfunction. If possible, dogs should be exercised outdoors in walkers, dog carts, or slings. Limbs should be massaged vigorously to stimulate muscle tone and delay muscle contracture. Muscle massage with warm mineral oil is also helpful. Proper exercise seems to encourage dogs to walk and improves their mental status.

Bladder Care

Many neurologic lesions disrupt voluntary micturition, resulting in urinary incontinence, retention cystitis, and bladder atony. Urinary bladders should be expressed or emptied by intermittent catheterization at least three times a day. Urinary tract infections should be treated with appropriate antibiotics.

Cage Care

Paralyzed dogs must be turned frequently and must be kept on soft beds to prevent decubital ulcers and wound infections. Waterbeds, sealed foam mattresses, and air mattresses are helpful. The primary concern is to keep the cage clean and free of bacterial contamination. Paralyzed dogs, especially large-breed dogs, are predisposed to wound infections, respiratory infections, and urine soiling. They must be cleaned frequently and nursed compassionately in order to be rehabilitated.

REFERENCES

1. Murphy, F. K., Mackowiak, P., and Luby, J.: Management of infections affecting the nervous sytem. *In* Rosenberg, R. N.: A Textbook of the Treatment of Neurological Diseases. New York, SP Medical & Scientific Books, 1978.
2. Kornegay, J. N., Lorenz, M. D., and Zenoble, R. D.: Bacterial meningitis in two dogs. JAVMA 173:1334, 1978.
3. Lorenz, M. D.: Unpublished observations.
4. Kornegay, J. N., and Barber, D. L.: Diskospondylitis in dogs. JAVMA 177:337, 1980.
5. Sims, M. H., and Redding, R. W.: The use of dexamethasone in the prevention of cerebral edema in dogs. JAAHA 11:439, 1975.
6. Faupel, G., Reulen, H. J., Muller, D., and Schurmann, K: Double blind study on the effects of steroid in severe closed head injury. *In* Pappius, H. M., et al.: Dynamics of Brain Edema: Proceedings. New York, Springer-Verlag, 1977.

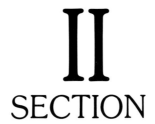

SECTION II

CLINICAL PROBLEMS
Signs and Symptoms

The term *monoparesis,* or *monoparalysis,* denotes partial or complete loss of motor function in one limb resulting from neurologic dysfunction. With mild neurologic dysfunction, the clinical signs may suggest lameness or pain from musculoskeletal disease. With more severe neurologic disease, paresis or paralysis is usually obvious, and the clinician's attention is immediately directed to the nervous system. Thus, when movement disorders occur in only one limb, the initial step in diagnosis is to localize the problem to either the musculoskeletal system or the nervous system (see Chapters 3 and 4). In a few cases, electrodiagnostic techniques are necessary in order to differentiate musculoskeletal disorders from primary neurologic disorders.

Physical injury to the peripheral or spinal nerves is a significant cause of movement disorders involving one limb and often results from skeletal fractures or luxations. Thus, careful evaluation of both systems is extremely important, since injury to the musculoskeletal system may produce injury or dysfunction of nerves. In general, the prognosis for recovery is better with skeletal injuries than with neurologic injuries.

ANATOMIC DIAGNOSIS: LOCALIZATION

The basic anatomic and physiologic principles that enable a clinician to localize lesions based on motor or sensory deficits have been presented in Chapter 4. A brief review of these concepts as they relate to the localization of lesions producing monoparesis or monoparalysis will be presented here (Fig. 8–1).

Monoparesis usually is caused by disease or injury to the lower motor neurons (LMNs) innervating the affected limb (see Chapter 4). Thus, dysfunction of the neuron (motor nerve cell body), the axon (ventral root, spinal nerves, peripheral nerves), or the neuromuscular endplate results in motor dysfunction and denervation atrophy. Disruption of the axon (especially the spinal and peripheral nerves) is the most common cause of monoparesis, although in rare circumstances, selective disease of motor neurons in the ventral gray matter of the spinal cord also may produce this problem. In most cases, unilateral spinal cord lesions rostral to T3 produce signs of hemiparesis, and bilateral lesions produce tetraparesis. Unilateral spinal cord lesions caudal to T3 may produce paresis or paralysis of the ipsilateral pelvic limb. Obviously, bilateral lesions caudal to T2 produce bilateral pelvic limb paresis. Thus,

when lesions are localized in cases of neurologic dysfunction of one thoracic limb (with the rest of the limbs normal), primary consideration is given to the brachial plexus or the peripheral nerves (Table 8–1). Spinal cord disease is not likely to be present, because disease in spinal cord segments C1–T2 affects the upper motor neurons (UMNs) to the ipsilateral pelvic limb. Rarely, lesions confined solely to ventral gray matter (C6–T2) result in thoracic limb monoparesis. Lesion locations for neurologic dysfunction of one pelvic limb may be in the ipsilateral spinal cord from T3–S1. More commonly, however, pelvic limb monoparesis results from damage to spinal or peripheral nerves. Unilateral spinal cord lesions (T3–L3) produce UMN signs in the ipsilateral limb, whereas lesions in the region L4–S2 or in the spinal or peripheral nerves result in LMN signs.

Disease of the spinal or peripheral nerves produces both sensory and motor dysfunction distal to the lesion, because these nerves contain both motor and sensory fibers. In contrast, lesions that originate in the spinal cord and are confined to the ventral gray matter (motor neurons only) do not produce sensory loss in the affected limbs. Also, unilateral spinal cord lesions (T2–L3) do not produce analgesia to the affected limb because of the bilateral, multisynaptic anatomy of the deep pain pathways (see Chapter 4). The presence of analgesia in the affected limb is very suggestive of peripheral or spinal nerve lesions. If sensory loss cannot be detected in the affected limb, lesions in the spinal cord gray matter or the ventral spinal roots are suspected. It should be remembered that unilateral spinal cord lesions involving segments T2–L3 produce paresis of the ipsilateral pelvic limb, but sensory

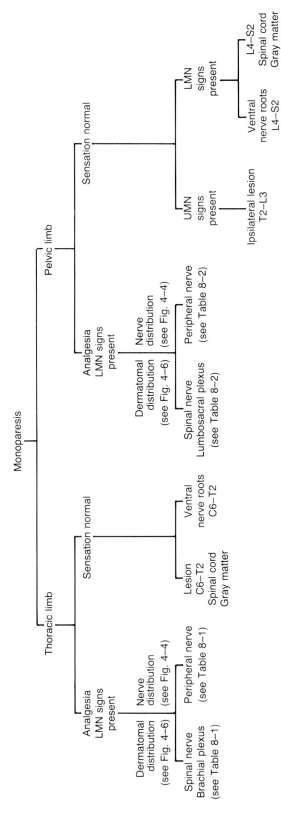

Figure 8–1. An algorithm for the localization of lesions that produce monoparesis.

loss usually is not detectable. However, lesions in this region of the spinal cord produce UMN signs in the affected limb, in contrast to the LMN signs produced by lesions in the L4–S2 segments. Figure 8–1 outlines the localization of lesions that produce monoparesis of the thoracic and pelvic limbs.

The distribution of sensory loss in an affected limb has great localizing value, because lesions can be pinpointed to a particular nerve or within two to three spinal cord segments (see Fig. 3–43). In addition, the degree of sensory loss influences the prognosis for functional recovery. The pattern of denervation atrophy also is helpful for the localization of lesions to a particular nerve or nerve group. Tables 8–1 and 8–2 outline the motor and sensory distribution of the brachial and lumbosacral plexus. The neurologic signs associated with lesions in each major nerve also are summarized in these tables.

Lesions in the gray matter of the spinal cord (T1–T3) or in the roots of the brachial plexus may injure the LMNs of the sympathetic nerve fibers that form the cranial sympathetic trunk. Loss of sympathetic stimulation to the ipsilateral eye produces signs of miosis, enophthalmos, and ptosis (Horner's sign). Horner's sign commonly is associated with traumatic injuries of the brachial plexus.

The term *mononeuropathy* refers to a disease or an injury of a specific peripheral nerve or its nerve roots. If a large nerve, such as the sciatic or radial nerve, is injured, a severe monoparesis may occur. In most cases, mononeuropathies result from physical injury secondary to compression, laceration, or contusion or from the intramuscular injection of

Table 8–1. NERVES OF THE BRACHIAL PLEXUS

Nerve	Spinal Cord Segments	Motor Function	Cutaneous Sensory Distribution	Signs of Dysfunction
Suprascapular	C6–C7	Extensors of the shoulder	—	Little gait abnormality, pronounced atrophy of supraspinatus and infraspinatus muscles (sweeny)
Axillary	C6–C7–C8	Flexors of the shoulder	Dorsolateral brachium	Little gait abnormality, decreased shoulder flexor reflex; analgesia on lateral side of arm
Musculocutaneous	C6–C7–C8	Special flexors of the elbow	Medial side of the forearm	Little gait abnormality, weakened flexion of the elbow; analgesia on medial surface of the forearm
Radial	C7–C8, T1–T2	Extensors of the elbow, the carpus, and the digits	Dorsal surface of the paw and dorsal and lateral parts of the forearm	Loss of weight bearing, paw and carpus knuckle over, weakened triceps reflex, analgesia of dorsal surface of paw and forearm
Median and ulnar	C8, T1–T2	Flexors of the carpus and the digits	Palmar surface of the paw; caudal forearm	Little gait abnormality, slight sinking of the carpus and the fetlock; loss of carpal flexion on withdrawal reflex; partial loss of sensation of the palmar surface of the paw
Sympathetic*	T1, T2, T3	Dilator of the pupil	—	Miosis, ptosis, and enophthalmos

*The sympathetic nerve is not considered a part of the brachial plexus; however, its nerve fibers travel along the roots of the brachial plexus as they exit from the vertebral column. Numbers in *italics* indicate the major cord segment that forms the peripheral nerve.

Table 8–2. NERVES OF THE LUMBOSACRAL PLEXUS

Nerve	Spinal Cord Segments	Motor Function	Cutaneous Sensory Distribution	Signs of Dysfunction
Obturator	L4, *L5*, L6	Adduction of pelvic limb	—	Little gait abnormality on normal surfaces, limb may slide laterally on slick surfaces
Femoral	L3, *L4*, *L5*, L6	Extension of the stifle and flexion of the hip	Saphenous branch: supplies the medial digit and the medial surface of the limb	Severe gait dysfunction, absence of weight bearing, decreased or absent knee jerk, loss of sensation of medial digit and medial surface of rear leg
Sciatic	*L6*, *L7*; *S1*, S2	Extension of the hip, flexion of the stifle—see *Tibial and Peroneal Branches*	Caudal and lateral sides of true leg—see *Tibial and Peroneal Branches*	Severe gait dysfunction; the paw is knuckled over, but weight bearing occurs; the hock cannot be flexed or extended, and the hip cannot be extended (in more central lesions, the hip is flexed and drawn toward the midline); cutaneous desensitization below the stifle except for areas supplied by the saphenous nerve; absent withdrawal reflex
Peroneal	See *Sciatic Nerve*	Flexion of the hock, extension of the digits	Dorsal aspect of paw, hock, and distal leg	Hock is straightened, and paw tends to knuckle over; loss of sensation to the dorsal aspects of the paw, the hock, and the distal leg; poor hock flexion on withdrawal reflex*
Tibial	See *Sciatic Nerve*	Extension of the hock, flexion of the digits	Plantar surface of the paw	Hock is dropped, loss of sensation of plantar surface of paw*

*Peroneal and tibial nerve paralysis commonly occur in association with each other. The signs of peroneal nerve damage tend to predominate.
Numbers in *italics* indicate the major cord segment that forms the peripheral nerve.

drugs. In addition to motor dysfunction and atrophy, variable degrees of sensory loss are encountered, because peripheral nerves innervating the limbs contain both motor and sensory fibers. The term *polyneuropathy* refers to a disease or an injury of several peripheral nerves or their nerve roots. In regard to monoparesis, the term polyneuropathy suggests an injury or a disease of the brachial plexus, the lumbosacral plexus, or the cauda equina. As is true for mononeuropathies, the most important category of disease resulting in monoparesis from polyneuropathies is physical injury. Occasionally, neoplasia of a specific peripheral nerve, nerve root, or nerve plexus is encountered. The incidence of this problem is low, however, and the clinical course is slowly progressive, in contrast to the acute nonprogressive course that tends to characterize physical injuries.

MONOPARESIS OF THE PELVIC LIMBS

Peripheral Nerve Injuries

SCIATIC NERVE INJURY

The sciatic nerve is a mixed nerve that arises from spinal cord segments L5–S2 (see Table 8–2). Since the spinal cord ends at the middle of the sixth lumbar vertebra in the dog, the sciatic nerve fibers travel caudally within the vertebral canal before exiting from the vertebrae. The course of these nerve fibers makes them particularly subject to injury from lumbosacral fractures, lumbosacral subluxations, and pelvic fractures. Sciatic nerve paralysis is a common calving injury in cattle. Damage to the fibers within the vertebral canal usually results in bilateral injury, producing pelvic limb paresis. Occasionally, the injury may be asymmetric, involving only the fibers of one sciatic nerve. Injuries of the lumbosacral area rarely result in a true mononeuropathy, because fibers forming the pudendal, pelvic, and caudal nerves are also injured. One therefore should consider injuries at this level as polyneuropathies.

After giving off branches within the pelvis, the major portion of the sciatic nerve exits at the greater ischiadic foramen and courses caudally to the coxofemoral joint. Branches of the sciatic nerve supply muscles that help extend the hip and flex the stifle. Proximal to the stifle (near the distal third of the femur), the sciatic

nerve branches into the peroneal and tibial nerves. These latter nerves supply all muscles below the stifle and provide sensation to all areas of the foot except for the medial digit, which is innervated by the saphenous branch of the femoral nerve. The proximal portion of the sciatic nerve is most frequently damaged by fractures of the shaft of the ilium, acetabular fractures, fractures of the proximal femur, and calving injuries in cattle. Injuries below the distal third of the femur produce signs from loss of function of the peroneal and tibial nerves. These injuries will be described later. Damage to the high sciatic nerve results in severe monoparesis, because the extensor muscles of the stifle are the only group that remains functional. Although the animal may bear weight, the stifle does not flex. The hock and the digits will not flex or extend because of tibial and peroneal nerve involvement. The animal stands "knuckled over," and the hock usually is dropped. Sensation below the stifle is severely compromised, but normal sensation is perceived from the medial leg surface or the medial digit (innervated by the femoral nerve). The dorsal surface of the foot frequently is ulcerated from the animal's dragging or walking on the knuckled-over paw (Fig. 8–2).

The sciatic nerve is the major nerve evaluated by the pelvic limb flexor reflex. In high sciatic nerve injuries, the digits, the hock, and the stifle do not flex when the toes are stimulated. Stimulation of the medial digit or the medial distal leg elicits a pain response and flexion of the hip, but the remainder of the joints of the affected limb do not flex. Atrophy of the caudal thigh muscles and the muscles below the stifle may be severe.

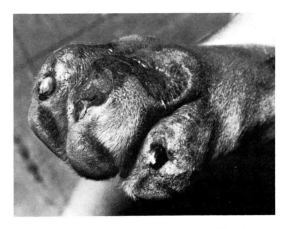

Figure 8–2. Ulcerated digits of the pelvic limb in a dog with peroneal nerve paralysis.

PERONEAL NERVE INJURY

The peroneal nerve supplies the muscles that flex the hock and extend the digits or the feet. It provides cutaneous sensory innervation to the dorsal aspect of the foot and the cranial surface of the hock and the tibia. This nerve is subject to injury where it crosses the lateral aspect of the stifle joint. In large animals, prolonged recumbency may injure the nerves at this site. In small animals, injuries usually result from the intramuscular injection of drugs into or near the nerve. The foot tends to "knuckle over," and the hock may be overextended. Loss of sensation occurs from the dorsal areas of the foot and the cranial surface of the hock and the tibia. The flexor reflex is severely depressed when the dorsal aspects of the foot or the digits are stimulated. Pinching the plantar surface of the digits or the foot elicits a definite pain response, and the flexor reflex is present, but the animal may not actively flex the hock joint. The examiner must exercise care in evaluating the flexor reflex, because some passive flexion of the hock may occur as the stifle actively flexes. Although the foot tends to knuckle over, the dorsal surface usually does not become abraded or ulcerated as severely as it does in higher sciatic nerve lesions (see Fig. 8–2). Dogs soon learn to place the foot by greater flexion of the hip and extension of the stifle.

TIBIAL NERVE INJURY

The tibial nerve supplies the muscles that extend the hock and flex the digits. It provides cutaneous sensory innervation to the plantar surface of the foot and the caudal surface of the leg. In a pure tibial nerve injury, the hock joint is dropped when the animal walks or supports weight (Fig. 8–3). Loss of sensation occurs from the plantar aspect of the foot. This problem may cause the formation of large ulcers in the digital pads of small animals. Apparently, the lack of sensation allows the pads to be ground into hard surfaces during weight bearing. The flexor reflex is severely depressed when the plantar surface of the foot is stimulated. Pinching the dorsal surface of the foot elicits a definite pain response, and the flexor reflex is present even though the toes are not flexed. In small animals, tibial nerve lesions usually occur in association with peroneal nerve injuries, and a mixture of neurologic signs is encountered.

FEMORAL NERVE INJURY

The femoral nerve arises from lumbar segments 4, 5, and 6 and supplies the extensor muscles of the stifle, which are the major weight-bearing muscles of the pelvic limb. Its saphenous branch is the sensory pathway from the skin on the medial surface of the foot, the leg, the stifle, and the thigh. Peripheral injuries to this nerve are not common, because it is well protected. Rarely, unilateral damage restricted to the ventral gray matter of lumbar segments 4, 5, and 6 results in a neuronopathy involving the femoral nerve. With femoral nerve lesions, the stifle cannot be fixed (extended) for weight bearing. The leg usually is carried, and the dog hops on the opposite limb. Lesions involving the peripheral femoral nerve produce analgesia in areas innervated by the saphenous nerve. Selective lesions involving the gray matter of the spinal cord produce mo-

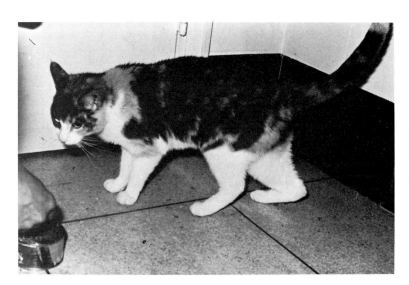

Figure 8–3. Tibial nerve paralysis in a cat, resulting from an injection injury. Note the dropped hock of the right pelvic limb, a result of paralysis of the gastrocnemius muscle.

tor dysfunction only. Sensation through the saphenous nerve is preserved. The knee-jerk (patellar) reflex is absent or diminished; however, the flexor reflex is normal. The hopping reaction is greatly decreased in the affected leg, because weight bearing is inhibited.

In large animals, femoral nerve paralysis results in a severe monoparesis. The affected limb is poorly advanced and collapses during weight bearing. In cattle, femoral nerve paralysis results from trauma to calves during parturition. Forced extraction of calves from the "hip-lock" position may hyperextend the hip and overstretch the nerve where it enters the quadriceps muscle. Apparently, there is an increased incidence in the heavy-muscled breeds of cattle.

OBTURATOR NERVE INJURY

Injuries to the obturator nerve in the dog or the cat do not result in monoparesis, although the affected leg may slide laterally when the animal stands on a smooth surface. Injuries to this nerve are not clinically important in small animals.

Obturator paralysis is a common calving injury in cattle. The obturator nerve innervates the adductor muscles of the limb, and injuries to this nerve produce marked pelvic limb ataxia, especially on slippery surfaces. The limbs may be placed in a wide-based stance, and this posture is exaggerated as the animal runs. Unilateral paralysis produces less of a gait abnormality, since the signs are associated with only one limb. Most calving injuries damage the branches to the sciatic nerve as well as the obturator nerve.

Spinal Cord Diseases

Unilateral spinal cord lesions involving segments L4–S2 result in monoparesis. Because these lesions may damage the motor neurons that form the nerves of the lumbosacral plexus, lower motor neuron dysfunction occurs. Occasionally, spinal cord trauma, neoplasia, or vascular occlusions have a unilateral distribution and produce monoparesis. Rarely, inflammatory disease of the spinal cord is restricted to one side, and monoparesis may be the presenting complaint. Some degree of sensory loss usually accompanies the motor dysfunction. In rare cases in which the spinal cord lesions are restricted to ventral gray matter, sensation will be normal. In most cases, several spinal cord segments are involved, and

dysfunction of several nerves (polyneuropathy) occurs.

Unilateral spinal cord lesions involving segments T2–L3 also result in monoparesis, but it is of the UMN type. Usual causes are trauma, vascular occlusion, neoplasia, and, occasionally, inflammation. Pertinent disorders that produce unilateral spinal cord lesions will be discussed in the chapters dealing with pelvic limb paresis and tetraparesis (Chapters 9 and 10).

MONOPARESIS OF THE THORACIC LIMBS

Peripheral Nerve Injuries

The nerves that innervate the muscles of the thoracic limbs and the clinical signs associated with injuries of these nerves are presented in Table 8–1. In this section, injuries to the brachial plexus, the radial nerve, and the suprascapular nerve are discussed, because they are of greatest clinical importance.

AVULSION OF THE BRACHIAL PLEXUS

The nerves of the brachial plexus have their origin from spinal cord segments C6–T2 (see Table 8–1). In addition, the sympathetic nerves that innervate the eye originate from neurons in the first three thoracic segments and travel along the roots of the brachial plexus as they exit from the vertebral column. Injuries to the brachial plexus result in monoparesis of the affected limb and, in some cases, an ipsilateral partial Horner's syndrome. Avulsion of the brachial plexus is a common traumatic injury in the dog and results from severe abduction of the limb. The nerve roots of the brachial plexus are torn or stretched from their spinal cord attachments.

The major signs of motor dysfunction are related to damage to the roots of the radial nerve and, to a lesser extent, to the other nerves of the plexus. The proximal radial nerve innervates the triceps muscle, which is the major weight-bearing muscle in the thoracic limb. The distal branches of the radial nerve innervate the extensors of the carpus and the digits. An injured animal bears little or no weight on the limb, and the paw is knuckled over and usually drags on the ground (Fig. 8–4). The dorsal aspect of the paw may become severely abraded and ulcerated. Sensory loss varies, depending upon the extent of the injury or the number of nerves in the plexus that are in-

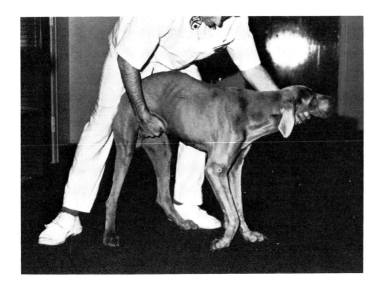

Figure 8–4. Brachial plexus injury in a dog, a result of a car accident. Note the knuckled paw and the inability to support weight on the limb. Atrophy is present in the scapular muscles.

volved in the injury. In many cases, both deep and superficial pain sensation are lost in the paw. The hopping and proprioceptive positioning reactions are decreased or absent. The flexor, extensor carpi radialis, and triceps reflexes are weak or absent. Muscle atrophy of the thoracic limb may be severe, depending upon the number of nerve roots injured. Because sympathetic nerve roots may be injured, an ipsilateral partial or complete Horner's syndrome is present in over 50 per cent of the cases. In addition to the neurologic examination, an electromyographic (EMG) examination of the thoracic limb is useful for assessing the extent of brachial plexus damage and can be helpful for establishing a prognosis for functional recovery. The utility of this examination is discussed in this chapter in the section dealing with therapy for peripheral nerve injuries and in Chapter 6.

The prognosis for use of the affected limb is poor if a proximal radial nerve injury is present. The more proximal branches of the radial nerve innervate the triceps muscle, which must be functional for weight bearing. Corrective orthopedic procedures such as carpal arthrodesis or tendon transplantation are not indicated when the nerves to the triceps muscle are injured. These procedures may be helpful in selected cases in which the injury has spared the proximal branches of the radial and the musculocutaneous nerve. An EMG examination is useful for evaluating these muscles for evidence of denervation when corrective surgery is contemplated.

Occasionally, bilateral brachial plexus injuries are encountered. These injuries have been observed in animals that have fallen from great heights and have landed in a sternal position, severely abducting both thoracic limbs. In addition to the signs of bilateral plexus injury, the diaphragm may be paralyzed if the roots of the phrenic nerve are damaged. The phrenic nerve arises from cervical segments 5, 6, and 7 but is not considered part of the brachial plexus. Rarely, the injury may involve these nerve roots; however, dyspnea resulting from diaphragmatic paralysis is uncommon.

RADIAL NERVE INJURY

The entire radial nerve may be injured by fractures of the first rib or in avulsion of the brachial plexus. Fractures of the humerus may injure the nerve distal to the branches that supply the triceps muscle. In large animals, radial nerve injuries occur most commonly during anesthetic procedures or when the animal is in lateral recumbency on a hard surface for extended periods. Distal radial injuries produce less severe gait abnormalities than do brachial plexus injuries. The elbow can be extended; however, the foot tends to knuckle over when the animal walks, because the extensors of the carpus and the digits are paralyzed. Sensation is lost from the dorsal and cranial aspects of the limb below the elbow.

SUPRASCAPULAR NERVE INJURY

Suprascapular paralysis occurs most frequently in large animals secondary to trauma or fracture of the scapula. The nerve innervates the supraspinatus and infraspinatus muscles. These muscles may atrophy severely, resulting in sweeny. Weight bearing is usually unaffected; however, the stride may be shortened and the shoulder abducted when weight is borne on the leg. Cattle may be injured in malfunctioning chutes or from striking the head gate with the shoulders. Work horses may be injured from poorly fitting collars.

Contracture of the infraspinatus muscle occurs in dogs and results in a thoracic leg lameness. The elbow and the foreleg are abducted as the dog runs. The forward stride of the limb may be slightly shortened. Characteristically, the foot is moved laterally as the limb is advanced. The cause is unknown. Cutting the insertion of the infraspinatus muscle is beneficial.

Spinal Cord Diseases

Unilateral spinal cord lesions restricted to the ventral gray matter (C6–T2) may destroy the motor neurons of the brachial plexus, resulting in LMN monoparesis. Unlike peripheral nerve injuries, which involve both motor and sensory nerve fibers, lesions in this area result in paresis or paralysis, but sensation to the leg is preserved. Vascular occlusions that infarct this area of the spinal cord and, rarely, inflammatory diseases produce this problem. Lesions in the spinal cord at this level usually involve the motor and proprioceptive pathways to the ipsilateral pelvic limb. Unilateral spinal cord lesions (C6–T2), therefore, usually result in hemiparesis with UMN signs in the ipsilateral rear limb and LMN signs in the thoracic limb. Avulsion of the brachial plexus may be associated with paresis or paralysis of the ipsilateral pelvic limb if the spinal cord is compressed, contused, or otherwise damaged at the time of trauma. Spinal cord diseases will be discussed in the chapters dealing with pelvic limb paresis and tetraparesis.

PROGNOSIS

The prognosis of peripheral nerve injuries depends upon the type of damage and the severity of neurologic dysfunction. Nerve fibers that have been contused, compressed, or stretched may regain function slowly. Nerves that have been lacerated or avulsed from their spinal cord attachments, however, seldom regain function. Unfortunately, in routine practice it sometimes is difficult to establish which of these situations has occurred at the time of the initial examination. In order for nerve fibers to regenerate, the nerve sheath must remain intact. Axonal regeneration occurs slowly; however, an intact sheath must be present in order to guide the axon to the denervated muscle. Motor function in affected muscles may be regained by the sprouting and innervation of these muscle fibers by adjacent intact neurons. Regardless of the repair process involved, return to function may take several months and may never be complete.

In general, the prognosis for functional recovery for animals with severe motor dysfunction and complete analgesia is poor. These lesions are usually severe and may involve complete disruption of nerve fibers. Some animals regain function; however, the outcome is often unsatisfactory. The prognosis is better for animals with partial loss of motor or sensory function, because the damage to the axons may be transitory, and reinnervation from adjacent, intact nerve fibers is more predictable. In addition, animals with partial dysfunction may learn to compensate for their problem by using other, uninvolved muscle groups. In most cases, the distribution and the severity of sensory loss are considered when a prognosis is established.

If available, an EMG examination is useful for formulating a prognosis and assessing the recovery of peripheral nerve injuries. This technique helps the clinician to establish the severity and the distribution of the nerve injury. A total lack of voluntary motor potentials, an absence of responses to nerve stimulation, and evidence of diffuse denervation are highly correlated with a poor prognosis. The presence of some motor unit activity and patchy denervation suggests that the lesion is not complete and that a better chance for nerve regeneration exists. EMG examinations can be repeated periodically over several months in order to determine if reinnervation is occurring. If tendon transplant surgery is contemplated, an EMG examination of the involved muscles is performed. The muscles should be free of fibrillation potentials and positive sharp waves.

TREATMENT

The initial therapy for a nerve injury consists of corticosteroid administration to relieve inflammation and immobilization of the limb to prevent further trauma. Nerve decompression or anastomosis is indicated if the site of injury is accessible for surgical manipulation.

Long-term management consists of physical therapy to help prevent muscle atrophy and trauma to the foot. Tendon transplantation and joint arthrodesis are performed primarily for distal radial nerve and peroneal injuries. Probably the most important aspect of long-term management is prevention of trauma to the distal extremity. There are commercially available boots that help protect the paw, are easily applied by the owner, and are well tolerated by the dog. Owners frequently request amputation of the affected limb because of distal extremity trauma. Prevention of this problem spares the limb for a period that is sufficient for the veterinarian to see if nerve regeneration will occur. Generally, amputation of the limb should be delayed for 6 months, unless traumatic complications can-

not be prevented. The owner should be warned that recovery is slow and that amputation is an irreversible solution to the problem. A "wait-and-see" approach should be recommended.

Many peripheral nerve injuries can be avoided by proper management of large animals placed in lateral recumbency. Adequate padding must be provided at all times, and recumbent animals should be turned frequently (at least 3 times a day). Excessive traction on limbs should be avoided during anesthesia, animal movement, or fetal extraction. Injured limbs should be protected by bandages, splints, or casts. Cattle with obturator paralysis must be kept on good footing. Hobbles on the pelvic limbs may be helpful. Recumbent animals should be supported with slings whenever possible.

CASE HISTORIES

Case History 8A

Signalment

Canine, Weimaraner, male, 6 years old.

History

Hit by a car 20 days ago. Since that day, the dog has been unable to use the right thoracic limb. He has been dragging the foot and is unable to advance the leg or bear weight. Open sores have developed on the dorsum of the foot.

Physical Examination

No abnormalities other than the neurologic problem described in the next section.

Neurologic Examination *

A. Observation
1. Mental status: Alert.
2. Posture: Normal, see *Gait*.
3. Gait: Severe paresis of right TL. Drags the leg and the foot. The paw knuckles over, and the dog can bear little weight on the limb.

B. Palpation
Atrophy of triceps, supraspinatus, infraspinatus, biceps, and flexor carpi radialis muscles of right TL.

C. Postural Reactions

Left	Reactions	Right
	Proprioceptive positioning	
+2	PL	+2
+2	TL	0
+2	Wheelbarrowing	0
+2	Hopping, PL	+2
+2	Hopping, TL	0
+2	Extensor postural thrust	+2
+2	Hemistand-hemiwalk	0
+2	Tonic neck	0
	Placing, tactile	
+2	PL	+2
+2	TL	0
	Placing, visual	
+2	TL	0
	Rear	

*Key: 0 = absent, +1 = decreased, +2 = normal, +3 = exaggerated, +4 = very exaggerated or clonus, PL = pelvic limb, TL = thoracic limb.

D. Spinal Reflexes

Left	Reflex Spinal Segment	Right
	Quadriceps	
+2	L4−L6	+2
	Extensor carpi radialis	
+2	C7−T1	0
	Triceps	
+2	C7−T1	0
	Flexion, PL	
+2	L5−S1	+2
	Flexion, TL	
+2	C6−T1	0
0	Crossed extensor	0
	Perineal	
+2	S1−S2	+2

E. Cranial Nerves

Left	Nerve + Function	Right
	C.N. II vision	
+2	menace	+2
Nor.	C.N. II + C.N. III pupil size	constricted
+2	Stim. left eye	+2
+2	Stim. right eye	+2
Nor.	C.N. II fundus	Nor.
	C.N. III, C.N. IV, C.N. VI	
0	Strabismus	0
0	Nystagmus	0
+2	C.N. V sensation	+2
Nor.	C.N. V mastication	Nor.
Nor.	C.N. VII facial muscles	Nor.
+2	Palpebral	+2
Nor.	C.N. IX, C.N. X swallowing	Nor.
Nor.	C.N. XII tongue	Nor.

F. Sensation: Location
Hyperesthesia _____ None _____
Superficial pain _____ 0 right TL _____
Deep pain _____ 0 to +1 right TL _____

Complete sections G and H before reviewing Case Summary.

G. Assessment (Anatomic diagnosis and estimation of prognosis)

H. Plan (Diagnostic)

Rule-outs	Procedure
1.	
2.	
3.	
4.	

Case History 8B

Signalment

Canine, boxer, male, 1 year old.

History

Hit by a car 10 months ago. Treated for shock and multiple pelvic fractures. Referred 2 days after initial injury because of severe dyspnea. Massive pleural effusion was treated with chest drains. Moderate paresis in right PL. Hypalgesia below the stifle. No treatment was given, and the dog was discharged 4 days later. Returned 10 months after initial injury for follow-up examination. No improvement in right PL.

Physical Examination

Negative except for the neurologic problem.

Neurologic Examination *

A. Observation
1. Mental status: Alert.
2. Posture: Normal.
3. Gait: Moderate paresis of right PL. Hyperflexion of the stifle. The paw does not knuckle over; however, the hock sinks when weight bearing occurs. All other limbs are normal.

B. Palpation
Atrophy of cranial tibial muscle and flexors and extensors of the hock and digits. Deep ulcers in the plantar surfaces of the middle two digital pads. These toes are swollen.

C. Postural Reactions

Left	Reactions	Right
	Proprioceptive positioning	
+2	PL	0
+2	TL	+2
+2	Wheelbarrowing	+2
+2	Hopping, PL	0
+2	Hopping, TL	+2
+2	Extensor postural thrust	0
+2	Hemistand-hemiwalk	0
+2	Tonic neck	+2
	Placing, tactile	
+2	PL	0 − +1
+2	TL	+2
	Placing, visual	
+2	TL	+2
	Rear	

*Key: 0 = absent, +1 = decreased, +2 = normal, +3 = exaggerated, +4 = very exaggerated or clonus, PL = pelvic limb, TL = thoracic limb.

D. Spinal Reflexes

Left	Reflex Spinal Segment	Right
+2	Quadriceps L4−L6	+2
+2	Extensor carpi radialis C7−T1	+2
+2	Triceps C7−T1	+2
+2	Flexion, PL L5−S1	Flexes hip and stifle—0 below stifle
+2	Flexion, TL C6−T1	+2
0	Crossed extensor	0
+2	Perineal S1−S2	+2

E. Cranial Nerves

Left	Nerve + Function	Right
+2	C.N. II vision menace	+2
Nor.	C.N. II + C.N. III pupil size	Nor.
+2	Stim. left eye	+2
+2	Stim. right eye	+2
Nor.	C.N. II fundus	Nor.
0	C.N. III, C.N. IV, C.N. VI Strabismus	0
0	Nystagmus	0
Nor.	C.N. V sensation	Nor.
Nor.	C.N. V mastication	Nor.
Nor.	C.N. VII facial muscles	Nor.
+2	Palpebral	+2
Nor.	C.N. IX, C.N. X swallowing	Nor.
Nor.	C.N. XII tongue	Nor.

F. Sensation: Location
Hyperesthesia _____ None _____
Superficial pain Blunted below stifle in right PL
Deep pain 0 from middle two digits in right PL

Complete sections G and H before reviewing Case Summary.

G. Assessment (Anatomic diagnosis and estimation of prognosis)

H. Plan (Diagnostic)

Rule-outs	Procedure
1.	
2.	
3.	
4.	

Case History 8C

Signalment

Feline, domestic, female, 7 years old.

History

Mild lameness noted in right TL 6 to 8 weeks ago. The cat has gotten slowly worse and now cannot bear weight on the leg. She holds the leg extended with the paw flexed and now is knuckling occasionally on the right PL.

Physical Examination

Negative except for the neurologic problem.

Neurologic Examination *

A. Observation
   1. Mental status: Alert.
   2. Posture: Normal.
   3. Gait: Severe paresis in right TL. The cat occasionally drags and knuckles the right pelvic paw.
B. Palpation
   Mild atrophy in right scapular muscles.

C. Postural Reactions

Left	Reactions	Right
	Proprioceptive positioning	
+2	PL	+1
+2	TL	0
+2	Wheelbarrowing	0
+2	Hopping, PL	+1
+2	Hopping, TL	0
+2	Extensor postural thrust	+1
+2	Hemistand-hemiwalk	0
+2	Tonic neck	0
	Placing, tactile	
+2	PL	+1
+2	TL	0
	Placing, visual	
+2	TL	0
	Rear	

*Key: 0 = absent, +1 = decreased, +2 = normal, +3 = exaggerated, +4 = very exaggerated or clonus, PL = pelvic limb, TL = thoracic limb.

D. Spinal Reflexes

Left	Reflex Spinal Segment	Right
	Quadriceps	
+2	L4–L6	+3
	Extensor carpi radialis	
+2	C7–T1	0–+1
	Triceps	
+2	C7–T1	0–+1
	Flexion, PL	
+2	L5–S1	+2
	Flexion, TL	
+2	C6–T1	0
0	Crossed extensor	0
	Perineal	
+2	S1–S2	+2

E. Cranial Nerves

Left	Nerve + Function	Right
	C.N. II vision	
+2	menace	+2
Nor.	C.N. II + C.N. III pupil size	Constricted
+2	Stim. left eye	+2
+2	Stim. right eye	+2
Nor.	C.N. II fundus	Nor.
	C.N. III, C.N. IV, C.N. VI	
0	Strabismus	0
0	Nystagmus	0
Nor.	C.N. V sensation	Nor.
Nor.	C.N. V mastication	Nor.
Nor.	C.N. VII facial muscles	Nor.
+2	Palpebral	+2
Nor.	C.N. IX, C.N. X swallowing	Nor.
Nor.	C.N. XII tongue	Nor.

F. Sensation: Location
   Hyperesthesia _____ None _____
   Superficial pain _____ Normal _____
   Deep pain _____ Normal _____
Complete sections G and H before reviewing Case Summary.
G. Assessment (Anatomic diagnosis and estimation of prognosis)

H. Plan (Diagnostic)
   Rule-outs   Procedure
   1.
   2.
   3.
   4.

ASSESSMENT 8A

Anatomic diagnosis: The dog has monoparesis affecting the right thoracic limb and a partial Horner's sign of the right eye. LMN signs with sensory deficits in several nerves suggest a lesion of the right brachial plexus. C6–T2 lesions are discounted because the right pelvic limb is normal.
1. A brachial plexus injury.
2. An injury to the roots of the right sympathetic nerve that causes Horner's sign.
   Diagnostic plan (rule-outs):
1. Low cervical trauma—radiographs (negative).
2. Brachial plexus injury—EMG (fibrillation potentials and positive sharp waves in several muscle groups).
   Therapeutic plan:
1. Protect the foot with a boot.
2. Perform physical therapy.
   Client education: The prognosis is very poor for functional use of the leg, since the nerve roots have been severely injured. Amputation may be needed in the future.
   Case summary:
1. Diagnosis: Brachial plexus injury.
2. Result: The dog regained partial use of the leg in 6 months; however, he must wear a boot continually to protect the foot. Persistent mild pupil constriction is present in the right eye.

ASSESSMENT 8B

Anatomic diagnosis: The dog has monoparesis of the right pelvic limb. LMN signs with sensory deficits below the stifle localize the lesion to the lower sciatic nerve.

A lower sciatic nerve (peroneal and tibial nerves) injury was diagnosed.
Diagnostic plan (rule-outs):
1. Pelvic fracture—pelvic radiographs (multiple pelvic fractures that are now healed but are displaced).
2. Injection injury—EMG (diffuse denervation below the stifle; few fibrillation potentials and positive sharp waves in the gastrocnemius, the semitendinosus, and the semimembranosus muscles; evidence of reinnervation in some muscles).

Therapeutic plan:
1. Physical therapy should be performed.
2. The middle two digits are infected and require antibiotic therapy.
3. A boot should be fitted on the dog to prevent further trauma.
   Client education: Because the sciatic nerve injury is partial and evidence of reinnervation is present, the dog may regain functional use of the limb.
   Case summary: One must debate the cause of the nerve injury, i.e., a pelvic fracture versus a needle (injection) injury. The neurologic examination is more consistent with the diagnosis of a needle (injection) injury, because nerve damage usually occurs at the origin of the peroneal and the tibial nerves. The EMG, however, provides evidence that the lesion is more central. Denervation of the semitendinosus and semimembranosus muscles probably is a result of the pelvic fractures.
   Final diagnosis: Sciatic nerve injury from a pelvic fracture.
   Result: The dog regained good use of the leg, and the boot eventually was removed.

ASSESSMENT 8C

Anatomic diagnosis: LMN signs are present in the right thoracic limb, and UMN signs are present in the right rear leg. In addition, there is a mild Horner's sign in the right eye. A unilateral right C6–T3 lesion would explain these signs. The history suggests that the lesion may have begun in the brachial plexus and moved centrally.
Diagnostic plan (Rule-outs):
1. Neoplasia—radiology (survey films negative), myelogram (swelling at the right side of the cord at C7–T1 intervertebral space).
2. Inflammation—CSF tap (0 cells, 20 mg/dl protein).
   Therapeutic plan: Administer dexamethasone to help relieve spinal cord edema. Surgical removal may be possible but probably will cause denervation of the limb requiring amputation.
   Case summary: A neurofibroma of the right brachial plexus is present with cord compression of C6, C7, C8, and T1. The history is typical for a neurofibroma of the brachial plexus.

9
CHAPTER

PELVIC LIMB PARESIS, PARALYSIS, OR ATAXIA

Bilateral motor dysfunction of the pelvic limbs is termed *paraparesis* or *paraplegia,* depending upon the severity of the motor loss. Loss of proprioception from the pelvic limbs results in sensory ataxia. In addition, loss of pain perception from the pelvic limbs may accompany the motor dysfunction. Lesion localization has been discussed in Chapter 4 and is summarized in Figure 9–1. A brief review follows.

LESION LOCALIZATION

Animals with pure pelvic limb paresis and ataxia have neurologic disease caudal to the second thoracic spinal cord segment. Lesions in the region T3–L3 produce paraparesis of the upper motor neuron (UMN) type. The pelvic limb lower motor neurons located in the segments L4–S2 remain intact and are capable of reflex motor activity; however, voluntary motor control from the brain is lost, because the motor pathways in the spinal cord are damaged. The spinal reflexes are normal or exaggerated. Exaggerated reflexes result when UMN inhibitory influence on the lower motor neurons (LMNs) is lost. Similarly, extensor hypertonus also may develop. Ataxia results from damage to the spinal cord proprioceptive pathways, which transmit position sense signals from receptors in the pelvic limbs to the brain. Hypalgesia or analgesia distal to the lesion results from disruption of pain pathways from the pelvic limbs to the brain. Deep pain sensation is lost only if the lesions are bilateral and severe. Voluntary visceral functions (see Chapter 5), such as micturition, may be lost when motor or sensory pathways in the spinal cord are damaged. Disuse atrophy may develop with time.

In summary, spinal cord lesions in the region T3–L3 result in paresis, ataxia, decreased or absent postural reactions, normal reflexes or hyperreflexia, impaired micturition, and variable degrees of sensory loss caudal to the lesion. Examination of the thoracolumbar dermatomes may be helpful in the localization of lesions to spinal segments within this spinal cord region (see Chapter 4).

Lesions in the area L4–S2 or those that involve the cauda equina produce pelvic limb paresis of the LMN type. Lesions involving spinal cord segments L4–S2 injure the motor neurons that form the lumbosacral plexus. Abnormalities related to femoral, sciatic, pudendal, and pelvic nerves are encountered in these patients. Pelvic limb reflexes are depressed or absent, and the muscles may be hypotonic. Neurogenic atrophy will develop. Sensory dysfunction (ataxia, hypalgesia, analgesia) results from an injury to the sensory neurons and the nerve fibers located in this region of the spinal cord. Abnormalities of visceral function result from an injury to the motor and sensory neurons that innervate the bladder and the anus. Lesions involving the coccygeal segments of the spinal cord and the cauda equina damage nerve fibers that form the sciatic, pudendal, pelvic, and coccygeal nerves. Because the femoral nerve is spared, the animal is able to support weight on the pelvic limbs. The knee-jerk reflex is normal, and pain is perceived from the medial digit and the thigh. The clinical signs relate to motor and sensory dysfunction of the involved nerves. Figure 9–2 summarizes lesion localization for the problem of pelvic limb paresis based on motor signs.

DISEASES

The disorders or diseases that affect the spinal cord segments T3–L3 are classified in Figures 9–3, 9–4, and 9–5. Disorders that affect spinal cord segments L4–S2 and the cauda equina are presented in Figures 9–6, 9–7, and 9–8. These figures are organized according to the logic used in the formulation of a neurologic diagnosis, which has been discussed in Chapter 2. After the lesion has been localized to a region or segment of the spinal cord or nerve root, consideration is given to the pos-

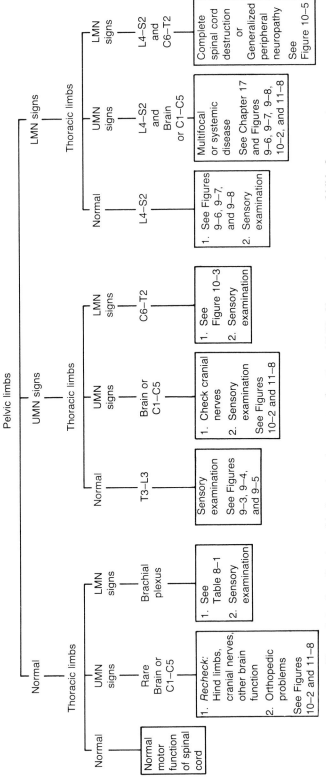

Figure 9–1. Localization of lesions based on motor function. *UMN* = Upper motor neuron. *LMN* = Lower motor neuron. *C* = Cervical. *T* = Thoracic. *L* = Lumbar. *S* = Sacral spinal cord segments. (Modified from Hoerlein, B.F.: Canine Neurology: Diagnosis and Treatment, 3rd ed. Philadelphia, W.B. Saunders Co., 1978.)

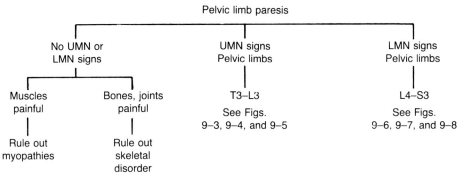

Figure 9–2. Algorithm for the localization of lesions causing pelvic limb paresis.

sible etiologic categories that could produce the lesion. The etiologic categories are listed in the left-hand column and follow the *DAMNIT* scheme that has been described in Chapter 2. The diseases are further divided into acute progressive, acute nonprogressive, and chronic progressive categories. The examiner should make these decisions based on historical information or by following the clinical course of the illness. Most diseases have been included in the figures; those in italics are of greatest clinical importance. The most impor-

T3–L3

| Etiologic Category | Acute | | Chronic |
	Progressive	Nonprogressive	
Degenerative	1. *Disk disease*** 2. Ascending, descending myelomalacia (hematomyelia)	None	1. *Degenerative myelopathy*** (degenerative radiculomyelopathy) 2. *Type II disk disease* ("slow disk") 3. Spondylosis deformans* 4. *Dural ossification** 5. *Hereditary myelopathy of Afghans* 6. Neuronopathy (hereditary canine spinal muscular atrophy) 7. Demyelinating diseases 8. Multiple cartilagenous exostosis
Anomalous	None	None	1. Hemivertebrae* 2. Spinal dysraphism (syringomyelia)
Neoplastic	Metastatic	None	1. Primary 2. Lymphoreticular 3. Skeletal 4. Metastatic
Nutritional			Hypervitaminosis A (cats)
Inflammatory			See *Acute Progressive*

Infectious	1. Distemper myelitis
	 2. Myelitis, bacterial
	   a. Meningomyelitis
	   *b. Secondary to spondylitis
	   *c. *Secondary to diskospondylitis***
	 3. Toxoplasmosis
	 4. Mycosis
	   a. Cryptococcosis
	   b. Blastomycosis
	   c. Histoplasmosis
	   d. Nocardiosis
	   e. Coccidioidomycosis
		None	1. Mycotic infections, toxoplasmosis, and *diskospondylitis* usually have a chronic progressive course
			 2. Noneffusive feline infectious peritonitis
			 3. Distemper myelitis

Traumatic	Ascending, descending myelomalacia (hematomyelia)	1. Fractures 2. Subluxations 3. Traumatic disk herniation	None
Toxic	See *Seizures,* Tables 15–2 and 15–3.		

*Indicates disease is not always associated with neurologic signs.
**Indicates increased incidence of nonselective disease at particular site.

Figure 9–3. Thoracolumbar spinal cord diseases. Differential diagnosis of T3–L3 spinal cord disease based on its clinical course and etiologic categories. *Italics* indicate most important diseases clinically.

T3–L3

Etiologic Category	Acute Progressive	Acute Nonprogressive	Chronic
Degenerative	Degenerative myelopathy		
Anomalous	None	None	Vertebral anomaly
Neoplastic	Metastatic	None	1. Primary 2. Lymphoreticular 3. Skeletal 4. Metastatic
Nutritional	None	None	None
Inflammatory	None	None	Vertebral abscess (Diskospondylitis) See *Acute Progressive*

Infectious	1. *Necrotizing myeloencephalitis* (Herpes 1 infection)
	2. *Protozoal encephalomyelitis* (*focal myelitis*)
	3. *Vertebral abscess*
	4. Mycotic myelitis
	  a. Cryptococcosis
	  b. Blastomycosis
	  c. Histoplasmosis
	  d. Coccidioidomycosis
	5. *Verminous migration*
	  a. *Micronema delethrix*
	  b. *Strongylus vulgaris*
	  c. *Hypoderma lineatum*
			1. Verminous migration
			  a. *Micronema delethrix*
			  b. *Strongylus vulgaris*
			  c. Hypoderma lineatum
			2. *Protozoal encephalomyelitis* (focal myelitis)

Traumatic	None	1. Fractures 2. Subluxations	None
Toxic			Cycad poisoning

Figure 9–4. Equine thoracolumbar spinal cord diseases. Differential diagnosis of T3–L3 spinal cord diseases based on their clinical course and etiologic categories. *Italics* indicate most important diseases clinically.

T3–L3

Etiologic Category	Acute Progressive	Acute Nonprogressive	Chronic
Degenerative	Aortic embolus-B	Aortic embolus-B Fibrocartilaginous embolus-B	Progressive ataxia of charolais cattle-B
Anomalous			Vertebral malformation-All Syringomyelia-P
Neoplastic			*Lymphosarcoma-B*
Nutritional			Copper deficiency-P,O
Inflammatory			Verminous migration-All

Infectious	1. Viral leukoencephalomyelitis-C
	2. Verminous migration
	  a. Cerebrospinal parelaphostrongylosis-C,O
	  b. Hypoderma-B
	  c. Stephanurus dentatus-P
	3. Vertebral abscess-All
			Vertebral abscess-All
			Mycosis-All

Traumatic		Fractures Subluxations } All	
Toxic	Organophosphate-B,P,O *Astragali* poisoning-B,C,O Cycad poisoning-B,P,O		Organophosphate-B,P,O Astragali poisoning-B,C,O Cycad poisoning-B,P,O

Figure 9–5. Food animal thoracolumbar spinal cord diseases. Differential diagnosis of T3–L3 spinal cord diseases based on their clinical course and etiologic categories. *B* = Bovine. *C* = Caprine. *P* = Porcine. *O* = Ovine. *Italics* indicate most important diseases clinically.

	L4–S2 and Coccygeal		
Etiologic Category	*Acute*		*Chronic*
	Progressive	*Nonprogressive*	
Degenerative	1. Disk disease 2. Ascending, descending myelomalacia (hematomyelia)	*Fibrocartilaginous*† *embolization*	1. *Degenerative myelopathy* (Degenerative radioculomyelopathy) 2. *Type II disk disease* ("slow disk") 3. Lumbosacral malformation *4. Spondylosis deformans *5. Dural ossification 6. Neuronopathy (Hereditary canine spinal muscular atrophy) 7. Stockard's paralysis

Anomalous	None	None	1. *Spinal dysraphism*
			  a. Weimaraners
			  b. Bulldogs
			  c. Boston terriers
			2. *Spina bifida* (often associated with myeloschisis)
			  a. Brachycephalic breeds
			  b. Manx cats
			3. *Hypoplasia of coccygeal segments and cauda equina*
			  a. Manx cats
			  b. Brachycephalic breeds
			4. Hemivertebrae

Neoplastic	Metastatic (prostatic carcinoma)	None	1. Primary 2. Metastatic 3. Lymphoreticular 4. Skeletal
Nutritional			Hypervitaminosis A (cats)

Inflammatory
Infectious
	1. Distemper myelitis/ myoclonus
	2. Bacterial myelitis
	  a. Meningomyelitis
	  *b. Secondary to spondylitis
	  *c. Secondary to diskospondylitis
	3. Toxoplasmosis
	4. Mycosis
	  a. Cryptococcosis
	  b. Blastomycosis
	  c. Histoplasmosis
	  d. Nocardiosis
	  e. Coccidioidomycosis
		None	See *Acute Progressive*
			1. Mycotic infections, toxoplasmosis, and diskospondylitis usually have a chronic progressive course
			2. Noneffusive feline infectious peritonitis
			3. Distemper myelitis/ myoclonus

Traumatic	Ascending, descending myelomalacia (hematomyelia)	1. *Fractures, subluxations* Pelvic fractures and *lumbosacral subluxations* are very common 2. Traumatic disk herniation	None
Toxic	See *Seizures*, Tables 15–2 and 15–3.		

*Indicates disease is not always associated with neurologic signs.
†Indicates increased incidence of nonselective disease at a particular site.

Figure 9–6. Lumbosacral spinal cord and cauda equina diseases. Differential diagnosis of L4–S2 and coccygeal spinal cord diseases based on their clinical courses and etiologic categories. *Italics* indicate most important diseases clinically.

	L4–S2		
	Acute		**Chronic**
Etiologic Category	*Progressive*	*Nonprogressive*	
Degenerative	None	None	None
Anomalous	None	None	Vertebral anomaly
Neoplastic	None	None	1. Primary
			2. Lymphoreticular
			3. Metastatic
			4. Skeletal
Nutritional			
Inflammatory	1. *Necrotizing myeloen-*	None	1. *Neuritis of the cauda*
Infectious	*cephalitis* (Herpes 1 in-		*equina*
	fection)		2. *Vertebral abscess*
	2. *Protozoal encephalomy-*		
	elitis (focal myelitis)		
	3. *Vertebral abscess*		
Traumatic	None	1. *Fractures (Sacral, low*	None
		lumbar)	
		2. Subluxations	
Toxic			1. *Lathyrism* (sorghum cystitis)
			2. Triorthocresyl phosphate
			tester intoxication

Figure 9–7. Equine lumbosacral spinal cord diseases. Differential diagnosis of L4–S2 and coccygeal spinal cord diseases based on their clinical courses and etiologic categories. *Italics* indicate most important diseases clinically.

tant disorders will be described in subsequent sections of this chapter. They will be reviewed briefly, with emphasis on diagnosis and treatment. Interested readers should consult other veterinary texts for more detailed information.

Acute Progressive Diseases, T3–L3

THORACOLUMBAR INTERVERTEBRAL DISK DISEASE

Intervertebral disk disease is one of the most common disorders producing pelvic limb pa-

resis in the dog. In one study, an approximate incidence rate of 23 cases per 1000 dogs was reported.[1] Degenerative changes within the disk tend to lead to protrusion or herniation of the disk substance into the vertebral canal. Basically, two types of disk degeneration that result in different clinical syndromes have been described (Fig. 9–9). Hansen Type I disk degeneration occurs primarily in the chondrodystrophoid breeds (small poodle, dachshund, beagle, cocker spaniel, pekingese, or mixed chondrodystrophoid breeds). It develops when the animal is young (2 to 9 months), and clin-

	L4–S2		
	Acute		**Chronic**
Etiologic Category	*Progressive*	*Nonprogressive*	
Degenerative	Aortic embolus-B	1. Aortic embolus-B	Spastic paresis-B
		2. Fibrocartilaginous embolus-P	
Anomalous			1. Vertebral malformation-All
			2. Syringomyelia-P
Neoplastic			1. Lymphosarcoma-B
			2. Neurofibroma-B
Nutritional			
Inflammatory	1. Verminous migration-All		1. Verminous migration-All
	2. *Vertebral abscess-All*		2. *Vertebral abscess-All*
			3. Mycosis-All
Traumatic		1. Fractures	
		2. Subluxation	
		3. *Calving injuries* (see Chapter 8)	

Figure 9–8. Food animal lumbosacral spinal cord diseases. Differential diagnosis of L4–S2 and coccygeal spinal cord diseases based on their clinical courses and etiologic categories. *B* = Bovine. *P* = Porcine. *Italics* indicate most important diseases clinically.

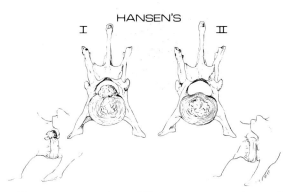

HANSEN'S
I   II

Figure 9–9. Drawings of Hansen's Type I and Type II disk protrusions. (From Hoerlein, B.F.: Canine Neurology: Diagnosis and Treatment, 3rd ed. Philadelphia, W.B. Saunders Co., 1978. Used by permission.)

ical signs are present by the time the animal is 3 to 6 years of age. The disk degeneration is basically a chondroid metaplasia of the nucleus pulposus with degeneration and weakening of the annulus fibrosus. The weakened annulus cannot restrain the degenerative nucleus, and normal movements of the vertebral column are sufficient to initiate acute disk prolapse. These extrusions of disk material result primarily in an acute focal compressive myelopathy. In some cases, a severe progressive myelopathy, known as ascending-descending myelomalacia, follows acute "blowouts" of the nuclear material.

Hansen Type II disk degeneration occurs in nonchondrodystrophoid breeds, such as German shepherds and Labrador retrievers. It develops at a slower rate, and clinical signs occur when the animal is 5 to 12 years of age. The disk degeneration is basically a fibroid metaplasia that may result in the gradual protrusion of disk material contained within an intact, but degenerate, annulus. True extrusion of free nuclear material into the epidural space does not occur. Compression from this protrusion results in a slowly progressive focal myelopathy. This syndrome has been termed geriatric disk disease or slow disk disease and will be discussed in the section dealing with chronic progressive spinal cord disorders.

Compressive myelopathy has been attributed primarily to the mechanical derangement of nerve tissue. Vascular factors that result in ischemia undoubtedly play a role in the development of more severe spinal cord degeneration and the syndrome of ascending-descending myelomalacia. The severity of the spinal cord lesion is influenced by the magnitude of the protrusion and its rate of development. The inflammatory reaction induced by the extruded material and the diameter of the vertebral canal are also related to the severity of the clinical signs. Acute protrusions produce more severe spinal cord lesions than chronic progressive protrusions, and less severe lesions occur in areas in which the vertebral canal is large (such as the cervical area).

Ascending-descending myelomalacia (also known as progressive hematomyelia) has an unknown pathogenesis, but vascular lesions leading to severe ischemia probably are important. This syndrome follows severe acute spinal cord trauma of any cause and results in nearly complete nervous tissue destruction. The clinical signs result from necrosis of the motor neurons and the sensory fibers. LMN signs develop in the muscles supplied by the affected spinal cord segments. Analgesia develops caudal to the cranial edge of the lesion. This syndrome should be suspected in all animals that develop ascending or descending signs of LMN dysfunction and ascending analgesia following spinal trauma. Affected animals usually die of respiratory failure 2 to 4 days after the onset of clinical signs. The lesion is irreparable, and euthanasia should be performed on affected animals in order to prevent needless suffering.

Clinical Signs

In addition to the neurologic signs that characterize lesions in this region of the spinal cord, disk disease is associated with considerable pain in the area of the protrusion. The extruded material irritates the nerve roots and the meninges, resulting in severe pain and hyperesthesia when the vertebral column is manipulated. An animal may arch its back and tense its abdominal muscles—motions that are suggestive of acute abdominal disorders, such as pancreatitis. Sensory examinations, such as pin pricking the skin and palpating the vertebra, are important, because they allow the clinician to localize the lesion to two or three spinal cord segments. Lesions that affect the superficial pain pathways will abolish the panniculus reflex caudal to the lesion. This reflex is normally most apparent when the skin over the thoracolumbar junction is stimulated. Students incorrectly believe that this apparent exaggeration of the skin twitch represents hyperesthesia and thus correlates with lesion location. Hyperesthesia is an exaggerated cerebral response to painful stimuli. Cooperative animals that cry out or try to bite when an area is palpated or pin pricked may be experiencing hyperesthesia, and the lesion is usually one or two segments cranial to the point at which the response was induced. In animals that are analgesic in the pelvic limbs, the level of analgesia along the spine should be found. The lesion is usually one or two segments cranial to the point at which the animal first feels painful stimuli.

Thoracolumbar disk disease may develop at intervertebral disk spaces T9–T10 to L7–S1. The intercapital ligament usually prevents protrusion of the cranial and midthoracic disks. Over 65 per cent of disk protrusions occur at sites T11–T12, T12–T13, T13–L1, and L1–L2. These areas should be evaluated carefully in animals with suspected thoracolumbar disk disease. Less frequently, disk protrusions occur in sites caudal to L3–L4. Protrusions at these sites produce LMN signs in the pelvic limbs, because the compressive myelopathy affects the motor neurons that form the lumbosacral plexus. These cases must be differentiated from those of descending myelomalacia as the result of a more cranial lesion.

Animals that develop progressive myelomalacia have ascending or descending signs of progressive LMN dysfunction and ascending levels of analgesia. Typically, affected dogs develop hypotonic abdominal muscles and hypotonic, areflexic pelvic limbs. The anus may be dilated, and the perineal reflex is weak or absent. The bladder is usually distended and easily expressed because of poor tone in the urethral sphincter.

Ascending signs of LMN paralysis include a loss of intercostal respirations and an inability to remain sternal because of paralysis of the paraspinal muscles. The thoracic limbs may be rigidly extended, and hyperesthesia may develop in the feet a few hours before the necrosis affects the lower cervical cord. Animals die of respiratory failure when the necrosis ascends to the level of the fifth and sixth cervical cord segments and thus destroys the neurons of the phrenic nerves. This syndrome apparently occurs with greatest frequency in dogs that develop acute paralysis and sensory loss. Owners should be warned of this possibility, particularly in cases in which surgical therapy is contemplated.

Diagnosis

A tentative diagnosis of thoracolumbar disk disease is based on an assessment of the clinical signs, a knowledge of the typical breed involvement, and the results of the neurologic evaluation. The diagnosis can be confirmed by a conventional radiographic examination of the spine with the x-ray beam centered over the probable lesion site, which is established with the neurologic examination (Figs. 9–10, 9–11, and 9–12). In most cases, general anesthesia is required for making diagnostic radiographs. In our hospital, radiographs are taken when the animal is treated surgically. For cases treated by conservative medical procedures, radiographs are not routinely made. It is difficult to justify the expense and the risk of anesthesia in a dog that probably has this disease if medical therapy is contemplated. In some cases, myelography is needed in order to detect the site of the compression, particularly in animals that have several potential sites on survey radiographs. The major value of spinal radiographs is to confirm the lesion site and, possibly, to indicate which surgical pro-

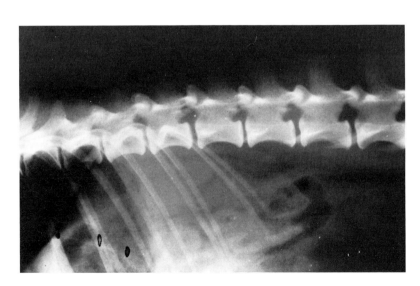

Figure 9–10. Lateral thoracolumbar (TL) radiograph with narrowed space at L1–L2. A common radiographic lesion in intervertebral disk (IVD) disease.

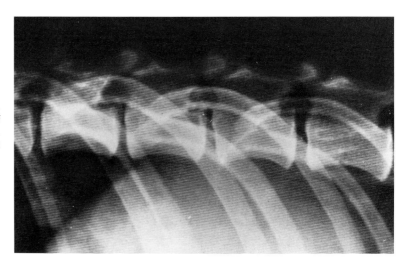

Figure 9–11. Lateral TL radiograph demonstrating wedging of the vertebral bodies at T12–T13. This is another radiographic lesion indicative of disk protrusion.

cedure is best suited for the patient in question.

Treatment

Many dogs with intervertebral disk disease respond at least temporarily to attentive nursing care that allows their spontaneous healing processes to operate. Because of this finding, it is extremely difficult to cite clear-cut evidence of the superiority of one therapy versus another. The major treatment controversy centers on the benefit of surgery versus conservative medical management. In addition, the relative benefits of the various surgical procedures still are being debated. During the past 8 years, we have evaluated those procedures in which benefits have been documented in both clinical and experimental trials. Various authors have attempted to classify disk disease by the severity of clinical signs and have developed treatment protocols for the animals in each class. We remain unconvinced that complex classification schemes have been useful for establishing the superiority of any treatment. The important aspects of these

studies are the trends that have surfaced. Table 9–1 summarizes the indications for treatment and the forms of management used at the teaching hospital of the University of Georgia.

Medical Therapy. Medical therapy is indicated for animals that are experiencing an initial episode of mild neurologic dysfunction or pain. Therapy should support the normal healing processes but should not totally relieve pain or totally inhibit the beneficial inflammatory process induced by the extruded disk material. Analgesics and anti-inflammatory drugs (aspirin, meperidine, phenylbutazone, corticosteroids) should be used with caution so that complete relief of pain is not produced. Total relief of pain may allow overactivity of the animal, which may result in further disk extrusion and rapidly worsening clinical signs. The most important aspect of therapy is enforced cage rest, preferably under direct veterinary supervision.

Owners often are told to place the animal in a baby crib or playpen. In our opinion, this is poor advice, because this form of confinement encourages the animal to jump in an attempt

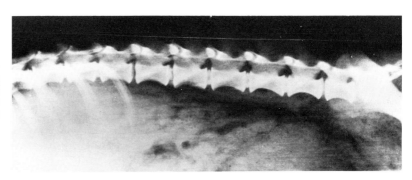

Figure 9–12. Lateral TL radiograph demonstrating numerous calcified disks. The active site of disease is L1–L2, where the disk space is narrowed. Calcified disks seldom cause clinical disease.

Table 9–1. SUMMARY OF THE THERAPY AND THE INDICATIONS FOR THERAPY FOLLOWED AT THE SMALL ANIMAL TEACHING HOSPITAL AT THE UNIVERSITY OF GEORGIA

Therapy	Indications Based on the History and the Clinical Signs
Medical	Pain only—first episode. *Mild* ataxia and paresis—first episode. Paralyzed—deep pain response absent 48 hours or longer.
Surgical	
Fenestration only	Multiple episodes of pain only.
Decompression (hemilaminectomy) with fenestration	Paresis and ataxia—second episode. Deterioration of signs with medical therapy. Moderate paresis or paralysis—deep pain response present—first episode. Paralysis—deep pain response absent for less than 48 hours (very guarded prognosis).

to get out. Confinement at home should be in a small airline crate placed in a quiet room where the animal will not be disturbed. The animal should be exercised twice a day on a leash, away from other dogs or cats. Analgesics or other anti-inflammatory drugs should not be used at home unless the client agrees to cooperate fully with the instructions for strict cage rest. The most common mistake made by the veterinarian is to administer corticosteroids and send the animal home. Predictably, these animals return in 36 to 48 hours with severe neurologic signs. Generally, dogs should be hospitalized for one week. Prednisolone, 0.25 mg per lb, is given every 12 hours for 72 hours and then discontinued. The animal is sent home with instructions for cage confinement of 3 weeks' duration. If satisfactory progress is made, exercise is restricted to a leash for an additional 3 weeks. If followed closely, these procedures result in considerable improvement; however, the owner must be aware that further attacks will occur in over 50 percent of the cases. If the animal's signs deteriorate at any time, surgery should be performed immediately.

Paralyzed animals with deep pain sensation that is absent for 48 hours or longer have a grave prognosis (less than 5 percent chance) for recovery with or without surgery. The absence of deep pain perception represents a severe, usually irreparable spinal cord injury. Unless the owner definitely wants to try surgery in the face of these odds, the animal should be treated medically. Dexamethasone, 2 mg per kg, is given intravenously upon presentation, and this dosage is repeated in 4 to 6 hours. Thereafter, 0.1 mg per kg is given intramuscularly every 12 hours for 48 to 72 hours and then discontinued. Physical therapy then is initiated. No improvement in clinical signs in 3 weeks is an indication for euthanasia. Corticosteroid therapy, particularly the administration of dexamethasone, if continued longer than 5 to 7 days, may result in gastrointestinal ulceration and may aggravate urinary tract infection in those dogs with urine retention from a paralyzed detrusor muscle.

Surgical Therapy. The various forms of surgical therapy have been reviewed extensively by Hoerlein.[2] There appears to be general agreement that disk fenestration is indicated for those animals with recurrent pain or minimal paresis and ataxia. Although there is little decompressive effect, fenestration helps prevent further protrusion. This surgical procedure also may produce an acute inflammatory process that stimulates phagocytosis, the resorption of necrotic disk material, and the formation of fibrosis, which helps to stabilize the disk.[3]

In dogs with moderate to severe paresis and ataxia, decompressive surgery should be performed immediately. This finding has been supported by clinical and experimental studies comparing the speed and the duration of spinal cord compression with the rate of recovery. Tarlov and coworkers have demonstrated that acute spinal cord compression with a force sufficient to produce complete sensorimotor paralysis results in complete recovery if the compression is less than 2 hours in duration.[4] Furthermore, the rate of recovery in Tarlov's study was directly correlated with the duration of compression. Following 10 minutes of acute compression, 2 to 3 days were required for initial improvement in neurologic function. With 50 to 120 minutes of acute compression, 20 to 30 days were required for initial improvement. Gradual compression of the spinal cord was better tolerated, and irreversible changes developed at a slower rate in these animals. Gradual compression to paralysis in 75 minutes resulted in full recovery if the compressive force was removed within 9 hours. One to three days was required for initial improvement. Thus, early decompressive surgery may have a positive influence on both the return to function and the rate of recovery. *When indicated, spinal cord decompression should be performed without delay.* The common practice of medically treating dogs with moderate to severe paresis or paraplegia for 24 to 48 hours and then performing surgery if no improvement occurs should be condemned. This procedure discounts the experimental data regarding the effects of spinal compression over variable periods.

Dogs with acute paralysis and no deep pain responses should be decompressed within 2 hours for predictable functional recovery. Surgery is recommended for dogs with absence of deep pain sensation for up to 48 hours; however, the rate and degree of recovery are much less predictable. After 48 hours, the chance for recovery is probably less than 5 percent. These dogs are surgically treated only at the owner's insistence.

Dexamethasone, 2 mg per kg body weight, is given intravenously in the early preoperative period. Thereafter, dexamethasone can be given at a dosage of 0.1 mg per kg body weight every 12 hours for 48 hours. Dexamethasone reduces inflammation and edema of the spinal cord associated with the disk protrusion and surgical trauma.

Supportive Care of the Paraplegic. Supportive care of the "downer dog" is directed at prevention of decubital ulcers, urinary tract infection, and muscle atrophy. Animal compartments should be well padded with sealed foam rubber, air mattresses, or waterbeds. The animals should be exercised frequently, and the skin and perineal areas must be kept clean. Whirlpool baths are very beneficial because they keep the skin clean, reduce muscle spasticity, improve circulation, and help reduce muscle atrophy.

Urine retention is a major problem in most paraplegics and commonly predisposes to urinary tract infection. Intermittent catheterization should be performed three times a day with a soft, atraumatic rubber catheter. Indwelling catheters are recommended by several authors; however, these retention catheters may increase the risk of urinary tract infection. Antibiotic solutions, such as nitrofurazone or neomycin, can be flushed into the bladder after the urine is evacuated. Unlike normal dogs, paraplegics tend to retain these antibiotic solutions for longer periods, which increases the effectiveness of the agents in the prevention of infection. If urinary tract infection develops, the urine should be cultured, and the animal should be treated with the appropriate systemic or urinary antibiotic. Manual bladder expression should be used whenever this procedure is effective in decompressing the bladder without trauma. Manual bladder expression is easier to perform in female dogs. The procedure also may stimulate the micturition reflex in some dogs. Many owners can be taught this technique, and in these cases, the animal can be discharged from the hospital prior to the return of voluntary micturition.

Tailing exercises, body slings, and exercise carts are used to stimulate motor activity of the pelvic limbs. Muscle massage, passive manipulation of the limbs, and whirlpool therapy help delay disuse muscle atrophy. Dogs should not become dependent on exercise carts for mobility. They should be encouraged to walk or to stand unassisted. In this regard, owners are best suited to participate in the rehabilitation process.

The rate of return to acceptable pelvic limb function and micturition is highly correlated with the duration and rate of the spinal cord compression. Generally, micturition and normal pain responses return within 2 to 3 weeks. Voluntary motor activity should return within 4 to 5 weeks, and the unassisted ability to support weight usually is restored within 6 to 8 weeks. Proprioception is the last function to return. Once again, it must be stressed that *early* decompression hastens the return of neurologic function.

The remainder of the small animal diseases listed in the second column (acute progressive diseases) of Figure 9–3 will be described in other sections of this book.

NECROTIZING MYELOENCEPHALITIS

Necrotizing myeloencephalitis is an acute progressive neurologic disease that usually affects older horses, but disease in foals also has been reported.[5] The cause of this disease appears to be equine herpes 1 virus. Multifocal neurologic lesions, primarily a severe vasculitis and necrosis, occur in the brain and the spinal cord;[6] however, the spinal cord lesions usually produce the majority of clinical signs. The pathogenesis of this disease is not related to direct viral infection of the CNS. An immune-mediated reaction involving a viral antigen and an antibody may induce the severe neurologic vasculitis characteristic of this disease.

Clinical Signs

This disease usually occurs within 1 to 2 weeks after outbreaks of upper respiratory infections or abortions. Respiratory infections seldom are observed in affected animals. Pregnant mares may be more susceptible to the development of severe spinal cord lesions and may abort if infected in the last trimester of pregnancy. Neurologic signs develop acutely; however, progression of the signs is variable depending upon the severity of the initial spinal cord lesions. Affected horses may recover in 24 to 48 hours, or they may progress rapidly to severe tetra- or paraplegia. Neurologic signs vary according to the area of the spinal cord involved. Usual neurologic signs include dysuria, ataxia of the pelvic limbs, and a flaccid anus and tail. Signs may progress to severe pelvic limb paresis or paralysis. Tetraparesis may be severe if cervical cord lesions are extensive. In a few cases, involvement of the cortex or the brain stem may produce seizures, cranial nerve dysfunction, or vestibular signs. In most cases, the clinical signs are those of thoracolumbar cord dysfunction. One must remember that both UMN and LMN signs may develop relative to the site of development of vascular lesions in the spinal cord. In addition, neurologic signs may be symmetric or lateralizing, depending upon the site of involvement.

Diagnosis

This is a sporadic disease of horses and must be suspected when neurologic disease appears to follow outbreaks of respiratory infection or abortion. Analysis of the cerebrospinal fluid (CSF) reveals significant elevations of protein (150 mg/dl or greater) with normal or slightly elevated cell counts. The CSF may be xanthochromic. Definitive diagnosis is made by isolation of the virus from nervous tissue or by serologic methods. Since viral isolation is difficult, comparison of antibody titers at the onset of clinical signs and during convalescence is the preferred method for confirming a clinical diagnosis. In experimental studies, a sharp rise in serum neutralization titers occurs within 5 to 7 days after inoculation.

Treatment

There is no definitive treatment for this disease. Because an immune mechanism may be responsible, some authors have suggested the use of immunosuppressive dosages of corticosteroids (2.2 mg per kg dexamethasone). The benefits of this therapy are hard to document, since many animals recover if given supportive nursing care. A killed intramuscular vac-

cine is available that may protect the nervous system against equine herpes 1 infection.

PROTOZOAL ENCEPHALOMYELITIS (FOCAL MYELITIS-ENCEPHALITIS)

Focal myelitis-encephalitis is a neurologic syndrome in horses characterized by a *sudden* or a *gradual* onset of pelvic limb paresis and ataxia. Since lesions may be multifocal in the spinal cord, neurologic signs may develop in the thoracic limbs. Originally, the disease was associated with moldy corn poisoning;[7] however, more recently, many cases have been associated with a protozoan organism similar to *Toxoplasma gondii.*[8] Apparently, many cases of focal myelitis-encephalitis are caused by this unnamed protozoal organism; hence, the disease is more commonly called protozoal encephalomyelitis.

Lesions within the CNS are focal or multifocal and usually are asymmetric. The histopathologic lesion is a nonsuppurative myelitis affecting both gray and white matter. The disease apparently is most common in young to middle-aged standard-breed horses.

Clinical Signs

Clinical signs usually develop suddenly and progress slowly over days to weeks. Asymmetric ataxia and paresis of the pelvic limbs are the usual predominant manifestations. Because lesions may be multifocal, however, a mixture of UMN and LMN signs may be present in the pelvic and thoracic limbs. If the lesion occurs in the brachial intumescence, the thoracic limb signs may be worse than the pelvic limb signs. The clinical signs resemble those observed in the equine wobbler syndrome and necrotizing myeloencephalitis; however, the asymmetry that is seen helps in the clinical differentiation of protozoal myelitis-encephalitis from the other two diseases.

Diagnosis

In protozoal myelitis-encephalitis, unlike necrotizing encephalomyelitis, there are few abnormalities in the CSF. Mild increased concentrations of monocytes and proteins occasionally are found. Cervical radiographs are normal (differentiating this disease from equine wobbler syndrome).

Treatment

Although no definitive therapy is known, pyrimethamine, 3 gm per 450 kg intramuscularly over a 2-week period, and triple sulfas,

2.2 grains per kg intravenously over several weeks, have been suggested. Many of these patients have irreversible neural damage and usually require euthanasia.

VERMINOUS MIGRATION

Equine

The migration of several parasites through the spinal cords of horses has been described. The most important of these organisms include *Micronema deletrix, Strongylus vulgaris,* and *Hypoderma lineatum.* The clinical features of this disease closely resemble those of protozoal encephalomyelitis in that the progressive signs may be acute or chronic in onset. In addition, depending upon the site of migration, the distribution of signs may be asymmetric, focal, or multifocal. Embolization of *Strongylus vulgaris* larvae into spinal arteries may produce severe acute progressive or nonprogressive clinical signs. In this regard, the clinical signs are very similar to those observed in necrotizing myeloencephalitis.

A confirmed clinical diagnosis is difficult to make. The CSF may contain increased concentrations of eosinophils and red blood cells. It is not xanthochromic, in contrast to the CSF of animals with necrotizing encephalomyelitis.

No definitive therapy is known. In suspected cases, levamisole, 8.8 mg per kg, or thiabendazole, at ten times the therapeutic dose, has been recommended. Corticosteroids can be used to decrease the inflammatory response to the dying worms.

Bovine

The larvae of *Hypoderma bovis* migrate through the epidural space of cattle, usually during the months of July through October. If the larvae die or are killed while in the epidural space, a severe immunologic reaction occurs, resulting in spinal cord injury. The clinical signs usually appear in cattle treated with pour-on insecticides during the period of epidural larvae migration. Clinical signs develop acutely within one day of treatment and usually are caused by thoracolumbar spinal cord injury. Prominent signs include pelvic limb ataxia and paresis. If the lumbosacral cord is involved, LMN signs may be detected in the pelvic limbs. The signs are usually asymmetric. The diagnosis is based on the history and the clinical signs. The CSF changes reflect signs of degeneration (moderate increases in protein and cell concentrations). Eosinophils may not be present in the CSF. Affected animals should be treated with corticosteroids in or-

der to reduce the inflammatory reaction. Pour-on topical insecticides should not be used during periods of larvae migration in the epidural space.

Ovine, Caprine

Sheep and goats may serve as aberrant hosts for the meningeal worm of white-tailed deer, *Parelaphostrongylus tenuis.* Migration of this parasite through the central nervous system (CNS) produces a variety of clinical signs, including pelvic limb paresis and ataxia. The clinical course is variable and may include progression, stasis, or improvement in clinical signs. Affected animals have a history of grazing in pastures that have been exposed to white-tailed deer. The CSF of these animals usually contains increased concentrations of protein and cells. A mononuclear and eosinophilic pleocytosis is usually encountered. Treatment with diethylcarbamazine, levamisole, or thiabendazole is recommended. The prognosis is guarded.

Porcine

The kidney worm of swine, *Stephanurus dentatus,* may migrate through the spinal cord, producing pelvic limb paresis and ataxia. This organism must be considered in individual swine that are found on farms in the southeastern United States and that develop acute paraparesis. No effective treatment is known.

VIRAL LEUKOENCEPHALOMYELITIS OF GOATS

This disease affects goats 2 to 4 months of age and probably is caused by a virus that results in a perivenous demyelination and nonsuppurative leukomyelitis. As in other viral diseases, lesions may develop anywhere in the spinal cord, producing focal or multifocal asymmetric neurologic signs. The clinical signs of this disease closely resemble *Parelaphostrongylus* migration in the spinal cord. The CSF usually contains markedly increased concentrations of mononuclear cells and modestly increased concentrations of protein; however, an eosinophilic pleocytosis is not present. There is no effective treatment.

Acute Nonprogressive Diseases, T3–L3

SPINAL CORD TRAUMA

Spinal cord trauma, usually the result of automobile accidents, is a common neurologic injury. The incidence is much greater in areas where leash laws are poorly enforced. Spinal cord trauma is more frequent in large animals when they are young but may occur in mature animals as a result of falls, trailer accidents, or overcrowding in chutes. The management of spinal cord trauma has been discussed extensively by other authors.[2,9,10] This section provides a concise review of the management of this problem. Veterinarians have two primary obligations. They first must diagnose and treat shock, major abdominal or thoracic hemorrhage, visceral rupture, or ventilation abnormalities. Second, they must be able to give owners accurate prognoses for the recovery of neurologic function.

First Aid and Emergency Medical Treatment

An injury of sufficient force to produce spinal cord trauma usually results in another life-threatening injury.[10,11] The maintenance of a patent airway is of the utmost importance. The mouth is cleared of fluid or blood, the tongue is pulled forward, and the unconscious animal is intubated. Adequate ventilation is of great importance, since hypoxia aggravates CNS edema. Shock, if present, must be treated. Lactated Ringer's solution is given intravenously to restore vascular volume. Corticosteroids, such as dexamethasone, are given intravenously at a dosage of 2 mg per kg body weight over a 10-minute period. This drug also is beneficial in the prevention and treatment of CNS edema. Fluid therapy must be carefully monitored to prevent overhydration, which may aggravate CNS edema.

After providing first aid and treating shock, the veterinarian must perform a thorough physical examination. Abdominal or thoracic trauma may be difficult to appreciate immediately after an injury; therefore, visceral function must be monitored for several days.[10] There is little benefit in successfully repairing the spinal fracture only to have the animal die several days later from a diaphragmatic hernia or a ruptured urinary bladder. However, spinal cord trauma must be treated without delay in order to improve the odds of recovery. Once circulatory problems are corrected, mannitol therapy is instituted (see Chapter 7).

During the period of early evaluation and treatment, the animal must be restrained in order to prevent further spinal cord injury. Animals should be transported on a rigid stretcher or a board. Movement should be discouraged, especially if vertebral fractures or subluxations are suspected.

Neurologic Examination

Most spinal cord injuries are the result of vertebral fracture, vertebral luxation, or traumatic disk extrusion and are likely to produce severe permanent neurologic deficits, especially if early treatment has not been provided. The localization of the spinal cord lesion and the prognosis based on the severity of the injury are determined by the neurologic examination. The spinal column should not be manipulated vigorously during the examination; however, gentle palpation for alterations in vertebral conformation should be attempted, because these changes have good localizing value. The principles of lesion localization have been reviewed previously. Table 9–2 summarizes the signs of complete spinal cord transection at various levels of the cord.

The prognosis of a spinal cord injury depends on the suddenness of the injury, the duration of the compressive force, and the extent of secondary vascular responses to the injury. The bottom line is reversibility. The spinal cord may be anatomically or physiologically transected. In most cases, physiologic transection is the most common cause of irreversibility. As previously stated in the section dealing with disk disease, sudden compression of the spinal cord is far worse than gradual compression. Acute experimental compression of the spinal cord with a force sufficient to produce paralysis and analgesia results in irreversible spinal cord injury if the duration of compression exceeds 4 hours. The key to prognosis is the *perceptual response* to noxious stimuli applied caudally to the lesion. In the absence of deep pain perception, the duration of the injury becomes the critical factor related to prognosis. The absence of deep pain perception is a very unfavorable sign, especially if the injury has been present for longer than 4 hours. Other neurologic signs that correlate with severe thoracolumbar spinal cord injury include spinal shock, crossed extensor reflexes, and the Schiff-Sherrington phenomenon. The presence of these signs does not always indicate that the lesion is irreversible, since these signs may occur in the presence of deep pain perception.

Assuming that the skeletal lesion can be stabilized, injured animals are categorized as shown in Table 9–3.

Special Examinations

Radiographs of the spinal column are necessary if surgical treatment is contemplated.

Table 9–2. SIGNS OF COMPLETE SPINAL CORD TRANSECTION*

Spinal Cord Segments	Signs Caudal to Lesion		
	Motor	*Sensory*	*Autonomic*
C1–C4	Tetraplegia with hyperreflexia	Anesthesia	Apnea, no micturition
C5–C6	Tetraplegia with hyperreflexia, LMN suprascapular nerve	Anesthesia, hyperesthesia—midcervical	Apnea—phrenic nerve, LMN, no micturition
C7–T1	Tetraplegia or paraplegia with hyperreflexia, LMN brachial plexus	Anesthesia, hyperesthesia—brachial plexus	Diaphragmatic breathing only, no micturition
T2–L3	Paraplegia with hyperreflexia, Schiff-Sherrington syndrome	Anesthesia, hyperesthesia—segmental	Diaphragmatic, some intercostal and abdominal respiration, depending on level of lesion; no micturition
L4–S1	Paraplegia with LMN lumbosacral plexus	Anesthesia, hyperesthesia—segmental	No micturition; S1 = anal sphincter may be atonic
S1–S3	Knuckling of hind foot, paralysis of tail	Anesthesia, hyperesthesia—segmental	No micturition; sphincters atonic
Cy1–Cy5	Paralysis of tail	Anesthesia, hyperesthesia—segmental	None

*C = cervical; T = thoracic; L = lumbar; S = sacral; Cy = coccygeal; LMN = lower motor neuron signs.

Radiographs define the precise location and type of skeletal lesion (Fig. 9–13). These findings dictate the surgical procedure needed to decompress and stabilize the injury. Spinal radiographs are not useful for evaluating the functional status of the spinal cord. The amount of displacement that is viewed on radiographs is frequently the least displacement that occurred at the time of the injury. The functional status is determined by the neurologic examination. In some institutions, somatosensory-evoked potentials are used to define spinal cord integrity more precisely (see Chapter 6).

Medical Therapy. Corticosteroids are given as part of the emergency treatment for shock. Dexamethasone should be given initially at a dosage of 2 mg per kg body weight intravenously. This dosage is repeated in 6 hours. Thereafter, the dosage is reduced to 0.1

mg per kg body weight every 12 hours for 48 to 72 hours. A hypertonic osmotic diuretic, such as 20 per cent mannitol solution, should be administered immediately after hypovolemia has been corrected. Mannitol acts very quickly to reduce spinal cord edema and is indicated in addition to dexamethasone, since the full beneficial effects of corticosteroids may not occur for 4 to 6 hours. Mannitol is given at a dosage of 2 gm per kg body weight (10 ml per kg of a 20 per cent solution) as rapidly as possible. Vomiting may occur if the rate of administration is too rapid. The mannitol therapy is repeated in 2 to 3 hours and then is discontinued. Thereafter, the antiedema effects of the dexamethasone are believed to be sufficient.

Surgical Therapy. There are two major indications for spinal surgery in the animal with a traumatic injury: decompression and im-

Table 9–3. PROGNOSIS OF ACUTE SPINAL CORD INJURIES

	Signs	Duration of Injury	Prognosis
Group 1	Good pain response	Less than 24 hours	Fair to good
Group 2	No pain response	Less than 4 hours	Poor
Group 3	No pain response	Greater than 4 hours	Grave

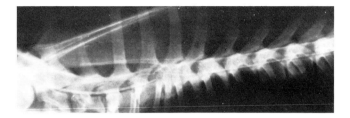

Figure 9–13. Myelogram of a dog with a compressive fracture of T3. The compressive nature of the fracture was not apparent on survey films.

mobilization of the vertebra. The decision for decompression is based on the clinical signs. Animals with paralysis almost always require decompression and usually require stabilization. Animals with mild paresis and ataxia may require stabilization, but decompression usually is not indicated. Decompression must be performed within 4 to 6 hours on an animal with complete paralysis in order to prevent permanent damage. Animals in Groups 1 and 2 (see Table 9–3) should have early surgery. Surgery is not recommended for animals in Group 3.

The decision for the method of immobilization is based on the findings of clinical and radiographic examinations and on observations made during the operation. Flexible plates, body plates, and vertebral body cross-

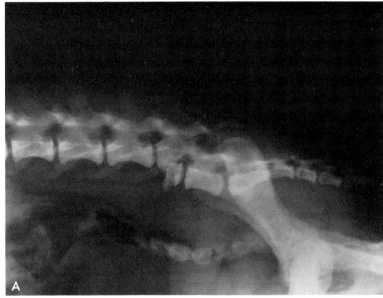

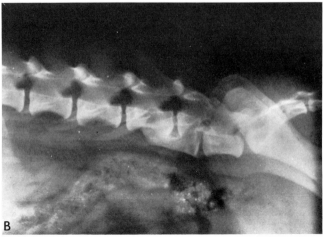

Figure 9–14. *A.* Lumbosacral lateral radiograph demonstrating a fracture of L6 and L6–L7 luxation. These injuries entrap the roots of the sciatic, pelvic, pudendal, and coccygeal nerves. *B.* Follow-up postsurgical radiograph of the same dog. The fracture site was decompressed, and the nerves in the vertebral canal were freed from compression. A callus had bridged the fracture site, although no internal stabilization had been provided.

pinning are the most commonly used methods and usually are superior to any form of external support. Compressive fractures of the vertebral body and fractures of the transverse spinous processes without displacement may be stable. Fractures of the vertebral body with luxation or fractures involving several articular facets require reduction and stabilization. When decompression and stabilization are simultaneously indicated, hemilaminectomy is the favored approach for decompression, because any method of fixation can be used with this procedure (Fig. 9–14). The reader is referred to other texts for in-depth descriptions of the various surgical techniques.[2,9]

Supportive Care and Rehabilitation. Very few animals become ambulatory during the first week after surgery following severe trauma. The majority remain paretic or paralyzed and require attentive nursing care, physical therapy, and a rehabilitation period. In general, the procedures for supportive care of the paraplegic in cases of disk disease also should be followed after spinal surgery. Animals should improve within 6 weeks. Failure to show improvement during this time is strongly correlated with permanent spinal cord damage; however, every clinician encounters a few dogs that regain functional use of the pelvic limbs when the initial outlook has seemed hopeless. Unfortunately, in veterinary medicine, the outcome of the case often depends upon the enthusiasm and financial cooperation of the owner.

Chronic Progressive Diseases, T3–L3

These diseases are characterized by an insidious onset and slow progression of the neurologic signs. Degenerative, neoplastic, and inflammatory diseases are the most important of the various etiologic categories. Although the diseases listed in the right-hand column of Figures 9–3, 9–4, and 9–5 may start in the T3–L3 spinal cord segments, progression into other regions may occur. With longstanding disease, cervical cord involvement may cause tetraparesis or hemiparesis. These problems will be discussed in Chapter 10.

DEGENERATIVE MYELOPATHY

Degenerative myelopathy is a slowly progressive degenerative disease involving primarily the long tracts of the canine thoracolumbar spinal cord. The disease was first described by Averill in 1973, and subsequent

authors have reported various clinical and pathologic findings.[12] The disease appears to be most prevalent in older German shepherd dogs and has been termed *diffuse degenerative myelopathy* in aging German shepherds.[2,13] Griffiths and coworkers have termed this disorder *degenerative radiculomyelopathy* because of dorsal root involvement in several of their cases.[14] A degenerative myelopathy also has been described in horses. Unlike the canine disease, the equine syndrome is characterized by an acute progressive course and involves primarily the cervical cord, although thoracolumbar lesions also occur. The equine disease will be discussed in Chapter 10.

Pathologic Findings

In Averill's study, 22 dogs with progressive ataxia and paresis had diffuse degeneration of spinal cord myelin and axons in all spinal cord funiculi.[12] These changes were most extensive in the midthoracic region and were not associated with intervertebral disk extrusion, spondylosis deformans, or dural ossification. Griffiths and Duncan reported their findings in 16 dogs.[14] In addition to confirming many of Averill's observations, these authors reported extensive lesions in the lumbar dorsal columns and involvement of the dorsal nerve roots. They reported that the lesions suggested a "dying back" process of axons confined to the central nervous system. In another study, Braund and Vandevelde studied 14 German shepherds affected with this disease.[13] Although this study reconfirmed many of the earlier observations, it did not support the "dying back" hypothesis. The condition should be regarded as a primary spinal cord degeneration of unknown cause.[2,12] The predisposition of German shepherd dogs to this syndrome suggests that genetic factors may be involved in the pathogenesis.

Clinical Signs

Clinical signs generally are first recognized in affected dogs at 6 to 9 years of age, although the disease has been documented in a few 4-year-old dogs. It occurs almost exclusively in large breeds, predominantly German shepherds or shepherd dog crossbreeds. Early clinical signs include mild ataxia and paresis of the pelvic limbs. The onset is insidious, and an owner may not seek veterinary assistance for several months, believing that the dog has mild coxofemoral arthritis. The outstanding clinical sign is pelvic limb ataxia. Knuckling of the feet, dragging of the toes, and dysmetria are common signs. The pelvic limbs may cross when the animal walks, and swaying movements of the rear quarters are apparent. If forced to turn quickly, many dogs will fall in an outward direction. Clinical signs are bilateral; however, they may not be symmetric. One limb may be affected more severely than another. Urinary or fecal incontinence are uncommon findings. Most animals appear healthy in other respects. In chronic cases, atrophy of the caudal paraspinal and pelvic limb muscles may occur.

The neurologic examination usually suggests a lesion in spinal cord segments T3–L3. Postural reactions, such as proprioceptive positioning, hopping, placing, and the extensor postural thrust, are deficient. The degree of proprioceptive dysfunction is usually greater than the degree of motor dysfunction. Flexor (withdrawal) reflexes are normal and, in more advanced cases, may be clonic. Crossed extensor reflexes may be present. In many dogs, the knee-jerk reflex is normal or exaggerated. In some dogs, the knee-jerk reflex is depressed or absent, even though the leg can be extended readily at the stifle and pain normally is perceived from areas innervated by the saphenous branch of the femoral nerve. It is believed that involvement of the dorsal roots of the femoral nerve may inhibit sensory impulses from stretch receptors located in the quadriceps muscle. Electrophysiologic and pathologic studies have not detected abnormalities in the lower motor neuron, thus confirming clinical observations that the motor reflex pathways are intact.[14] When present, this clinical finding is highly suggestive of degenerative myelopathy (radiculomyelopathy).

Pain perception is normal from the pelvic limbs. Abnormalities of micturition are uncommon. Occasionally, in advanced cases, the perineal reflex is weak, and fecal incontinence has been observed. The tail may be severely paretic or paralyzed, and this abnormality may result in soiling of the perineal region. Muscle atrophy develops slowly and is clinically apparent only in long-standing cases. Hyperesthesia is absent. Although mild lesions occur in the cervical spinal cord, the thoracic limbs usually retain normal function.

Diagnosis

The clinical signs and the neurologic findings suggest a slowly progressive compression of the spinal cord. In fact, this disease originally was attributed to spinal cord compression from dural ossification, Type II disk protrusions, or thoracolumbar spondylosis. Degenerative myelopathy must be differentiated radiographically from Type II (slow) disk protrusions and spinal neoplasia. Survey radiographs and myelographic examinations should be performed in order to rule out the presence of compressive (potentially surgically correctable) diseases. CSF is collected at the time of myelography in order to help eliminate the presence of inflammatory diseases. Vertebral spondylosis and dural ossification are common radiographic findings in older large-breed dogs. They seldom cause neurologic dysfunction, and their presence does not correlate with the clinical signs or pathologic findings in dogs affected with degenerative myelopathy.[12] The presence of a Type II disk does not rule out degenerative myelopathy, so the prognosis is guarded, especially for German shepherd dogs.

Treatment

Since the cause is unknown, no specific treatment is available. The animal responds poorly, if at all, to corticosteroids, phenylbutazone, indomethacin, salicylates, or B-complex vitamins. The owner must be warned as to the hopeless prognosis for cure; however, with supportive care, many dogs can be maintained for several months before euthanasia becomes necessary.

TYPE II DISK DISEASE

Pathophysiology

Type II disk disease occurs primarily in large-breed, nonchondrodystrophoid dogs. It occurs in older dogs (at 5 to 12 years of age), hence the synonym *senile disk disease*. The pathologic change within the intervertebral disk is a fibroid degeneration and a weakening of the dorsal annulus (see Fig. 9–9). Recurrent partial disk protrusion produces a dome-shaped mass that eventually becomes large enough to compress the spinal cord or to irritate meninges and nerve roots. Pain, paresis and, occasionally, paralysis develop. The spinal cord changes are those of a compressive myelopathy.

Clinical Signs

The clinical signs are similar to those of degenerative myelopathy, in that Type II disk protrusions result in slowly progressive signs of ataxia and paresis. With Type II disk protrusions, regional hyperesthesia in the area of the protruded disk may be present, in contrast with the lack of hyperesthesia in degenerative myelopathy. In addition, voluntary micturition may be affected by the compressive myelopathy, whereas micturition usually remains normal in cases of degenerative myelopathy.

Neurologic abnormalities in the pelvic limbs reflect the level of the disk protrusion and can be very similar to the findings in dogs with degenerative myelopathy or spinal neoplasia. Disk protrusions involving cord segments T3–L3 result in UMN signs, whereas protrusions involving segments caudal to L3 can produce a mixture of UMN and LMN signs. Dogs are evaluated critically for spinal pain or hyperesthesia. The presence of these signs has great localizing value and helps to differentiate Type II disk disease from degenerative myelopathy. The response to deep pain stimuli is usually normal in both diseases.

Diagnosis

Type II disk disease is differentiated from degenerative myelopathy by radiography of the spine. Plain radiographs may reveal the lesion; however, a myelographic examination is usually required to demonstrate the compressive nature of the disk in question (Fig. 9–15). As in cases of degenerative myelopathy, dural ossification and spondylosis are common radiographic findings. These radiographic lesions should not be construed as the cause of the dog's neurologic dysfunction.

Treatment

Early cases may respond temporarily to anti-inflammatory drugs, such as corticosteroids, phenylbutazone, or salicylates; however, the signs soon recur and progressively worsen. Dogs with pain as the only clinical sign can be treated medically, but decompressive surgery

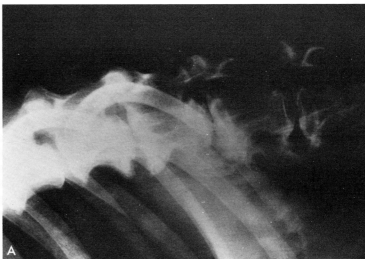

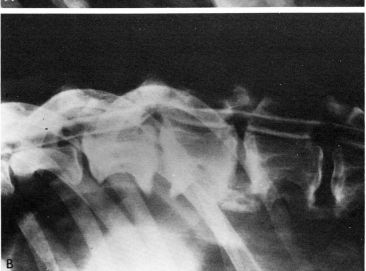

Figure 9–15. *A.* Survey lateral TL radiograph of a dog with slowly progressive paraparesis. Note the extensive hypertrophic spondylosis. This radiographic finding is common in older large-breed dogs; however, it is seldom a clinical problem. *B.* Myelogram of the same dog. Note the prominent extramedullary compression at T13–L1 from a Type II disk protrusion. (From Kneller, S.K., et al.: Differential diagnosis of progressive caudal paresis in an aged German shepherd dog. JAAHA 11:414, 1975. Used by permission.)

with removal of the protruded disk is more satisfactory in most cases. Decompressive surgery is indicated for all dogs with paresis and ataxia. Surgery should be performed early, so that further neurologic deterioration can be prevented. The prognosis with surgery is good, in that most dogs regain normal neurologic function, unless the condition is complicated by degenerative myelopathy.

NEOPLASIA

Pathophysiology

Tumors affecting the vertebra, the meninges, the nerve roots, or the spinal cord may result in neurologic signs. These tumors are classified as primary, metastatic, lymphoreticular, or skeletal. In general, the more common tumors affect structures that house the spinal cord and produce a compressive myelopathy when the mass expands upon or around the cord. Most tumors slowly compress the spinal cord, resulting in signs that are quite similar to those of degenerative myelopathy and Type II disk disease.

Skeletal (Vertebral) Tumors

Vertebral tumors may be primary or may arise from metastases. The latter case is more common. Generally, as the tumors grow into the vertebral canal, the spinal cord is compressed slowly, producing signs of a slowly progressive myelopathy. Occasionally, the tumor produces considerable vertebral destruction without cord compression. These vertebrae are weakened and may fracture, resulting in acute spinal cord compression. Vertebral tumors are usually painful because of periosteal and, perhaps, meningeal irritation. Primary vertebral tumors include osteomas, osteosarcomas (Fig. 9–16), chondromas, chondrosarcomas, and plasma cell myelomas (Fig. 9–17). A variety of carcinomas and sarcomas metastatic to vertebrae has been reported. Plain radiographs of the spine are usually diagnostic. Treatment is usually palliative,

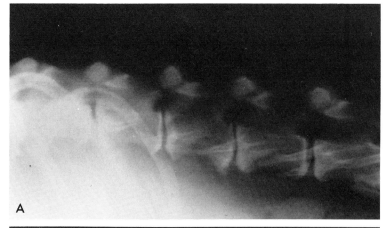

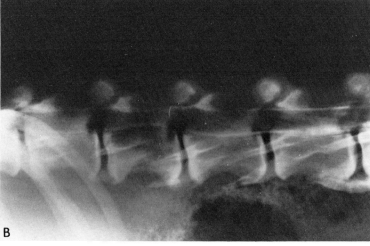

Figure 9–16. *A.* Osteogenic sarcoma of L2 in a dog with paraplegia and severe back pain. *B.* Myelogram of the thoracolumbar area of the same dog demonstrating extradural compression at L2.

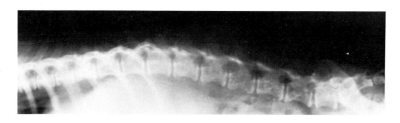

Figure 9–17. Lateral TL radiograph demonstrating multiple areas of bone lysis in several vertebrae. These changes are characteristic of plasma cell myeloma.

although total vertebral removal with spinal column fixation has been advocated for certain benign tumors.

Lymphoreticular Tumors

These tumors grow in the vertebral canal and are considered epidural. They do not arise from a vertebra or from the meninges. Lymphosarcoma involving the spinal canal is frequently encountered in cats and cattle but is uncommon in the dog and the horse. Tumor growth within the vertebral canal produces a compressive myelopathy. Several segments of the spinal cord may be involved, but lesions in the feline and the bovine are most common in thoracolumbar segments. Spinal lymphosarcoma must be considered in any cat or in older cows with a history of progressive neurologic dysfunction of the pelvic limbs. In addition to pelvic limb ataxia and paresis, regional hyperesthesia may be present. Plain radiographs are usually normal. A myelographic examination may reveal extensive compression, because the tumor may fill the spinal canals of several vertebrae. CSF analysis yields variable results. The CSF is normal when the tumor is outside the meninges. In some animals, the CSF may contain malignant lymphocytes and may have increased protein concentrations. In the feline, lymphosarcoma must be differentiated from the neurologic form of feline infectious peritonitis, which also affects the thoracolumbar spinal cord and results in progressive pelvic limb paresis and ataxia. In feline infectious peritonitis, the CSF usually contains a marked increase in protein, neutrophils, and some mononuclear cells. Therapy for spinal lymphosarcoma is palliative at best. Corticosteroids may alleviate some of the clinical signs temporarily. Specific antilymphosarcoma therapy is usually not effective. Euthanasia should be performed on affected cats in order to prevent further suffering.

Metastatic Tumors

Malignant tumors may metastasize to the vertebra and, rarely, to the spinal cord. Neurologic signs result from spinal cord compression secondary to vertebral instability. Malignant mammary tumors, prostatic adenocarcinomas, and hemangiosarcomas are tumors that most frequently metastasize to a vertebra. The rare tumor, multiple myeloma, also may involve a vertebra. Spinal radiographs are usually diagnostic (see Fig. 9–17). The tumor type is confirmed by histopathology. Treatment is palliative.

Primary Tumors

Primary tumors affecting the spinal cord may be medullary or extramedullary.[15] Extramedullary tumors may arise from nerve roots (neurofibromas, neurofibrosarcomas) or from the meninges (meningiomas). Neurofibromas that arise from nerve roots may be extradural, intradural, or even intramedullary. Early extra-

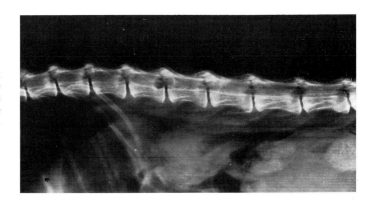

Figure 9–18. Lateral TL radiograph of a cat with progressive paraparesis. Note the enlarged intervertebral foramen at L2–L3 suggesting a mass in this area. These changes are characteristic of neurofibromas (the eventual diagnosis in this case).

medullary neurofibromas result in clinical signs that are restricted to the distribution of the affected nerve root. These early signs may go undetected if nerve roots T3–L3 are affected. These nerve roots innervate the muscles of the trunk, which are difficult to examine for neurologic dysfunction. If the nerve roots forming the brachial or lumbosacral plexus are involved, neurologic signs of monoparesis develop. As these tumors grow, they usually invade or compress the spinal cord, resulting in more symmetric neurologic signs caudal to the lesion. Plain radiographs and myelographic examinations are useful for pinpointing the lesion (Fig 9–18). Many of these tumors are inoperable, because the tumor either has invaded the spinal cord or involves multiple nerve roots that cannot be sacrificed at surgery. In some cases, the tumor and the affected nerve root can be removed.

Meningiomas usually grow slowly and produce progressive compression of the spinal cord. The site of the lesion may be painful. The clinical course usually resembles Type II disk disease or degenerative myelopathy. Plain spinal radiographs and myelographic examinations are necessary for detection of extramedullary spinal cord compression. These lesions should be surgically explored, since many meningiomas can be completely removed if detected early.

Medullary tumors of the spinal cord are rare. Initial signs may be unilateral; however, as the tumor grows, bilateral signs develop. Myelographic examinations are helpful for differentiating extramedullary compression from intramedullary tumors (Figs. 9–16B and 9–19A). The prognosis is poor, because these tumors are inoperable (Fig. 9–19B).

SPINAL DURAL OSSIFICATION

Dural ossification, also known as ossifying pachymeningitis, is a common radiographic or necropsy finding in middle-aged or older dogs.

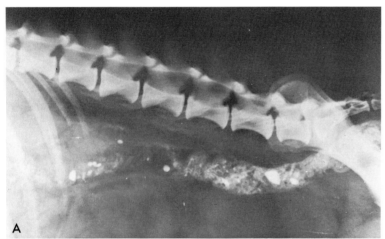

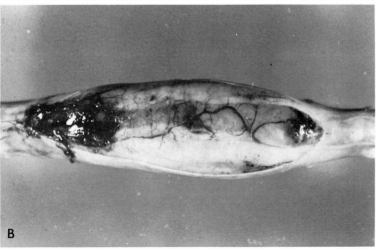

Figure 9–19. *A.* Lateral lumbar radiograph of a dog with progressive lower motor neuron (LMN) paraparesis, constipation, and urinary incontinence. Note the enlarged vertebral canal from L3–L6. These changes are characteristic of expanding intramedullary tumors. *B.* Spinal cord from the same dog, which was affected with an intramedullary tumor. The expanding tumor produced the radiographic changes found in *A.*

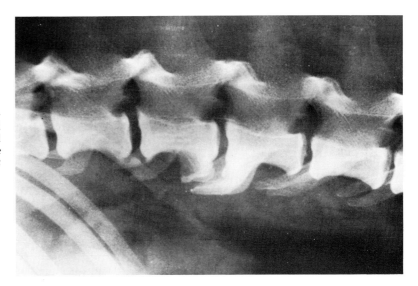

Figure 9–20. Severe spondylosis of the lumbar vertebrae and dural ossification were incidental findings in this dog. These changes seldom cause neurologic signs.

(Fig. 9–20). Plaques of bone develop on the inner dural surface in response to an unidentified factor. The lesion is most common in large-breed dogs and is often identified in association with vertebral spondylosis. The disease most commonly affects the cervical and lumbar areas. At one time, the clinical signs of degenerative myelopathy and canine wobbler syndrome were attributed to dural ossification. Later studies have demonstrated no relationship between the bony plaques and the clinical signs. The bony plaques are of little clinical importance, except in rare cases in which they entrap a nerve root or cause pain. We have observed one dog with extensive dural ossification that developed clinical signs of pelvic limb paralysis following trauma. No antemortem or necropsy evidence of vertebral fracture or luxation was found. At necropsy, a large subdural hematoma was present, which apparently resulted from a fracture of a large dural bony plaque. It was believed that spinal cord compression from this hematoma produced the neurologic signs.

Rarely, large dural plaques may cause local spinal cord edema, necrosis, or fibrosis. Radiographs are useful for establishing an antemortem diagnosis. Myelographic evidence of compression warrants exploratory decompression of the lesion. Medical treatment is nonspecific and is directed at the relief of pain. Clinicians should make every attempt to find other causes for the neurologic signs before assuming that dural ossification is the etiology.

SPONDYLOSIS DEFORMANS (HYPERTROPHIC SPONDYLOSIS)

This noninfectious, nonseptic condition is a common finding during routine radiographic or necropsy examinations. It is characterized by the formation of bony spurs and bridges at the intervertebral spaces (see Figs. 9–15A and 9–20). The term *spondylitis* originally was used to describe this condition, because investigators believed that inflammation produced the bony reaction. Later work suggested that the condition was a noninflammatory process associated with degeneration of the annulus fibrosus of the intervertebral disk.[16] The term *spondylosis* is therefore preferred. Although degeneration of the annulus may be important in the pathogenesis, nuclear degeneration and disk protrusion are not. The presence of spondylosis at a disk space is not proof of disk protrusion. The condition may be present anywhere in the spine but is most common in the caudal thoracic and caudal lumbar vertebrae. Spondylosis occurs in dogs, cats, bulls, and human beings.

Morgan found that osteophyte formation within the spinal canal is very rare and seldom, if ever, results in spinal cord compression.[16] In addition, the osteophyte formation does not constrict spinal nerves and usually is present without detectable clinical signs. This condition is rarely the cause of neurologic signs; however, occasionally it may produce spinal pain. As is true with dural ossification, clinicians must search for other causes of the neurologic signs before assuming that spondylosis is the etiology. Radiographic examinations can differentiate this condition from the true inflammatory spinal disorders (osteomyelitis, diskospondylitis) that produce severe neurologic and musculoskeletal signs. Aspirin, phenylbutazone, and corticosteroids may be required in some cases to help alleviate spinal discomfort in those animals with severe ankylosing spondylosis.

MULTIPLE CARTILAGINOUS EXOSTOSES

Multiple cartilaginous exostoses (MCE), also known as osteochondromatosis, osteocartilaginous exostoses, and multiple osteochondroma, is a condition that occurs in dogs and cats. The disease is a benign proliferation of cartilage and bone that affects the bones that are formed by endochondral ossification. In addition to the appendicular skeleton, lesions may develop in the vertebral bodies or the dorsal spinous processes (Fig. 9–21A). The ribs are also commonly affected (Fig. 9–21B). A small percentage of MCE may undergo malignant transformation into chondrosarcoma.

Clinical evidence indicates that MCE may be inherited in the dog.[17]

Clinical signs are manifested during the period of active bone growth. Pain or loss of function develops when adjacent structures are compressed or distorted by the bony lesions.[18] Vertebral involvement is frequent in the dog. Spinal cord compression with neurologic deficits caudal to the lesion is common (Fig. 9–21C). In the majority of dogs studied, progressive paraparesis was the most common neurologic finding; however, compressive lesions in the cervical spine may produce progressive tetraparesis. Radiographically, the bony exostoses are characterized as variably sized radiopaque densities with large radiolucent areas. Vertebral lesions tend to be circular in shape. Radiography provides strong supportive evidence of the diagnosis; however, a definitive diagnosis of MCE is based on typical biopsy findings. A microscopic examination of a tissue specimen is necessary in order to differentiate MCE from malignant vertebral neoplasia.

The exostoses apparently stop growing after

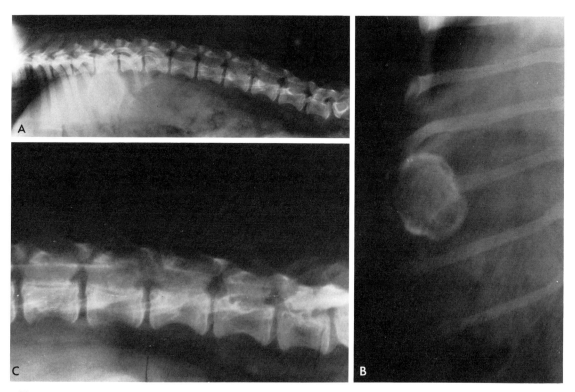

Figure 9–21. *A.* Multiple cartilaginous exostoses (osteochondromatosis) affecting the spine of a young dog. Note the cyst-like structures within the vertebrae. *B.* Radiograph of a cyst-like bone lesion in the rib of the same dog. These bone, bulla-like structures are very diagnostic of multiple cartilaginous exostoses. *C.* Myelogram of part *A* demonstrating severe spinal cord compression from L4–L6. Occasionally, these lesions undergo malignant transformation to chondrosarcoma.

physeal closure. Surgical removal of the lesion should be attempted if skeletal or neurologic dysfunction is present. Spinal cord compression should be surgically removed. Prata and coworkers have reported the successful surgical decompression of MCE vertebral lesions in two young dogs.[19] Both dogs regained neurologic function postoperatively. One dog was neurologically normal 1 year after surgery, and the second dog had mild proprioceptive dysfunction in one rear limb 9 months post surgery.

AFGHAN HOUND MYELOPATHY

In 1973, Cockrell and coworkers described a demyelinating malacic spinal cord disease in related young Afghan hounds.[20] The age of onset varied from 3 to 13 months, and the clinical course was 2 to 6 weeks. Affected dogs developed progressive pelvic limb ataxia and paresis. Spinal reflexes were usually normal or exaggerated. In some dogs, mild thoracic limb deficits were detected. The disorder progressed to tetraplegia and death from respiratory failure in 2 to 6 weeks. Severe malacic changes were found in the ventromedial portion of spinal cord segments C5–L3. The most severe changes were found in the cranial thoracic spinal cord.

The pathogenesis is unknown, although a genetic basis may be important. deLahunta proposes that the lesion is a primary leukodystrophy with a heriditary basis.[27] There is no effective treatment.

DISKOSPONDYLITIS AND VERTEBRAL ABSCESS

Pathologic Findings

Diskospondylitis is an intervertebral disk infection with concurrent osteomyelitis of con-tiguous vertebrae (Fig. 9–22). Various causes are known, including foreign body migration and bacterial or fungal infection. In dogs, the most common causes are *Staphylococcus aureus* and, occasionally, *Brucella canis*. Diskospondylitis is associated with urinary tract infection and bacteremia. Infection of the intervertebral disks and the vertebrae usually occurs secondarily to one of these primary foci. The infection may involve cervical or thoracolumbar vertebrae; however, it most frequently develops in the vertebrae of the back.

Vertebral abscesses are formed primarily in young or debilitated large animals. There is often an association with omphalophlebitis (navel ill) in calves and foals, tail docking in lambs, tail biting in pigs, and enteric salmonella infections in horses. The bacteria producing vertebral abscesses in horses include *Corynebacterium pyogenes* and *equi, Streptococcus equi* and *zooepidemicus, Escherichia coli,* and salmonella. In food animals, *Corynebacterium pyogenes* is the bacteria most commonly isolated, but *Fusobacterium necrophorum* in cattle and streptococci in swine are also common.

Neurologic signs develop in two ways. The spread of the infection to adjacent meningeal structures results in severe pain and, occasionally, in dysfunction of the spinal nerves in the diseased area. Destruction of the vertebrae may cause spinal instability with secondary compression of the spinal cord (Fig. 9–23). Paresis or paralysis and ataxia caudal to the lesion result from the spinal cord compression.

Clinical Signs

Diskospondylitis may affect dogs of any age but is more common in adults. In a recent study, the mean age was 5.1 years.[21] The in-

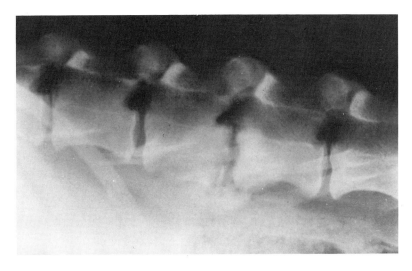

Figure 9–22. Lateral lumbar radiograph of a dog with fever, depression, and severe back pain. There is lysis of the L3–L4 disk space, with involvement of the vertebral bodies in this area. New bone production is also present. This lesion is characteristic of diskospondylitis.

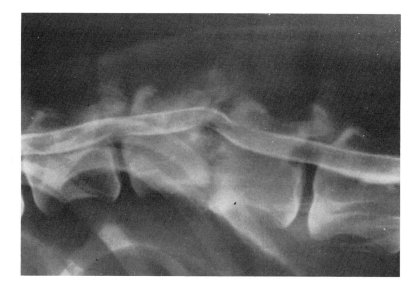

Figure 9–23. Myelogram of lumbar diskospondylitis demonstrating spinal cord compression secondary to lumbar vertebral instability. This dog had acute pelvic limb paralysis, although other signs had been present for several weeks.

cidence of this disease is apparently more frequent in male dogs than in female dogs (in a ratio of 2:1). In all animals, clinical signs may develop acutely and progress rapidly; however, the usual course is chronic and progressive. Most animals have systemic signs, including anorexia, depression, and pyrexia. In dogs, signs of urinary tract infection or endocarditis-myocarditis occasionally are detected. Dogs with brucellosis may have signs suggesting this disease (orchitis, epididymitis, abortion, infertility, and so forth). Systemic signs, however, usually are not localizing to any body system.

Frequently encountered clinical signs are directly referable to the musculoskeletal and nervous systems. These signs include hyperesthesia in the area of vertebral involvement, a stiff gait, and paresis or paralysis if spinal cord compression occurs. The syndrome is quite similar to intervertebral disk disease, except that animals with diskospondylitis frequently are systemically ill and have a more chronic course of disease. Specific neurologic signs relate to the site of involvement. Cervical lesions may cause tetraparesis and severe neck pain. Thoracolumbar lesions cause back pain and pelvic limb paresis and ataxia.

Diskospondylitis and vertebral abscesses always are suspected in animals with fever, depression, anorexia, vertebral pain, and pelvic limb ataxia or paresis.

Diagnosis

A definitive diagnosis is made with conventional radiography of the spine. Occasionally, radiographic abnormalities are not detected in early lesions, even though typical clinical signs

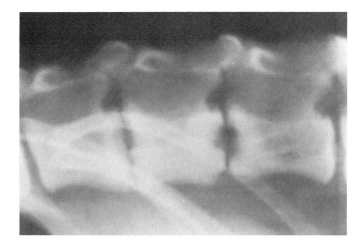

Figure 9–24. Brucella diskospondylitis affecting T13–L1 and L1–L2.

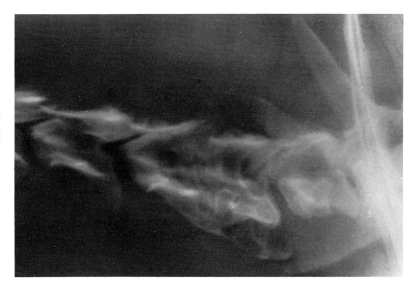

Figure 9–25. Chronic disko-spondylitis at C5–C6. Note the extensive vertebral destruction and exostosis. A large amount of fibrous tissue was surgically removed. The dog responded to surgical decompression and antibiotic therapy.

are present.[21] Radiographic lesions may lag behind the onset of clinical signs for up to 3 weeks. Typical radiographic findings include concentric lysis of adjacent vertebral end-plates (Fig. 9–24) and varying degrees of vertebral lysis and bone production (Fig. 9–25). Vertebral bodies may be shortened, and intervertebral disk spaces may be narrowed. Severely destructive lesions may cause vertebral luxation and spinal cord compression (see Fig. 9–23).

Affected dogs occasionally have leukocytosis and pyuria. Leukocytosis is more common in dogs with associated endocarditis. The CSF is usually normal, although occasionally, elevations in protein concentration and mononuclear cells are encountered. Blood cultures are usually positive, and *Staphylococcus aureus* is the most common bacteria isolated. Urine cultures also may be positive, and *S. aureus* usually is isolated in these tests as well. The tube agglutination test is usually positive in dogs affected with *Brucella canis*.

Treatment

Antibiotic therapy is based upon sensitivity testing of bacteria isolated from urine or blood or from around infections (see Chapter 7). Results of one study suggest that dogs with minimal neurologic dysfunction respond best to vertebral curettage and antibiotic therapy for 4 to 6 weeks.[21] Antibiotic therapy alone is suggested for dogs with multiple disk involvement or lesions not accessible to surgery. Compressive lesions require decompression, curettage, and stabilization in addition to long-term antibiotic therapy. Brucellosis is difficult to resolve and warrants a poor prognosis (see

Chapter 7). In large animals, antibiotic therapy is based on culture and sensitivity testing. In horses, surgical curettage and drainage of infected vertebrae are beneficial.

Acute Progressive Diseases, L4–S3

The acute progressive diseases affecting the caudal lumbar and sacral spinal cord segments are listed by etiologic category in Figures 9–6, 9–7, and 9–8. Most of these diseases have been discussed in the previous sections dealing with T3–L3 disorders. It must be remembered that some of these diseases initially may present as pelvic limb paresis but may progress to involve the cervical spinal cord. Tetraparesis (tetraplegia) may develop as the disease progresses (see Chapter 10).

Acute Nonprogressive Diseases, L4–S3

In this section, two diseases will be described: fibrocartilaginous embolization (FCE) and lumbosacral trauma. Although FCE can affect any spinal cord segment, it occurs most frequently in the caudal lumbar area. For this reason, we have elected to discuss it with the other L4–S3 disorders. FCE has a brief progressive course (a few hours) and then becomes nonprogressive. We therefore have classified it as a nonprogressive disease.

FIBROCARTILAGINOUS EMBOLIZATION
Pathophysiology

The cause of this disease is uncertain. It occurs in dogs and pigs. Fibrocartilaginous ma-

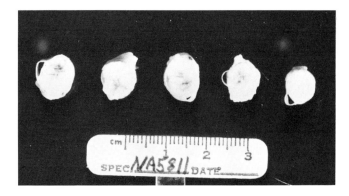

Figure 9–26. Severe lumbar cord necrosis secondary to fibrocartilaginous embolization and vessel infarction. These signs developed acutely in a 5-year-old Great Dane.

terial found in spinal cord arterioles and veins apparently results in an ischemic necrotizing myelopathy (Fig. 9–26). Exactly how this material is distributed into the spinal cord circulation is not known, but several theories have been proposed. Most of these hypotheses are based on the belief that fibrocartilaginous emboli originate from the intervertebral disks. One popular theory is that disk material is herniated directly into the vertebral venous sinus.[22] The material may be driven in a retrograde direction through the arcuate veins into the small veins of the spinal cord. The presence of arterial emboli is more difficult to explain. The presence of arteriovenous malformations has been suggested. During periods of raised pressure, such as straining, coughing or, perhaps, vigorous exercise, the disk material could enter the arterial circulation. Regardless of the mechanism, vigorous exercise often precedes the onset of clinical signs. This observation suggests that trauma to the intervertebral disk may be important in the pathogenesis.

Clinical Signs

The clinical signs develop acutely and progress rapidly within 1 to 2 hours from initial pain to unilateral or bilateral paralysis. Vigorous exercise may precede the development of signs; however, known trauma is absent. The clinical syndrome is characteristic of acute spinal cord compression from herniated intervertebral disks or vertebral fractures, except that hyperesthesia is absent. Lateralization of signs is very suggestive of FCE. The degree of neurologic deficit corresponds to the site and the extent of the spinal cord infarction. In giant-breed dogs, such as the Great Dane, lesions in the caudal lumbar spinal cord are most frequent. Lesions in this area produce LMN signs in the pelvic limbs, the urinary bladder, and the anal sphincter. Pain is not perceived

when the lesion is moderately severe and bilateral.

Lesions in the cervical spinal cord resulting in hemiparesis or tetraparesis have been reported in other breeds.[23,24] The clinical signs suggest acute cervical cord compression.

Diagnosis

The presence of FCE must be suspected in dogs, particularly giant breeds, that develop acute neurologic signs without evidence of trauma. Lateralizing signs and lack of hyperesthesia are quite suggestive. There is no definitive antemortem diagnostic procedure for FCE. The diagnosis is supported by evidence that rules out the presence of spinal cord compression. Plain radiographic and myelographic examinations are usually negative. The hemogram and the biochemistries are normal. The CSF may contain a slight increase in protein.

Treatment

The therapy for FCE is largely aimed at reducing spinal cord edema and inflammation with corticosteroids. The benefit of anticoagulants is unknown. Affected dogs should rest for 1 to 2 weeks. Dexamethasone, 2 mg per kg body weight, is given intravenously, and the dosage is repeated in 6 hours. Thereafter, the dosage is decreased to 0.1 mg per kg body weight every 12 hours for 3 days. Affected dogs should improve within a few days, but functional recovery may require several weeks. The clinical signs of complete paralysis, analgesia, or LMN involvement are associated with a very poor prognosis. Euthanasia should be recommended for these cases.

TRAUMA

Pelvic fractures, caudal lumbar fractures, and lumbosacral subluxations are very common skeletal injuries in animals. Traumatic lesions

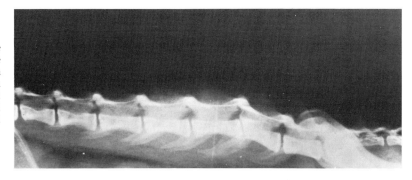

Figure 9–27. Compressive fracture of L6 produced severe paraplegia and loss of deep pain caudal to the lesion. Although little displacement is appreciated radiographically, the fracture had functionally severed the spinal cord and the nerves in this area.

in this area may involve the termination of the spinal cord or the cauda equina. These injuries may compress or entrap the roots of the sciatic, pelvic, and pudendal nerves, resulting in severe neurologic dysfunction of the pelvic limbs, the urinary bladder, and the anal sphincter (Fig. 9–27). The assessment of pelvic fractures or lumbosacral subluxations must include a neurologic evaluation of the pelvic limbs, the external anal sphincter, and the urinary bladder. The prognosis for recovery is much better in animals with normal neurologic function. The diagnosis and management of sciatic nerve injury have been discussed in Chapter 8.

Chronic Progressive Diseases, L4–S3

LUMBOSACRAL SPONDYLOPATHY

Compression of the cauda equina at the lumbosacral articulation has been reported in several dogs of varying ages and breeds. In one study, older German shepherd dogs or crossbred German shepherd dogs were affected more frequently.[25]

Pathogenesis

The cause of this syndrome is not known; however, developmental, traumatic, or degenerative etiologies have been suspected. The majority of the dogs studied had massive ventral spondylosis of the L7–S1 vertebrae (Fig. 9–28) that frequently extended laterally to the intervertebral foramen. Fifty per cent of affected dogs had subluxation of the L7–S1 vertebrae as measured by ventral displacement of the body of S1 relative to L7 (see Fig. 9–28). Direct examination of the lumbosacral spinal canal at surgery or necropsy revealed severe compression of the nerve roots by the dorsal laminae of S1 in 11 of 15 cases. In four dogs, the cranial foramen of S1 appeared stenotic, and this ab-

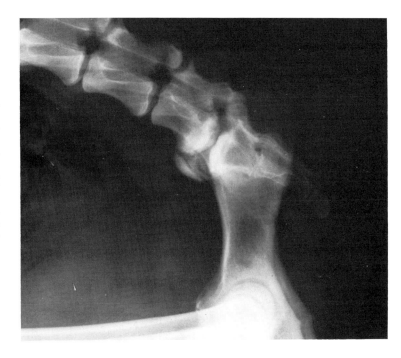

Figure 9–28. Lateral lumbosacral radiograph of a dog with urinary incontinence, mild paraparesis, and sacral pain. There is extensive exostosis of the lumbosacral area and ventral displacement of the sacrum, producing compression of the cauda equina at the lumbosacral articulation. (From Oliver, J.E., Jr., et al.: Cauda equina compression from lumbosacral malarticulation and malformation in the dog. JAVMA 173:207, 1978. Used by permission.)

normality was demonstrated radiographically in two other cases. Type II disk protrusions were present in three dogs, but this finding appeared to be significant in only one case. The ventral spondylosis, present in most dogs, apparently was the primary problem in only one dog, in which the bony proliferation entrapped the L7 nerve root as it left the intervertebral foramen.

This syndrome appears to have several similarities to canine wobbler syndrome (cervical spondylopathy—see Chapter 10). Both syndromes are characterized by a narrowing of the spinal canal as a result of subluxation or stenosis of the vertebral foramen. Altered soft tissue structures and Type II disk herniations may narrow the vertebral canal further. Cervical spondylopathy results in spinal cord compression, whereas lumbosacral spondylopathy produces compression or entrapment of the cauda equina or the L7 nerve root. Remodeling of the cranial vertebral foramen of the sacrum may occur in the same manner as has been hypothesized for the cervical malformation. The high incidence in the German shepherd dog suggests a developmental predisposition, even though the clinical signs occur in older dogs.

Clinical Signs

Early clinical signs are related to lumbosacral pain. Affected dogs become sensitive over the hindquarters, particularly in those areas innervated by the L7 dermatome. Dogs may experience difficulty rising, and at this stage, the clinical signs are easily confused with hip dysplasia. Pressure on the dorsal spinous process of the L7 or S1 vertebra usually elicts a painful response. Mild to moderate paresis and ataxia may develop in one or both pelvic limbs. Affected dogs can bear weight, because the femoral nerve is not involved. The paresis is related to motor dysfunction of the muscles innervated by the sciatic nerve (see Chapter 8). Paralysis of the tail may occur if the coccygeal nerves are affected. The knee-jerk reflexes are normal; however, the flexor reflexes may be depressed, even though pain sensation is usually preserved.

Urinary and fecal incontinence are common associated clinical signs and result from compression of the pudendal and pelvic nerve roots. The anal sphincter may be atonic, and the perineal reflex may be weak or absent. The urinary incontinence is of the LMN type, resulting in a poor detrusor reflex and a weak urethral sphincter. The bladder usually is easily expressed.

Diagnosis

Lumbosacral spondylopathy must be differentiated from disease syndromes with similar clinical signs. These disorders include Type II disk protrusion, lumbosacral neoplasia, degenerative myelopathy, and hip dysplasia. Localization of LMN signs to the L7–S1 region will rule out all of these conditions except neoplasia or Type II disk protrusion at L7–S1. Electromyography can be a valuable tool for mapping the distribution of denervation and localizing the lesion to specific nerve roots. Radiography is useful for establishing whether the skeletal lesions are compatible with stenosis, subluxation, or spondylosis. Transosseous vertebral sinus venograms and caudal epidurograms are usually abnormal and help to confirm that the vertebral lesions are compressive (Fig. 9–29). In certain cases, surgical

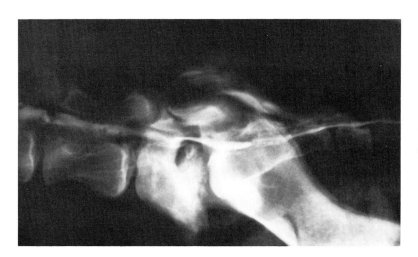

Figure 9–29. Caudal lumbosacral epidurogram of a dog with lumbosacral instability resulting from a fracture of L7. Note the compression of the dye column at L7–S1.

exploration may be necessary in order to establish a final diagnosis.

Treatment

The management of lumbosacral spondylopathy is based on an evaluation of the severity and the duration of the clinical signs. Rest for 4 to 6 weeks and analgesics are recommended for dogs with pain only or for those with mild motor deficits. Progression of clinical signs is a strong indication for surgery.

Dorsal laminectomy is recommended if signs progress or if urinary and fecal incontinence develop. Evidence of L7 nerve root entrapment warrants foraminotomy in addition to laminectomy. Unstable lumbosacral articulations should be fused surgically. Postoperative care includes scrupulous attention to the maintenance of bladder functions. The urinary bladder should be expressed or catheterized three times each day. Lower urinary tract infections should be treated with the appropriate antibiotics. The results with surgery are generally good in over 60 per cent of the cases.

DYSRAPHIC CONDITIONS

The dysraphic conditions affecting the spine or the spinal cord in animals include spinal dysraphism, syringomyelia, spina bifida with or without myelomeningocele, and coccygeal hypoplasia. The term *dysraphism* is commonly used to describe those conditions that result from defective closure of the neural tube or the vertebral arch.

Spinal Dysraphism

This condition results from failure of the primary neural tube to close during embryonic development. The condition occurs in several breeds of dogs and pigs but has been documented most frequently in the Weimaraner dog. Changes within the spinal cord include an absence, a distention, or a duplication of the central canal. Other changes include hydromyelia, syringomyelia, and anomalies of the ventral median fissure. Fluid-filled cavitations are commonly observed in dysraphic spinal cords, and spinal dysraphism, particularly in the Weimaraner breed, has been called syringomyelia. The fluid-filled cysts in the dysraphic spinal cords of Weimaraner dogs probably result from abnormal vascularization that produces ischemia, degeneration, and cavitation. The thoracic spinal cord is most commonly affected. Since dysraphic lesions are the cause of the clinical signs, the term *spinal dysraphism* is preferred to the term *syringomyelia*.

The clinical signs are usually apparent at 6 to 8 weeks of age, although in mild cases, the dog may not be presented for examination until it is several months old. The classical clinical signs include a symmetric hopping gait with the pelvic limbs (bunny hopping), a crouching posture, and a wide-based stance. Position sense in the pelvic limbs is depressed, and the animal may occasionally knuckle over. The postural reactions are depressed. The spinal reflexes are usually normal, and exaggerated scratch reflexes may be present. Pain perception is usually intact. The neurologic signs are nonprogressive but become more obvious as the animal matures. Less common clinical signs include abnormal hair streams or hair whorls in the dorsal cervical area, kinking of the undocked tail, scoliosis, and depression of the chest.

The diagnosis is based on the typical clinical

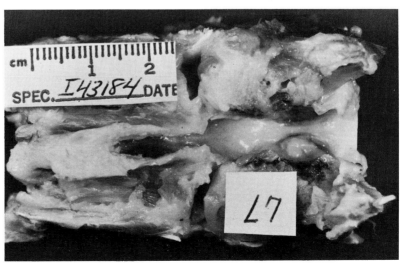

Figure 9–30. Necropsy specimen of L7 and sacrum from a bulldog puppy with spina bifida. The arch of L7 has been removed. Note the defect in the dorsal arch of the sacrum.

signs and the breed involvement. The clinical signs are nearly pathognomonic in the Weimaraner. Spinal radiographs and CSF analysis are useful for establishing that a potentially treatable disease is not present. There is no effective treatment. Since the syndrome is probably inherited in the Weimaraner, owners are advised to cease breeding animals that have produced affected puppies.

Spina Bifida

Spina bifida is the incomplete closure or fusion of the dorsal vertebral arches (Fig. 9–30). In many cases, it occurs in association with protrusion of the meninges (meningocele) or the spinal cord and the meninges (myelomeningocele) through the vertebral defect (Fig. 9–31). Often, these meningeal or spinal cord protrusions are adhered to the skin where the neural ectoderm failed to separate from the other ectodermal structures (see Fig. 9–31). These adhesions may produce a small depression or dimple in the skin at the site of attachment. In some cases, this defect may be open, and spinal fluid then leaks onto the skin, producing epidermal ulceration. Since the meninges are exposed in this situation, meningitis may develop. Spina bifida may affect any vertebra but is most common in the lumbar area. This defect has been observed in the thoracic and lumbar vertebrae in a litter of kittens. Spina bifida is most common in the manx cat and the bulldog.

Clinical signs may be minimal or extensive, depending upon the severity of the involvement of the spinal cord or the cauda equina. Some animals have signs similar to spinal dysraphism. In the bulldog, clinical signs often are related to dysfunction of the areas that are innervated by the cauda equina. Mild to moderate pelvic limb ataxia and paresis may be present. Affected dogs consistently have fecal incontinence. Urinary incontinence and pelvic limb ataxia are usually present. Pain perception may be decreased in the perineal area and from the distal regions of the pelvic limbs. In some animals, spina bifida is not associated with any neurologic deficits.

Spina bifida is confirmed radiographically. The presence of meningocele and myelomeningocele can be determined myelographically (Fig. 9–32). There are no specific treatments available for spina bifida. Meningoceles can be closed surgically to prevent the leakage of CSF.

Sacrococcygeal Hypoplasia in Manx Cats

The manx cat has been bred selectively to have a bobtail; however, numerous spinal and neural anomalies are encountered in the breed. The manx factor, or taillessness, is apparently inherited as an autosomal dominant trait. The anomalies are caused by incomplete penetrance of the dominant genes for taillessness. In addition to coccygeal dysgenesis, sacral hypoplasia may occur. Spina bifida is also commonly encountered in this breed. Spinal cord anomalies include dysraphism, syringomyelia, meningocele, and myelomeningocele.

The neurologic signs are related to abnormal development of the nerves in the cauda equina. These signs include LMN deficits to the anus, the urinary bladder, and the pelvic limbs. Urinary and fecal incontinence as well as fecal re-

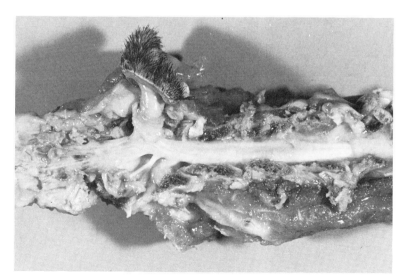

Figure 9–31. Myelomeningocele in a puppy with spina bifida. The lesion is caused by failure of the neural ectoderm to separate from the rest of the ectoderm completely during fetal development.

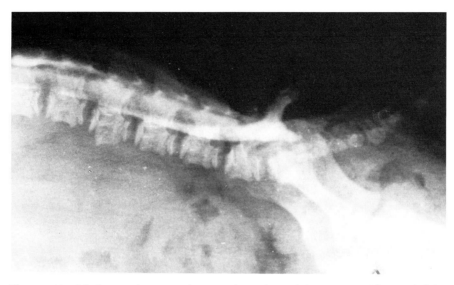

Figure 9–32. Myelogram demonstrating a myelomeningocele in a puppy with spina bifida.

tention are major problems. A bunny-hopping gait is characteristic of the breed and is not considered abnormal by manx breeders. Undoubtedly, a certain degree of spinal dysraphism is present in these so-called normal cats. Severely affected cats have pelvic limb paresis or paralysis and ataxia. Primary uterine inertia also has been observed. The clinical signs are present from birth and are nonprogressive. The diagnosis is based on the breed, the clinical signs, and radiographic evidence of sacrococcygeal abnormalities (Fig. 9–33). Therapy is directed at relieving urine and fecal retention.

SPASTIC PARESIS

This disease appears to be caused by a combination of inherited and environmental factors. It occurs in cattle 6 months of age or older. The pathogenesis of the neurologic disease is unknown; however, dysfunction of modulating internuncial neurons within the lumbosacral spinal cord is thought to cause the clinical signs.

Clinical Signs

Signs develop slowly at 6 months of age and may involve one or both pelvic limbs. At rest, the affected limb is rigidly extended backward with the heel raised. Spasticity of the limb is severe; however, proprioception and the spinal reflexes are normal. As the animal walks, the tarsus and the stifle do not flex, causing the limb to swing back and forth like a pendulum. As the disease progresses, the gluteal muscles

atrophy, the limb is held in rigid extension, and the gastrocnemius muscle and the Achilles tendon are visibly tense. Tarsal degenerative joint disease and flexor tendon contracture occur.

Diagnosis

The diagnosis is made from the clinical signs. Carrier animals can be detected by stimulation of the tibial nerve and measurement of the refractory period of the gastrocnemius muscles. Increased periods of refractivity suggest that the animal is a carrier of this trait.

Treatment

Several surgical treatments are advocated, including (1) resection of the deep digital flexor tendon; (2) neurectomy of the tibial nerve branches that supply the gastrocnemius muscles; and (3) dorsal rhizotomy of L4, L5, and L6. Overall, the prognosis is fair to poor.

NEURITIS OF THE CAUDA EQUINA

This is a severe, slowly progressive granulomatous LMN disease of older horses, usually restricted to the sacral spinal cord nerves and nerve roots. The etiology is unknown.

Clinical Signs

Early signs include pruritus and alopecia of the perineal area. LMN paresis or paralysis of the tail, the bladder, and the anal sphincter soon develop, causing fecal and urinary incontinence. Decreased sensation in the peri-

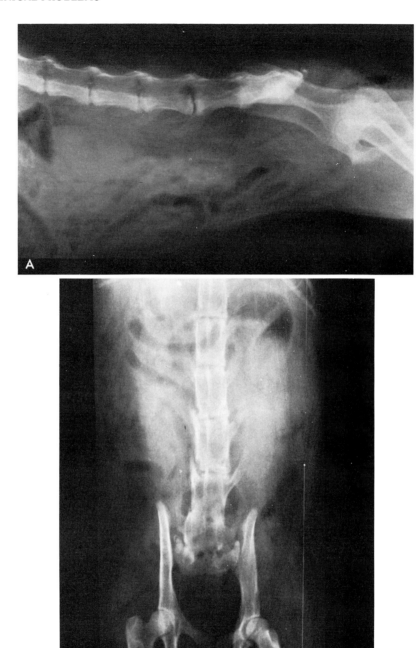

Figure 9–33. Lateral lumbosacral (*A*) and ventrodorsal (*B*) radiographs of a manx cat with sacrococcygeal abnormalities. Note the short malformed sacrum and the absence of coccygeal vertebrae.

neal area also occurs and becomes more severe as the disease progresses. In male horses, pudendal paralysis results in a dropped penis or an inability to retract the penis. Analgesia to the penis also may occur. Later signs include lameness, pelvic paresis and ataxia, myodegeneration, and stifle lock. Lesions may be multifocal. In addition to LMN signs in the pelvic limbs, cranial nerve signs, such as head tilt, nystagmus, and facial paralysis may occur in some horses.

Diagnosis

The clinical signs are very similar to those of lathyrism. Procurement of spinal fluid at the lumbar cisternae is often diagnostic of cauda equina neuritis. Lumbosacral taps reveal significantly increased concentrations of protein (100 to 300 mg/dl) and cells (more than 100 cells per cu mm). The cytologic composition is mainly macrophages, neutrophils, and a few eosinophils.

Treatment

No treatment is known.

LATHYRISM (SORGHUM CYSTITIS)

Lathyrism is a chronic progressive LMN disease that occurs in horses that ingest sorghums or Sudan grass. Lesions develop primarily in the lumbar, sacral, and coccygeal spinal cord segments. Histopathologically, these lesions are characterized by focal axonal degeneration and demyelination with associated lipid-laden macrophages.[26] It is thought that these lesions result from chronic sublethal doses of hydrocyanic acid found in plants of the genus *Sorghum.*

History

Enzootics of this disease occur in all ages of horses grazing in sorghum or Sudan grass pastures. The disease usually occurs when the plants are young and rapidly growing, but mature and second-growth pastures also have been incriminated. Apparently, the toxins do not persist in cured hay or silage.

Clinical Signs

Although the signs of urinary incontinence are most noticeable in many horses, neurologic signs usually develop first. They include flaccidity of the anus and the tail and pelvic limb ataxia. Occasionally, severe LMN paralysis of the pelvic limbs develops within 24 hours after the onset of neurologic signs. In the female horse, clinical signs include continual opening and closing of the vulva, perineal paresis, and dribbling of urine. Urine scalds and thick urine deposits occur on the buttocks, the thighs, and the hocks. Male horses drip urine from a relaxed and extended penis. Urinary incontinence is intensified when the animal is forced to move suddenly. Hyporeflexia and proprioceptive deficits are detectable in the pelvic limbs. Clinical signs rarely extend to the thoracic limbs, even though brain stem and cortex lesions have been reported.

Pregnant mares may abort, and aborted foals may have severe ankylosis (arthrogryposis). Arthrogryposis also may occur in full-term foals when the dam has grazed hybrid Sudan plants.

Diagnosis

The diagnosis is suspected from the history and the clinical signs. Affected horses have a severe fibrinopurulent cystitis secondary to neurogenic urine retention. Several different bacteria have been isolated from the urine of affected horses. Some animals develop severe ascending pyelonephritis from the chronic cystitis.

Mild changes in the CSF are found. Protein elevations are slight (60 to 80 mg/dl), and the cell counts range from 5 to 10 mononuclear cells per cu mm. Urine or serum can be tested for high levels of thiocyanate, the major detoxification product of cyanide.

Treatment

No definitive treatment is known. Horses should not be allowed to graze in sorghum pastures while the plants are rapidly growing or are stunted by drought. Plants are generally safe if they are yellow in color, are more than 2 feet tall, or have formed fruiting heads. Pastures can be checked periodically in order to determine the amount of cyanide present when toxic forage is suspected.

CASE HISTORIES

Case History 9A

Signalment

Canine, Saint Bernard, female, 6 years old.

History

Six days ago, the dog suddenly cried out in pain and developed paresis in the pelvic limbs. Within 2 hours, she became totally paralyzed in the pelvic limbs. No possibility of trauma. The dog developed signs under the owner's observation in the back yard.

Physical Examination

No abnormalities other than the neurologic problem described in the next section.

Neurologic Examination*

A. Observation
   1. Mental status: Alert.
   2. Posture: Normal, See *Gait.*
   3. Gait: Bilateral pelvic limb paralysis.
B. Palpation
   Hypertonus in right pelvic leg. Hypotonus in left pelvic leg.
C. Postural Reactions

Left	Reactions	Right
	Proprioceptive positioning	
0	PL	0
+2	TL	+2
+2	Wheelbarrowing	+2
0	Hopping, PL	0
+2	Hopping, TL	+2
0	Extensor postural thrust	0
0	Hemistand-hemiwalk	0
+2	Tonic neck	+2
	Placing, tactile	
0	PL	0
+2	TL	+2
	Placing, visual	
+2	TL	+2

---

*Key: 0 = absent, +1 = decreased, +2 = normal, +3 = exaggerated, +4 = very exaggerated or clonus, PL = pelvic limb, TL = thoracic limb.

D. Spinal Reflexes

Left	Reflex Spinal Segment	Right
	Quadriceps	
+1	L4–L6	+2
	Extensor carpi radialis	
+2	C7–T1	+2
	Triceps	
+2	C7–T1	+2
	Flexion, PL	
+1	L5–S1	+3
	Flexion, TL	
+2	C6–T1	+2
Absent	Crossed extensor	Present
	Perineal	
+2	S1–S2	+2

E. Cranial Nerves

Left	Nerve + Function	Right
	C.N. II vision	
+2	menace	+2
Nor.	C.N. II + C.N. III pupil size	Nor.
+2	Stim. left eye	+2
+2	Stim. right eye	+2
Nor.	C.N. II fundus	Nor.
	C.N. III, C.N. IV, C.N. VI	
0	Strabismus	0
0	Nystagmus	0
+2	C.N. V sensation	+2
+2	C.N. V mastication	+2
+2	C.N. VII facial muscles	+2
+2	Palpebral	+2
Nor.	C.N. IX, C.N. X swallowing	Nor.
Nor.	C.N. XII tongue	Nor.

F. Sensation: Location
   Hyperesthesia _____ 0 _____
   Superficial pain _____ +2 _____
   Deep pain _____ +2 _____

Complete sections G and H before reviewing Case Summary.

G. Assessment (Anatomic diagnosis and estimation of prognosis)

H. Plan (Diagnostic)

Rule-outs	Procedure
1.	
2.	
3.	
4.	

Case History 9B

Signalment

Canine, dachshund, female, 7 years old.

History

Two days ago, the dog had a sudden onset of paraparesis and within 6 hours became paralyzed in both pelvic limbs. When the dog initially was examined, the pelvic limb reflexes were present, but pain perception was absent in both rear legs. The thoracic limbs were normal.

Physical Examination

Urinary incontinence, hematuria, and shallow abdominal respirations. The dog cries periodically as if in pain.

Neurologic Examination *

A. Observation
1. Mental status: Apprehensive.
2. Posture: Cannot maintain sternal recumbency.
3. Gait: No voluntary movements of pelvic limbs. Short, choppy steps with thoracic limbs.
B. Palpation
Hypotonus in both pelvic limbs. Abdominal muscles are flaccid.
C. Postural Reactions

Left	Reactions	Right
	Proprioceptive positioning PL	
0		0
+2	TL	+2
+1 to +2	Wheelbarrowing	+1 to +2
0	Hopping, PL	0
+2	Hopping, TL	+2
0	Extensor postural thrust	0
0	Hemistand-hemiwalk	0
+1 to +2	Tonic neck	+1 to +2
0	Placing, tactile PL	0
+2	TL	+2
+2	Placing, visual TL	+2

*Key: 0 = absent, +1 = decreased, +2 = normal, +3 = exaggerated, +4 = very exaggerated or clonus, PL = pelvic limb, TL = thoracic limb.

D. Spinal Reflexes

Left	Reflex Spinal Segment	Right
0	Quadriceps L4−L6	0
+2	Extensor carpi radialis C7−T1	+2
+2	Triceps C7−T1	+2
0	Flexion, PL L5−S1	0
+2	Flexion, TL C6−T1	+2
0	Crossed extensor	0
0	Perineal S1−S2	0

E. Cranial Nerves

Left	Nerve + Function	Right
+2	C.N. II vision menace	+2
Nor.	C.N. II + C.N. III pupil size	Nor.
+2	Stim. left eye	+2
+2	Stim. right eye	+2
Nor.	C.N. II fundus	Nor.
0	C.N. III, C.N. IV, C.N. VI Strabismus	0
0	Nystagmus	0
Nor.	C.N. V sensation	Nor.
Nor.	C.N. V mastication	Nor.
Nor.	C.N. VII facial muscles	Nor.
+2	Palpebral	+2
Nor.	C.N. IX, C.N. X swallowing	Nor.
Nor.	C.N. XII tongue	Nor.

F. Sensation: Location
Hyperesthesia ___Present at T2−T3___
Superficial pain Absent caudal to shoulders
Deep pain Absent caudal to shoulders
Complete sections G and H before reviewing Case Summary.
G. Assessment (Anatomic diagnosis and estimation of prognosis)

H. Plan (Diagnostic)
Rule-outs   Procedure
1.
2.
3.
4.

Case History 9C

Signalment

Canine, German shepherd, female, 1½ years old.

History

Six weeks ago, the dog became lame in the right pelvic limb. Since then, she gradually has developed paresis and ataxia in both pelvic limbs, but in the right side worse than in the left side. Three days ago she became totally paralyzed in both pelvic limbs.

Physical Examination

Negative except for the neurologic problem.

Neurologic Examination *

A. Observation
 1. Mental status: Alert.
 2. Posture: See Gait.
 3. Gait: Paraplegia, thoracic limbs normal.

B. Palpation
 Muscle atrophy from TL region caudally along spine. Extensor rigidity in both pelvic limbs.

C. Postural Reactions

Left	Reactions	Right
	Proprioceptive positioning PL	
0		0
+2	TL	+2
+2	Wheelbarrowing	+2
0	Hopping, PL	0
+2	Hopping, TL	+2
0	Extensor postural thrust	0
0	Hemistand-hemiwalk	0
+2	Tonic neck	+2
0	Placing, tactile PL	0
+2	TL	+2
+2	Placing, visual TL	+2

*Key: 0 = absent, +1 = decreased, +2 = normal, +3 = exaggerated, +4 = very exaggerated or clonus, PL = pelvic limb, TL = thoracic limb.

D. Spinal Reflexes

Left	Reflex Spinal Segment	Right
	Quadriceps	
+3	L4−L6	+3
	Extensor carpi radialis	
+2	C7−T1	+2
	Triceps	
+2	C7−T1	+2
	Flexion, PL	
+2	L5−S1	+2
	Flexion, TL	
+2	C6−T1	+2
0	Crossed extensor	0
	Perineal	
+2	S1−S2	+2

E. Cranial Nerves

Left	Nerve + Function	Right
	C.N. II vision	
+2	menace	+2
Nor.	C.N. II + C.N. III pupil size	Nor.
+2	Stim. left eye	+2
+2	Stim. right eye	+2
Nor.	C.N. II fundus	Nor.
	C.N. III, C.N. IV, C.N. VI	
0	Strabismus	0
0	Nystagmus	0
Nor.	C.N. V sensation	Nor.
Nor.	C.N. V mastication	Nor.
Nor.	C.N. VII facial muscles	Nor.
+2	Palpebral	+2
Nor.	C.N. IX, C.N. X swallowing	Nor.
Nor.	C.N. XII tongue	Nor.

F. Sensation: Location
 Hyperesthesia _____ L2−L3 _____
 Superficial pain _____ Absent _____
 Deep pain Blunted caudal to L2−L3

Complete sections G and H before reviewing Case Summary.

G. Assessment (Anatomic diagnosis and estimation of prognosis)

H. Plan (Diagnostic)
 Rule-outs   Procedure
 1.
 2.
 3.
 4.

Case History 9D

Signalment

Canine, bulldog, male, 7 weeks old.

History

Since he became ambulatory, the puppy has had a spastic, ataxic gait in the pelvic limbs. Urinary and fecal incontinence have been present for at least two weeks.

Physical Examination

Normal except for the neurologic problem. Urinary incontinence present.

Neurologic Examination *

A. Observation
 1. Mental status: Alert, responsive.
 2. Posture: See Gait.
 3. Gait: Paretic and ataxic in pelvic limbs. Wide-based stance; feet tend to slip from under the dog.
B. Palpation
 No tone in anal sphincter. Small depression in lumbar area just cranial to sacrum.
C. Postural Reactions

Left	Reactions	Right
	Proprioceptive positioning PL	
0	PL	0
+2	TL	+2
+2	Wheelbarrowing	+2
+1	Hopping, PL	+1
+2	Hopping, TL	+2
+1	Extensor postural thrust	+1
+1	Hemistand-hemiwalk	+1
+2	Tonic neck	+2
0	Placing, tactile PL	0
+2	TL	+2
	Placing, visual PL	
+2	TL	+2

D. Spinal Reflexes

Left	Reflex Spinal Segment	Right
+2	Quadriceps L4−L6	+2
+2	Extensor carpi radialis C7−T1	+2
+2	Triceps C7−T1	+2
0 to +1	Flexion, PL L5−S1	0 to +1
+2	Flexion, TL C6−T1	+2
0	Crossed extensor	0
0	Perineal S1−S2	0

E. Cranial Nerves

Left	Nerve + Function	Right
+2	C.N. II vision menace	+2
Nor.	C.N. II + C.N. III pupil size	Nor.
+2	Stim. left eye	+2
+2	Stim. right eye	+2
Nor.	C.N. II fundus	Nor.
0	C.N. III, C.N. IV, C.N. VI Strabismus	0
0	Nystagmus	0
+2	C.N. V sensation	+2
+2	C.N. V mastication	+2
+2	C.N. VII facial muscles	+2
+2	Palpebral	+2
+2	C.N. IX, C.N. X swallowing	+2
Nor.	C.N. XII tongue	Nor.

F. Sensation: Location
 Hyperesthesia _____ None
 Superficial pain ___ Absent in perineal area
 Deep pain ___ Present but decreased ___
Complete sections G and H before reviewing Case Summary.
G. Assessment (Anatomic diagnosis and estimation of prognosis)

H. Plan (Diagnostic)
 Rule-outs Procedure
 1.
 2.
 3.
 4.

---

*Key: 0 = absent, +1 = decreased, +2 = normal, +3 = exaggerated, +4 = very exaggerated or clonus, PL = pelvic limb, TL = thoracic limb.

ASSESSMENT 9A

Anatomic diagnosis: This dog has bilateral pelvic limb paralysis characterized by UMN signs in the right leg and LMN signs in the left limb. An asymmetric lesion in the midlumbar spinal cord is probably present (spinal cord segments L2–L5). The lesion has spared spinal cord sensory pathways. Acute nonprogressive diseases should be considered.

Diagnostic plan (Rule-outs—see Figs. 9–3 and 9–6):
1. Fibrocartilaginous embolization: absence of evidence of cord compression.
2. Intervertebral disk disease: spinal radiology and myelography (negative).

Therapeutic plan:
1. Dexamethasone. At 6 days after the injury, it is very doubtful that corticosteroids will be beneficial.
2. Supportive care of a paraplegic.

Client education: The prognosis is very poor, since the lesion is severe. The presence of pain sensation implies that some spinal cord integrity is present, however. Maintain the dog for one week. If there is no improvement, plan euthanasia.

Case summary:
1. Diagnosis: spinal cord infarction.
2. Result: no improvement. Euthanasia was performed.
   Spinal cord hemorrhage with infarction from L2–L4.

ASSESSMENT 9B

Anatomic diagnosis: The motor examination reveals severe bilateral LMN disease in both pelvic limbs and in the pudendal nerve. The symmetry of the signs suggests severe disease in segments L4–S2. The sensory examination reveals complete analgesia caudal to the shoulders. This finding suggests a severe lesion extending as far forward as T3. In addition, the LMN neurons to the abdominal and intercostal muscles are involved. Therefore, diffuse symmetric disease of the spinal cord caudal to T3 should be suspected. The history suggests a progression of the lesion, since spinal reflexes in the pelvic limbs were present 2 days ago. The lesion involves both gray and white matter throughout the spinal cord.

Diagnostic plan (Rule-out—see Figs. 9–3 and 9–6): Ascending—descending myelomalacia secondary to spinal cord compression.

Therapeutic plan: None.

Client education:
1. The prognosis is hopeless.
2. Recommend euthanasia.

Case summary: The diagnosis is severe ascending-descending myelomalacia secondary to a herniated disk at T13–L1.

ASSESSMENT 9C

Anatomic diagnosis: The neurologic examination reveals bilateral UMN disease to both pelvic limbs, suggesting a lesion in the segment T2–L3. The clinical course suggests a progressive disease. The hyperesthesia suggests a lesion at the segment L2–L3.

Diagnostic plan (Rule-outs—see Fig. 9–3):
1. Type II disk disease—spinal radiography (negative).
2. Neoplasia—Myelography (intramedullary compression of the dye column at L1–L2).
3. Chronic meningomyelitis—CSF (1 WBC, 13.5 mg/dl protein).
4. Diskospondylitis.

Therapeutic plan:
1. Dexamethasone.
2. Exploratory laminectomy.

Client education: The prognosis is very poor. The myelogram suggests an intramedullary spinal cord tumor. These tumors are usually inoperable.

Case summary:
1. Diagnosis: inoperable ependymoma at L1–L2.
2. Euthanasia was performed.

ASSESSMENT 9D

Anatomic diagnosis: LMN signs with blunted pain perception suggest a bilateral lesion in the segment L3–S2 or in the lumbosacral plexus. The urine and fecal incontinence is explained by a lesion in this region. The history and the breed suggest a developmental abnormality.

Diagnostic plan (Rule-outs—see Fig. 9–6):
1. Spina bifida—radiography (lumbosacral area).
2. Spinal dysraphism—myelography (EMG, perineal muscles).

Therapeutic plan: None.

Client education:
1. The prognosis is poor.
2. This congenital abnormality is a problem in certain lines of bulldogs.

Case summary:
1. Diagnosis: spina bifida with concurrent meningomyelocele.
2. Euthanasia was performed.

REFERENCES

1. Priester, W. A.: Canine intervertebral disk disease—occurrence by age, breed, and sex among 8117 cases. Theriogenol. 6:293, 1976.
2. Hoerlein, B. F.: Canine Neurology: Diagnosis and Treatment, 3rd ed. Philadelphia, W. B. Saunders Co., 1978.
3. Olsson, S. E.: Observations concerning disc fenestration in dogs. Acta Orthop. Scand. 20:349–356, 1951.
4. Tarlov, I. M., Klinger, H., and Vitale, S.: Spinal cord compression studies. I. Experimental techniques to produce acute and gradual compression. II. Time limits for recovery after acute compression in dogs. III. Time limits for recovery after gradual compression in dogs. Arch. Neurol. Psych. 70:813, 1950; 71:271, 1954; 71:588, 1954.
5. Little, P. B., and Thorsen, J.: Disseminated necrotizing myeloencephalitis: A herpes-associated neurological disease of horses. Vet. Pathol. 13:161–171, 1976.
6. Jackson, T. A., Osburn, B. I., Cordy, D. R., and Kendrick, J. W.: Equine herpesvirus 1 infection of horses: Studies on the experimentally induced neurologic disease. Am. J. Vet. Res. 38:709–719, 1977.

7. Rooney, J. R., Prickett, M. E., Delaney, F. M., and Crowe, M. W.: Focal myelitis-encephalitis in horses. Cornell Vet. 60:494–501, 1970.
8. Dubey, J. P., Davis, G. W., Koestner, A., and Kiryw, K.: Equine encephalomyelitis due to a protozoan parasite resembling *Toxoplasma gondii.* JAVMA 165:249–255, 1974.
9. Oliver, J. E., Jr.: Neurologic emergencies in small animals. Vet. Clin. North Am. 2:341–357, 1972.
10. Brasmer, T. H.: Evaluation and therapy of spinal cord trauma. *In* Kirk, R. W.: Current Veterinary Therapy VI. Philadelphia, W. B. Saunders Co., 1977.
11. Kolata, R. J., and Johnston, D. E.: Motor vehicle accidents in urban dogs: A study of 600 cases. JAVMA 167:938–941, 1975.
12. Averill, D. R., Jr.: Degenerative myelopathy in the aging German shepherd dog: Clinical and pathologic findings. JAVMA 162:1045–1051, 1973.
13. Braund, K. G., and Vandevelde, M.: German Shepherd dog myelopathy—a morphologic and morphometric study. Am. J. Vet. Res. 39:1309–1315, 1978.
14. Griffiths, I. R., and Duncan, I. D.: Chronic degenerative radiculomyelopathy in the dog. J. Small Anim. Pract. 16:461–471, 1975.
15. Luginbuhl, H., Fankhauser, R., and McGrath, J. T.: Spontaneous neoplasms of the nervous system in animals. Prog. Neurol. Surg. 2:85, 1968.
16. Morgan, J. P.: Spondylosis deformans in the dog, a morphological study with some clinical and experimental observations. Acta Orthop. Scand. (Suppl. 96):7–87, 1967.
17. Chester, D. K.: Multiple cartilaginous exostoses in two generations of dogs. JAVMA 159:895–897, 1971.
18. Gambardella, P. C., Osborne, C. A., and Stevens, J. B.: Multiple cartilaginous exostoses in the dog. JAVMA 166:761–768, 1975.
19. Prata, R. G., Stoll, S. G., and Zaki, F. A.: Spinal cord compression caused by osteocartilaginous exostoses of the spine in two dogs. JAVMA 166:371–375, 1975.
20. Cockrell, B. Y., Herigstad, R. R., Flo, G. L., and Legendre, A. M.: Myelomalacia in Afghan hounds. JAVMA 162:362–365, 1973.
21. Kornegay, J. N., and Barber, D. L.: Diskospondylitis in dogs. JAVMA 177:337, 1980.
22. Zaki, F. A., and Prata, R. G.: Necrotizing myelopathy secondary to embolization of herniated intervertebral disk material in the dog. JAVMA 169:222–228, 1976.
23. Griffiths, I. R.: Spinal cord infarction due to emboli arising from the intervertebral discs in the dog. J. Comp. Pathol. 83:225–232, 1973.
24. deLahunta, A., and Alexander, J. W.: Ischemic myelopathy secondary to presumed fibrocartilaginous embolism in nine dogs. JAAHA 12:37, 1976.
25. Oliver, J. E., Jr., Selcer, R. R., and Simpson, S.: Cauda equina compression from lumbosacral malarticulation and malformation in the dog. JAVMA 173:207–214, 1978.
26. Adams, L. G., Dollahite, J. W., Romane, W. M., et al.: Cystitis and ataxia associated with sorghum ingestion by horses. JAVMA 155:518–524, 1969.
27. deLahunta, A.: Veterinary Neuroanatomy and Clinical Neurology. Philadelphia, W. B. Saunders Co., 1977.

10

CHAPTER

TETRAPARESIS, HEMIPARESIS, AND ATAXIA

Motor dysfunction of all four limbs is called *tetraparesis* or *tetraplegia* (quadriparesis, quadriplegia), depending upon the severity of motor loss. The term *hemiparesis* refers to motor dysfunction of two limbs on the same side. Ataxia is a frequently associated problem. Lesion localization has been discussed in Chapter 4 and is summarized in Figure 10–1. It will be reviewed briefly in this chapter.

LESION LOCALIZATION

Animals with tetraparesis usually have neurologic disease. Diffuse muscle or skeletal diseases may result in tetraparesis, which at times is difficult to differentiate from true neurologic lesions. In addition, tetraparesis of neurologic origin must be differentiated from generalized muscle weakness or depression associated with severe metabolic disease (e.g., adrenal insufficiency, hypoglycemia). When initially presented with a tetraparetic animal, the clinician must decide which systems are involved (nervous, musculoskeletal, or generalized metabolic disorders). The history, physical findings, and laboratory tests usually provide sufficient evidence for the practitioner to make this differentiation. In this chapter, primary consideration is given to lesions involving the nervous and musculoskeletal systems.

Neurologic lesions that produce tetraparesis may involve the cerebral cortex, the brain stem, the cervical cord, or the lower motor neurons (LMNs). Lesion localization is based on the decisions outlined in Figure 10–1. Although the motor cortex is important for the performance of learned reactions (see Chapters 3 and 4), these areas do not maintain locomotion in domestic animals. Diffuse brain stem centers coordinate these functions with reinforcement from the cerebral cortex. Therefore, animals with diffuse (bilateral) cerebral cortex disease usually have little or no gait abnormality. The postural reactions are generally abnormal contralateral to the lesion. Other signs of cerebral dysfunction, such as altered mental status, seizures, or blindness, may be present and may help in the localization of the lesion.

Lesions involving the brain stem and the cervical cord result in an abnormal gait, because motor signals from brain stem centers to the LMNs of the spinal cord are disrupted. Tetraparesis develops if the lesion is bilateral, and hemiparesis (usually ipsilateral) occurs if the lesion is unilateral. Altered sensory function (ataxia, hypalgesia) frequently is associated with the motor dysfunction, because lesions are usually severe enough to disrupt the sensory pathways from the limbs and the body.

Lesions in the brain stem and C1–C5 spinal cord segments result in upper motor neuron (UMN) signs in the limbs. As has been explained in Chapter 4, disruption of UMN signals that inhibit the segmental spinal reflexes results in "release," or hyperactivity, of the LMNs. Brain stem and rostral cervical cord lesions are differentiated by an examination of the head, because lesions in either region can result in identical abnormalities in the limbs. The brain stem can be described as a cervical spinal cord that is modified by the presence of nuclei. Evidence of dysfunction in these nuclei provides documentation of brain stem disease. Paresis associated with vestibular signs, depression, altered mental status, endocrine dysfunction, or abnormal cranial nerve function strongly suggests a lesion in the brain stem.

Lesions involving cervical segments C6–T2 result in paresis, as has been explained previously. LMN signs may be present in the thoracic limbs if the motor neurons forming the brachial plexus are injured. In addition, a Horner's sign may develop if the LMNs that form the sympathetic nerve (located in the segment T1–T3) are injured. UMN signs develop in the pelvic limbs because both facilitory and inhibitory motor impulses are disrupted as they pass through the caudal cervical cord. Altered sensory function is invariably present with lesions in the region C6–T2.

Animals with tetraparesis associated with diffuse LMN signs (involvement of the thoracic and the pelvic limbs) can, at least theoretically, have lesions involving the motor

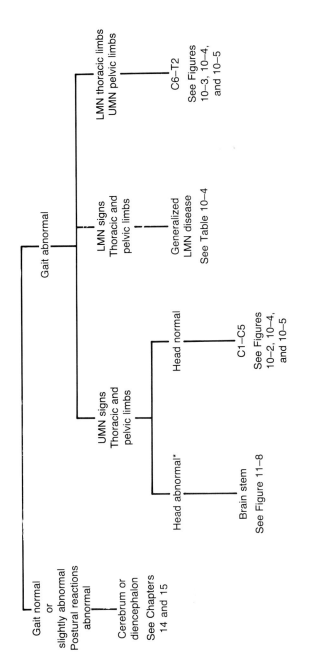

*Head involvement: one or more present—head tilt, head bob, tremor of head, nystagmus, cranial nerve signs, etc.

Figure 10–1. Algorithm for the diagnosis of tetraparesis, hemiparesis, and ataxia.

neurons located in the spinal cord, lesions of their axonal processes (ventral spinal root, spinal nerve, peripheral nerve), or diseases of the neuromuscular end-plate (motor end-plate). The last two conditions are commonly encountered in small animals, whereas the first condition is rare. Lesions involving the motor neurons, the ventral nerve root, or the neuromuscular end-plate do not produce sensory dysfunction, because sensory neurons or nerve fibers are not present in these areas. A disease that diffusely affects the peripheral nerves may cause sensory dysfunction, because most peripheral nerves contain both motor and sensory fibers. Animals with tetraparesis, LMN signs in the limbs, and normal pain perception usually have a disease involving the ventral nerve roots or the neuromuscular junction. Animals with neurologic signs that are episodic (that wax and wane with rest) usually have motor end-plate disease. It is important

to interject a note of caution at this point. Occasionally, animals with diffuse muscle disease develop clinical signs that are strongly suggestive of diffuse LMN disease. Careful muscle palpation and laboratory tests are necessary in order to separate primary muscle disease from primary neurologic disease.

DISEASES

The diseases discussed in this chapter include those that commonly affect the cervical spinal cord and those that diffusely affect the LMN system. The diseases that affect the cerebral cortex and the brain stem will be presented in Chapters 11 through 17. As has been the style in previous chapters, this section is organized according to the anatomic location of the lesion and the course of the disease (acute versus chronic, progressive versus non-

Etiologic Category	C1–C5		
	Acute		Chronic
	Progressive	Nonprogressive	
Degenerative	*Cervical disk disease**	1. *Fibrocartilaginous embolization*	1. *Storage diseases* (lipo- and leukodystrophies) 2. Demyelinating diseases 3. Neuronopathies (Brittany spaniels)
Anomalous	None	None	1. *Atlantoaxial subluxation* 2. *Vertebral malformation with subluxation* a. Basset hound b. Great Dane c. Doberman
Neoplastic	None	None	1. Primary a. Neurofibroma b. Glioma c. Meningioma 2. Metastatic 3. Lymphoreticular
Nutritional			Hypervitaminosis A
Inflammatory Infectious	1. *Distemper myelitis* myoclonus 2. Myelitis, bacterial a. Meningoencephalitis 3. Toxoplasmosis 4. Mycosis a. Cryptococcosis b. Blastomycosis c. Histoplasmosis d. Nocardiosis e. Coccidioidomycosis	None	See *Acute Progressive* 1. Mycotic infections and toxoplasmosis usually have a chronic progressive course 2. *Noneffusive feline infectious peritonitis* 3. Distemper myelitis
Traumatic	None unless progressive myelomalacia develops	1. Fractures 2. Subluxation 3. Traumatic disk herniation	None
Toxic	See *Seizures,* Tables 15–2 and 15–3		

*Indicates increased incidence of nonselective disease at a particular site.

Figure 10–2. Differential diagnosis of C1–C5 spinal cord diseases based on their clinical courses and etiologic categories. *Italics* indicate most important diseases clinically.

C6–T2

Etiologic Category	Acute		Chronic
	Progressive	Nonprogressive	

Degenerative	1. Cervical disk disease
	2. Hemorrhagic myelomalacia
		1. Vascular diseases
		  a. *Fibrocartilaginous embolization* *
		  b. Thrombosis, emboli, hemorrhage
			1. *Canine wobbler syndrome* (cervical spondylopathy)
			2. Cervical disk disease
			3. Hereditary myelopathy in Afghan hounds
			4. Neuronopathy (Canine hereditary spinal muscular atrophy)—Brittany spaniels
			5. Demyelinating diseases

Anomalous	None	None	Spinal dysraphism
Nutritional	None	None	Hypervitaminosis A of cats
Neoplastic	Metastatic (prostatic adenocarcinoma)	None	1. Primary 2. Lymphoreticular 3. Skeletal 4. Metastatic

Inflammatory Infectious	1. *Distemper myelitis* and myoclonus
	2. *Myelitis, bacterial*
	  a. *Primary bacterial with meningitis*
	  b. Secondary to spondylitis
	  c. *Secondary to diskospondylitis*
	3. *Toxoplasmosis*
	4. *Mycosis*
	  a. Cryptococcosis
	  b. Blastomycosis
	  c. Histoplasmosis
	  d. Nocardiosis
	  e. Coccidioidomycosis
		None	See *Acute Progressive*
			1. Mycotic infections, toxoplasmosis, and diskospondylitis usually have a chronic progressive course
			2. Noneffusive in feline infectious peritonitis
			3. Distemper myelitis

Traumatic	Ascending-descending myelomalacia (hematomyelia)	1. Fractures 2. Subluxations 3. Traumatic disk herniation	None
Toxic	See *Seizures,* Tables 15–2 and 15–3		

*Indicates increased incidence of nonselective disease at a particular site.

Figure 10–3. Differential diagnosis of C6–T2 spinal cord diseases based on their clinical courses and etiologic categories. *Italics* indicate most important diseases clinically.

progressive). The disorders that affect spinal cord segments C1–C5 and C6–T2 are presented in Figures 10–2 and 10–3, respectively. Equine cervical cord diseases are mentioned in Figure 10–4, and the cervical cord lesions of food animals are named in Figure 10–5. The diffuse LMN diseases are listed in Table 10–2. Although each list in Figures 10–2 to 10–5 is complete, the major diseases are written in italics; these disorders are emphasized in this chapter.

Acute Progressive Diseases, C1–C5

CERVICAL DISK DISEASE

The pathophysiology of intervertebral disk disease has been discussed in the previous chapter. Hansen Type I disk protrusions in the cervical area occur most frequently in the chondrodystrophoid breeds (small poodle,

dachshund, beagle, cocker spaniel) but also occasionally are encountered in certain large-breed dogs, such as the Doberman pinscher. The incidence of cervical disk disease is lower than that of thoracolumbar disk disease. Approximately 14 to 25 per cent of all disk lesions in the dog occur in the cervical area.[1-3] Intervertebral spaces C2–C3 and C3–C4 are most frequently involved.

Unlike thoracolumbar disk herniations, cervical disk herniations infrequently result in compressive myelopathy sufficient to cause paresis or paralysis. Although many factors may account for this finding, the larger diameter of the vertebral canal in the cervical area is probably the most important explanation. Because of the greater space surrounding the cervical cord, disk herniations in this area are less likely to result in focal compressive myelopathy. Likewise, the syndrome of ascend-

| Etiologic Category | Acute | | Chronic |
	Progressive	Nonprogressive	
Degenerative	Cervical spondylopathy *Degenerative myeloencephalopathy*		*Cervical spondylopathy* (cervical vertebral stenotic myelopathy) Degenerative myeloencephalopathy
Anomalous			Occipitoatlantoaxial (Arabian foals) malformation Atlantoaxial subluxation
Neoplastic	Metastasis		1. Primary 2. Metastatic 3. Skeletal
Nutritional			
Inflammatory Infectious	1. *Necrotizing myeloencephalitis* (see Chapter 9) 2. *Protozoal encephalomyelitis* (see Chapter 9) 3. *Vertebral osteomyelitis* (abscess) (see Chapter 9) 4. Toxoplasmosis 5. Mycotic myelitis 6. Verminous migration (see Chapter 9)		*Vertebral osteomyelitis* (see Chapter 9) See *Acute Progressive* 1. *Protozoal encephalomyelitis* 2. *Verminous migration*
Traumatic		Fractures Subluxations	
Toxic			

Figure 10–4. Equine cervical cord diseases. *Italics* indicate most important diseases clinically.

ing-descending myelomalacia rarely results from cervical disk herniation.

Clinical Signs

The most prominent sign in cervical disk protrusions is pain that arises from meningeal or nerve root irritation. The head is usually held low, and the neck may be extended rigidly. The dog may resist any attempt to move its head or neck. Occasionally, affected dogs develop a lameness of one thoracic limb. The paw may be held up intermittently as the animal stands or sits, and a slight limp may be present in the gait. A forced movement of the

| Etiologic Category | Acute | | Chronic |
	Progressive	Nonprogressive	
Degenerative			
Anomalous			
Neoplastic			
Nutritional			Copper deficiency-P,O

Inflammatory Infectious	1. *Viral leukoencephalomyelitis*-C
	2. Verminous migration
	  a. Cerebrospinal parelaphostrongylosis-C,O
	  b. Hypoderma-B
	  c. Stephanurus dentatus-P
	3. Vertebral osteomyelitis (abscess)-All (see Chapter 9 for discussion)
	4. Toxoplasmosis-All
			1. Verminous migration
			2. Vertebral osteomyelitis
			3. Mycotic myelitis-All
			4. Toxoplasmosis (see Chapter 9)

Traumatic		Fractures Subluxations (see Chapter 9)	
Toxic			

Figure 10–5. Food animal cervical cord diseases. B = Bovine. C = Caprine. O = Ovine. P = Porcine. *Italics* indicate most important diseases clinically.

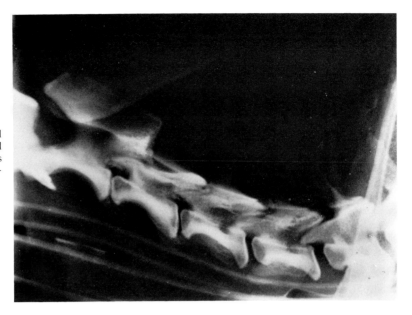

Figure 10–6. Lateral cervical radiograph of a dog with cervical disk disease. Note narrow spaces at C2–C3 and C3–C4. The dog responded to ventral fenestration.

limb may cause considerable pain. Dogs that are in pain have a stiff, short-strided gait and may cry or whine if forced to change direction suddenly. Most dogs are reluctant to, or refuse to, climb stairs or jump. The clinical signs resulting from pain are very similar to the signs associated with bacterial meningitis.

Occasionally, a cervical disk herniation may be large enough to compress the cervical cord, and paresis and ataxia of the thoracic and pelvic limbs will result. Rarely, a massive disk blowout will produce tetraplegia. Disk protrusions in the cervical cord may produce Horner's syndrome. Caudal cervical disk herniation may produce LMN signs in one or both thoracic limbs. The presence of neurologic signs other than pain strongly suggests spinal cord compression. Evidence of spinal cord compression is an indication for decompressive surgery.

Diagnosis

The clinical diagnosis of cervical disk disease is confirmed by radiographic examination of the cervical area (Figs. 10–6 and 10–7). Radiographs are taken for all surgical candidates. In most cases, anesthesia is required in order to achieve proper positioning when diagnostic radiographs are taken. If conventional radiographs fail to demonstrate a lesion,

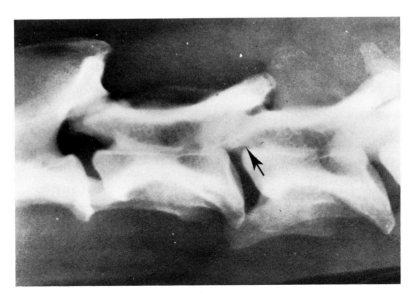

Figure 10–7. Lateral cervical radiograph. Note the massive disk herniation (*arrow*) at C3–C4. Decompressive surgery is indicated in this case.

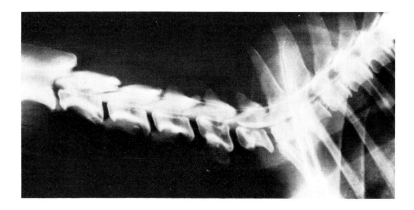

Figure 10–8. Cervical myelography of a dog with a caudal cervical disk protrusion at C6–C7. The lesion was not visualized on survey cervical radiographs. The dog responded to ventral decompressive surgery.

cerebrospinal fluid (CSF) should be obtained in order to rule out the presence of infectious meningomyelitis. If the spinal fluid is normal, a myelogram should be taken to demonstrate the spinal cord compression (Fig. 10–8). Dogs with an initial episode of pain may be treated medically, and in such cases conventional radiographs are not taken, since the risk of anesthesia largely outweighs the benefit of the procedure. If the diagnosis is not clear-cut, however, one should perform conventional radiography, CSF analysis, and myelography (if necessary) with the dog under anesthesia.

Treatment

Many dogs with cervical disk disease respond at least temporarily to nursing care that allows their spontaneous healing processes to operate. The risk of severe, permanent neurologic dysfunction is not as great in dogs with cervical disk disease as in those with thoracolumbar disk disease. Cervical disk disease therefore is usually not considered a major neurosurgical emergency.

There is a strong tendency to treat most patients with cervical disk disease medically, even though the majority of these cases relapse at a later date. Fenestration of the disks at an early stage in the disease prevents recurrences. Since severe herniations require decompression and recurrences are frequent, early fenestration is recommended. Decisions regarding medical or surgical therapy are based on the clinical signs and the chronicity of the problem.

Medical Therapy. Medical therapy for cervical disk disease, like that for thoracolumbar disk herniations, should be restricted to dogs with an initial episode of neck pain. Therapy must support normal healing processes but should not totally relieve the pain or inhibit any beneficial inflammatory processes. Anti-inflammatory drugs, such as glucocorticoids, are the mainstay of therapy. Prednisolone, 0.25 mg per lb every 12 hours, is given for 3 to 5 days. During this time, cage rest or total confinement is required. Collars and neck leashes should be avoided. A chest harness should be used when the animal is exercised on a leash. Analgesics and anti-inflammatory agents, such as aspirin with codeine or phenylbutazone, may be beneficial; however, one must be careful to enforce the instructions for strict cage confinement when these agents are used. Most dogs that are treated medically improve, only to relapse at a later date. Owners must be cautioned that medical therapy is seldom a total cure for cervical disk disease.

Surgical Therapy. The various forms of therapy have been reviewed extensively by Hoerlein.[1] There is general agreement that ventral fenestration is an effective procedure for dogs with recurrent cervical pain. The procedure is easy to perform and causes little postoperative reaction. This procedure will not remove disk material that is herniated into the vertebral canal. If the protrusion is large, the recovery will be slow or will not occur at all.[1]

Dogs with persistent pain following ventral fenestration or those with paresis, paralysis, and ataxia should undergo decompressive surgery. These clinical signs indicate that the disk material is compressing the cervical cord. The inflammatory process and the compression induced by the disk material seldom resolve with medical therapy. In addition, the disk material cannot be removed by ventral fenestration. Several decompressive techniques have been described, including partial spondylectomy and diskectomy with or without bone grafts (ventral slot, ventral decompression), dorsal laminectomy, and hemilaminectomy.[1] In most cases, the ventral slot technique is easiest to perform and affords nearly complete removal of the protruding mass with adequate decompression. The prognosis for functional recovery of most cervical disk patients following decompression is excellent. Occasionally, in large-breed dogs, recovery is slow and requires considerable physical therapy (see the section dealing with the management of canine wobbler syndrome).

CERVICAL MENINGOMYELITIS

Inflammation of the meninges by bacterial, viral, or fungal agents may produce clinical signs that are very similar to those of cervical disk disease. Cervical pain is frequent with meningitis. Involvement of the white or gray matter of the spinal cord results in paresis, paralysis, and sensory ataxia. These diseases usually are characterized by polysystemic signs and multifocal neurologic lesions. In many cases, the course becomes chronic and progressive following the acute development of neurologic signs. The diagnosis is primarily based on characteristic CSF abnormalities. These disorders will be discussed in Chapter 17.

EQUINE DEGENERATIVE MYELOENCEPHALOPATHY

Equine degenerative myeloencephalopathy (EDM) occurs in many breeds of horses (particularly Arabian) and zebras. It is characterized by an early onset (when the animal is 0 to 24 months old) of acute progressive symmetric ataxia and paresis. Chronic progressive forms of the disease have been described. Histopathologically, the disease is characterized by a diffuse myeloencephalopathy, with variations in the degree and the extent of the lesions.[4] There is consistent degeneration of white matter in all spinal cord funiculi, especially the dorsal spinocerebellar tracts in the thoracic segments. The etiology is unknown. The disease must be differentiated clinically from cervical spondylopathy and protozoal myeloencephalitis.

Clinical Signs

Signs develop in horses that are less than 2 years of age. In one study, this disease occurred five times more frequently in Arabian horses than in other breeds.[5] The signs are a symmetric UMN and a general proprioceptive deficit in all four limbs; however, the clinical signs are more severe in the pelvic limbs.[5] Although the disease is progressive, tetraplegia is rare. The early onset of signs (at a mean age of 0.4 year) and the marked disparity in the gait deficit between the thoracic and pelvic limbs help in the differentiation of EDM from focal cervical myelopathies.

Diagnosis

An antemortem diagnosis is difficult to confirm. Radiology of the cervical spine is useful for distinguishing EDM from cervical spondylopathy if rigid criteria are followed (see the section on cervical spondylopathy). There are few abnormalities in the CSF of horses with EDM, a feature that is useful for differentiating this disease from protozoal encephalomyelitis. Some horses with EDM have significantly increased concentrations of creatine phosphokinase in the CSF.[5]

Treatment

No effective treatment is known. The prognosis is poor, since recovery has not been reported.

Acute Nonprogressive Diseases, C1–C5

FIBROCARTILAGINOUS EMBOLIZATION

This syndrome was described in Chapter 9 because the disorder occurs most frequently in the caudal lumbar spinal cord; however, the disease also occurs in the caudal cervical cord. The clinical signs develop acutely and progress rapidly in 1 to 2 hours from initial pain to tetraparesis or hemiparesis (if only one side of the cord is involved). The signs suggest acute cervical cord compression; however, affected dogs experience much less pain than do dogs with cervical disk disease. Lesions in the caudal cervical cord frequently result in LMN signs in the thoracic limbs and UMN signs in the pelvic limbs. Lateralizing signs are suggestive of this disease. The diagnosis and management have been discussed in Chapter 9.

CERVICAL SPINAL CORD TRAUMA

Traumatic compression of the cervical cord, in contrast to the thoracolumbar spinal cord, is more likely to cause pain with little motor dysfunction; however, extensive compression will result in motor and sensory dysfunction. Injuries cranial to C5 may produce sudden death through disruption of the respiratory pathways to the phrenic and intercostal motor neurons. Therefore, tetraplegia with loss of deep pain sensation caudal to the lesion is rare, because affected animals die from respiratory failure. The pathophysiology, the diagnosis, and the management of spinal cord trauma have been discussed in Chapters 7 and 9.

Chronic Progressive Diseases, C1–C5

ATLANTOAXIAL SUBLUXATION

In 1967, a slowly progressive subluxation of the atlantoaxial articulation was described in ten small-breed dogs.[6] Since that time, a variety of lesions involving the atlas and the axis have been reported. Most of these lesions cause dorsal displacement of the axis into the spinal canal (Fig. 10–9A), resulting in compression of the cervical spinal cord.[7] These lesions include luxations with an intact dens, luxations with a congenital malformation of the dens (Fig. 10–9B), and fractures of the axis or the atlas.

Pathophysiology

Disorders of the atlantoaxial articulation usually result from a congenital malformation,

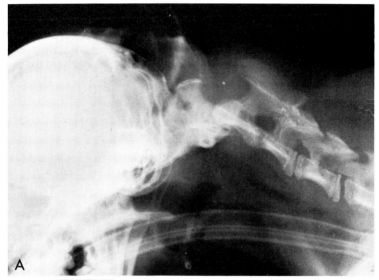

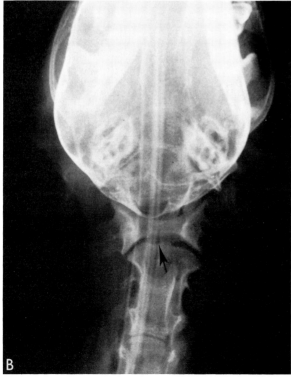

Figure 10–9. *A.* Lateral cervical radiograph of a dog with atlantoaxial subluxation. Note the dorsal displacement of C2, compressing the spinal cord at this level. *B.* Ventrodorsal radiograph of the same dog. Note the absence of a normal dens (*arrow*). (From Oliver, J. E., Jr., and Lewis, R. E.: Lesions of the atlas and axis in dogs. JAAHA 9:307, 1973. Used by permission.)

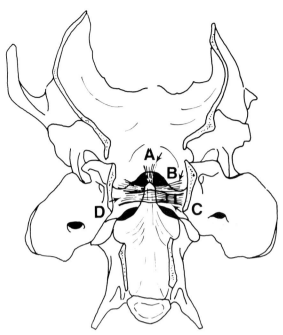

Figure 10–10. Drawing of the ligamentous attachments of the dens. *A* = Apical. *B* = Alar. *C* = Lateral. *D* = Transverse atlantal. (From Oliver, J. E., Jr., and Lewis, R. E.: Lesions of the atlas and axis in dogs. JAAHA 9:306, 1973. Used by permission.)

a traumatic fracture of the dens, or a traumatic tearing or stretching of the transverse atlantal ligament. The normal atlantoaxial articulation allows rotational movement. The dens projects from the body of the axis and is bound to the ventral arch of the atlas by a strong transverse ligament (Fig. 10–10). This attachment prevents flexion between the atlas and the axis (Fig. 10–11*A*). Disorders of this attachment allow the axis to rotate dorsally. The spinal cord is then compressed between the axis and the dorsal arch of the atlas (Fig. 10–11*B*). Cervical flexion accentuates the degree of spinal cord compression.

Atlantoaxial luxation with an intact dens results from traumatic rupture of the transverse atlantal ligament. Severe spinal cord compression occurs, because the cord is pinched between the intact dens and the dorsal atlantal arch (see Fig. 10–11*B*). Luxations caused by a fracture or a congenital malformation of the dens usually produce less severe neurologic signs, because less compression of the spinal cord occurs. Fractures of the body of the axis produce neurologic signs similar to those of acute traumatic luxation. Neurologic signs result from acute or chronic progressive com-

Figure 10–11. *A.* Drawing of the normal atlantoaxial articulation. *B.* Drawing of atlantoaxial subluxation resulting from separation of the dens from the body of the axis. Note the dorsal displacement of the axis pinching the spinal cord at this level.

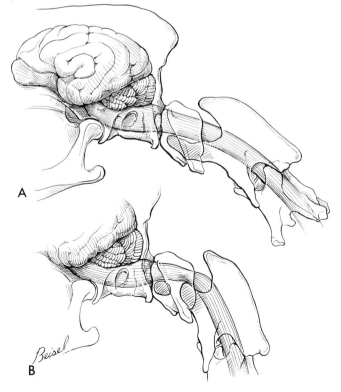

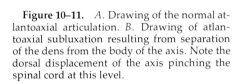

pressive myelopathy (see Chapter 9). The congenital disorders are usually more chronic with a gradual progression of neurologic signs. They occur most frequently in the toy or miniature breeds.

Clinical Signs

Traumatic luxations or fractures of C1, C2 result in acute compression of the cranial cervical spinal cord. Cervical pain and paresis, paralysis, and ataxia involving the thoracic and pelvic limbs are the usual signs. Neurologic signs develop acutely and may be asymmetric. Paresis or paralysis is of the UMN type. Dogs with congenital lesions usually develop signs before they are 1 year of age; however, older dogs also may develop signs. Some dogs may not develop clinical signs because adequate vertebral support by other fibrous and muscular structures prevents C1, C2 luxation. With age, these structures may weaken, allowing the axis to rotate dorsally and to compress the spinal cord. In the congenital form of the disorder, the initial clinical sign is usually cervical pain. The signs progress from pain to minor motor dysfunction to severe paresis or paralysis.[6,7]

The displaced axis may be palpated as a firm swelling just caudal to the occiput.[7] Flexing the neck results in severe pain and accentuates motor dysfunction. Neck flexion must be performed cautiously, because it can produce severe neurologic injury. Respiratory failure occurs when these pathologic events compromise respiratory pathways. *When atlantoaxial luxation or fractures are suspected, it is vital that extension of the neck be maintained.*[7]

Diagnosis

Atlantoaxial lesions must be suspected in all toy or miniature dogs with manifestations of rostral cervical pain, neck rigidity, and paresis or paralysis. Spinal radiography is useful for documenting the C1, C2 malalignment.[8] The survey spinal radiographs should be taken while the animal is awake. Anesthetized dogs do not maintain cervical muscle tension, which increases the possibility of neck flexion and severe spinal cord compression. In essence, an animal that is awake protects its injury. Lateral and ventrodorsal views should be taken. If the survey films demonstrate minor displacement, a definitive diagnosis can be formulated with the aid of radiographs taken with the dog anesthetized just prior to surgical fixation.[7] Careful neck flexion may be needed in order for the luxation to be demonstrated.

Treatment

Atlantoaxial luxations and most fractures require immediate surgical immobilization. Medical therapy is not beneficial and actually may increase the probability of more extensive spinal cord injury. Antiedema doses of dexamethasone and mannitol may be necessary for animals with traumatic lesions or during surgery to help control intraoperative spinal cord edema (see Chapter 7).

Several surgical techniques have been described.[6,7,9–11] The surgeon can stabilize luxations with or without fracture of the dens by wiring the arch of the atlas to the dorsal spinous process of the axis (Fig. 10–12). Most surgical techniques are based on modifications of this approach. Fractures of the atlas or the axis usually require decompression by hemilaminectomy in addition to stabilization. Pure C1, C2 luxations are usually adequately decompressed when the luxation is reduced. A hemilaminectomy may be required if the luxation cannot be reduced adequately.[7]

The prognosis for recovery is good if surgery is performed before irreversible spinal cord injury occurs.

EQUINE OCCIPITOATLANTOAXIAL MALFORMATIONS (OAAMs)

These congenital malformations can be divided into three clinical syndromes. Congenital asymmetric OAAM and asymmetric atlanto-occipital fusion have been reported in three breeds of horses.[5] Clinical signs include cervical scoliosis and a deviated head. Neurologic signs are uncommon. Familial occipitalization of the atlas with associated fusion of the axis and the atlas has been noted in Arabian foals.[5] Ataxia, tetraparesis, and a stiff neck may be found in neonates or in weanling foals. The abnormal cervical articulations usually can be palpated.

CERVICAL VERTEBRAL MALFORMATIONS

Cervical vertebral malformations with secondary spinal cord compression have been reported in young basset hounds, Great Danes, Doberman pinschers, and bullmastiffs and have appeared sporadically in other large breeds.[12–24] The syndrome is also reported in horses. Various names have been given to this syndrome, including *cervical spondylolisthesis*,[15] *cervical vertebral instability*,[16,17,24] *cervical vertebral malformation-malarticulation*,[19,22] and *cervical spondylopathy*.[18,20,21] *Canine wobbler syndrome* is a loosely applied name given

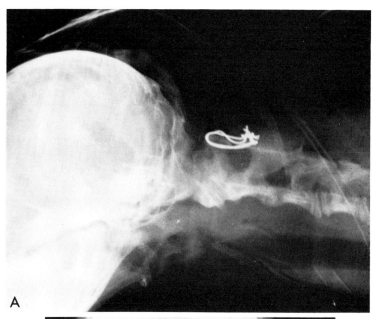

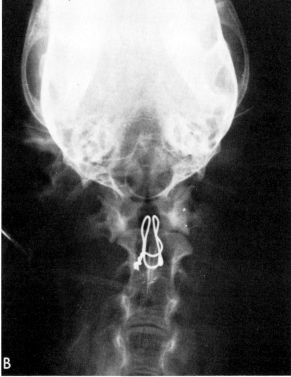

Figure 10–12. *A* and *B*. Lateral and ventrodorsal radiographs of a dog with atlantoaxial subluxation following reduction and wire stabilization. (From Oliver, J. E., Jr. and Lewis, R. E.: Lesions of the atlas and axis in dogs. JAAHA 9:310, 1973. Used by permission.)

to the neurologic phenomenon that results from cervical cord compression secondary to cervical spondylopathy. In most breeds, abnormalities are present in the caudal cervical region; however, cranial cervical vertebrae are involved in the basset hound. For this reason, the basset hound disease is discussed with the conditions that affect spinal cord segments C1–

C5. The disorders affecting other breeds of dog and those that affect horses will be discussed in subsequent sections of this chapter that deal with lesions involving spinal cord segments C6–T2.

In 1967, Palmer and Wallace first reported a form of paraparesis and tetraparesis in a family of basset hound puppies.[12] Clinical signs developed before the dogs had reached 6 months of age and were characterized as initial pelvic limb ataxia and paresis that progressed to the thoracic limbs. Some dogs developed tetraplegia, whereas others developed severe ataxia only. The neurologic signs resulted from progressive spinal cord compression at the C2–C3 and C3–C4 articulations. Radiographic and postmortem examinations revealed that a deformity of the body of the third cervical vertebra resulted in stenosis of the vertebral canal at C2–C3 and C3–C4. A compressive myelopathy that corresponded to these articulations was demonstrated. In addition, C2–C3 and C3–C4 malarticulations were present in three dogs. These vertebral changes are similar to the pathology encountered in other breeds that are affected with cervical spondylopathy. Pedigree analysis suggested an inherited basis for the disease. None of the puppies were treated.

Since the initial report in 1967, other workers have reported isolated cases of cervical spondylopathy in basset hounds.[20,21] In a survey of 35 dogs with cervical spondylopathy, Denny and coworkers found the disorder in three basset hounds.[20] One dog had radiographically demonstrated compression at C5, one at C3, and one at C3 and C5. A dorsal laminectomy was performed on the last dog at C2–C3 and C4–C5. Vertebral stabilization with screws placed in the bodies of C2–C3, C3–C4, and C4–C5 was attempted. The dog had normal neurologic function 6 weeks after surgery and was free of signs during the subsequent year of observation.

NEOPLASIA

Primary spinal cord tumors, such as neurofibromas, occasionally are encountered in the cervical spinal cord. The clinical signs are those of a slowly progressive myelopathy. Metastatic tumors to a cervical vertebra may result in a progressive myelopathy as the tumor grows into the vertebral canal. Mammary carcinomas, prostatic carcinomas, and hemangiosarcomas are some of the tumors that may spread to cervical vertebrae. Survey cervical radiographs or myelographic procedures are indicated to document the spinal cord compression or the vertebral lesion. The prognosis with or without surgery is poor.

NONEFFUSIVE FELINE INFECTIOUS PERITONITIS (FIP)

The noneffusive neurologic form of FIP may involve the cervical spinal cord. Affected cats develop asymmetric, progressive ataxia and tetraparesis. CSF analysis is helpful for confirming the diagnosis. This disease as well as other diffuse inflammatory conditions will be discussed in Chapter 17.

Diseases, C6–T2

The diseases affecting spinal cord segments C6–T2 are listed in Figures 10–3, 10–4, and 10–5. The acute progressive and acute nonprogressive disorders have been described previously in other sections. Of the chronic progressive disorders, only cervical spondylopathy is described here, because the other disorders are presented in other sections of this and other chapters.

CERVICAL SPONDYLOPATHY

The growing popularity of the giant-breed dogs and the performance horses during the past 20 years is probably responsible for the increased interest in this neurologic syndrome. The disorder appears with greater frequency in the Great Dane, the Doberman pinscher, and the Thoroughbred horse, but it has been recognized in several other breeds of dogs and horses. Controversy still exists regarding proper terminology for this syndrome. Presently, *cervical spondylopathy, cervical malformation-malarticulation*, and *cervical vertebral stenotic myelopathy* appear to be the most useful names, encompassing the forms of the disease in all affected animals. Some investigators prefer to lump all breeds together, whereas others prefer to split the disease into separate categories for each breed. Needless to say, each group of researchers has valid reasons for its decision. Our objective is to describe the similarities and the differences in the pathology and the management of each affected breed.

Pathophysiology

The pathology responsible for the clinical signs in the Great Dane, the Doberman pinscher, and the young Thoroughbred is the basic model with which the disease as it appears in other animals is compared. In affected animals, neurologic signs develop because of progressive spinal cord compression from surrounding vertebral structures. Abnormalities of the midcervical to the caudal cervical vertebrae or their articulations, or both, are the usual lesions that are demonstrated radiographically or at necropsy. Because the exact cause is unknown, the name *cervical spondylopathy* will be used as a broad term to encompass the various vertebral abnormalities.

Early studies suggested that excessive mobility of the caudal cervical vertebrae was primarily responsible for the cord compression. Subsequent studies demonstrated that malformation of the midcervical vertebrae resulted in stenosis of the vertebral canal.[25,26] These changes, which are more consistently present in the young Great Dane and the Doberman pinscher, include a narrowing and a dorsoventral flattening of the cranial vertebral foramen of C5, C6, and C7. The sixth cervical vertebra is usually most severely affected. In young Thoroughbred horses, these findings are more common at C3 and C4. Abnormalities in the size, the shape, or the position of the articular processes may be present. In some cases, hyperostosis of the articular facets may cause direct spinal cord compression. The malformation of the vertebrae tends to lead to malarticulation and vertebral instability. Instability without severe malformation often is seen in the Doberman pinscher. Apparently, in an attempt to correct the instability, soft tissues that support and strengthen the cervical articulations proliferate. In dogs and in some horses, hypertrophy of the interarcuate ligament, the dorsal longitudinal ligament, or the dorsal annulus may produce a soft tissue compression of the spinal cord at the vertebral articulations.

In the older Doberman pinscher, degeneration and protrusion of the lower cervical intervertebral disks are important in the development of clinical signs. In the reports in which primarily Doberman pinschers were studied, the majority of the radiographic, surgical, or necropsy findings in older dogs were highly suggestive of Type II disk disease.[16,17,21,24] Although there was other evidence of cervical spondylopathy in some dogs, it is not clear whether the disk changes were in fact caused by the cervical vertebral abnormalities. These findings have led to the speculation that the syndrome affecting the older Doberman pinscher is different from the syndrome affecting the young Great Dane. It has been demonstrated clearly that Type II disk disease must be ruled out carefully in older Doberman pinschers that have signs suggesting cervical spondylopathy. The management and the prognosis of the two conditions are considerably different in most cases.[24]

Although many factors, perhaps genetically controlled, may contribute to the development of cervical spondylopathy, the exact cause is unknown. Many of the large and giant breeds have been selected for their size and rapid growth. In horses, the disease occurs primarily in animals that are big for their age and breed. The very large head of certain breeds may exert an unusual force on structures that already have been genetically weakened (the midcervical to caudal cervical vertebrae). Great Danes, in particular, have been selected for a prancing, high-stepping gait that some consider to be a mild form of hypermetria. In selecting this gait, the breeder actually may have selected a neurologic-musculoskeletal disorder. One study of Great Danes established a relationship between excessive nutrition and several skeletal changes that also involved the cervical vertebrae.[27] Thus, nutritional factors also may be involved in the expression of clinical signs. The exact cause of the disorder awaits further clarification. The vertebral pathology is quite similar in the young Great Dane and the Thoroughbred horse.

Clinical Signs

In the majority of Great Danes and horses and in some Doberman pinschers, clinical signs develop at 3 to 18 months of age. In many Dobermans, clinical signs develop later in life (3 to 8 years of age). The disease usually occurs in horses that are less than 3 years of age.[28] Although most authors accept no sex predisposition, some studies report more affected male animals than female animals. This finding also has been noted in horses. Typical signs in dogs develop in the pelvic limbs and the pelvis as a mild lack of coordination that progresses to severe bilateral ataxia and hypermetria. The compression of ascending proprioceptive pathways is responsible for these neurologic signs. With increasing compression, the involvement of descending motor pathways produces paresis or paralysis of the UMN type. Although the site of compression is the cervical cord, clinical signs are usually more severe in the pelvic limbs. Ataxia and paresis in the thoracic limbs may be pronounced in some cases but are usually detectable only by certain neurologic examinations. Postural reaction deficits usually can be detected. Forcing the dog to wheelbarrow with its head extended (so that it cannot see the floor) accentuates proprioceptive deficits in the thoracic limbs. Some tetraparetic dogs and horses may have LMN signs in the thoracic limbs because of cervical gray matter involvement. Neck pain is usually absent unless the

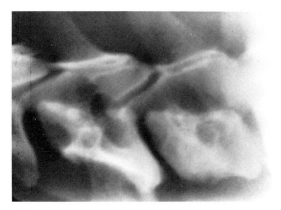

Figure 10–13. Lateral radiograph of a 6-year-old Doberman pinscher with tetraparesis and moderate caudal neck pain. The disk space at C5–C6 is narrowed, suggesting disk herniation.

disorder is also associated with cervical disk protrusion. Extension of the neck may elicit a pain response. The signs worsen progressively, and urinary incontinence is a common late manifestation in dogs. In some animals, trauma may precede the development of acute signs. Deep pain responses are usually preserved. Unlike the majority of dogs, most horses have an acute onset of ataxia, paresis, and spasticity of all four limbs. After an initial period of progression, the equine disease usually stabilizes. The abnormalities of the pelvic limbs are usually one grade worse than those of the thoracic limbs.[5,28]

Diagnosis

The diagnosis of cervical spondylopathy is confirmed radiographically. The radiographic findings have been reported extensively and will be summarized here. The changes ob-

served on survey radiographs, as classified by Chambers and Betts, include:

1. A change in shape or density, or both, in the intervertebral disk or the disk space, or both (Fig. 10–13). This change is more common in the older Doberman pinscher.
2. Changes in shape or density, or both, in the articular facets (sclerosis and exostosis) (Fig. 10–14).
3. Vertebral displacement (subluxation) (Fig. 10–15). This change is difficult to interpret when the cervical spine is in the flexed position, because the normal range of motion in these vertebrae is considerable.
4. Stenosis of the vertebral canal (See Fig. 10–15).
5. Malformed or misshaped vertebral bodies (Fig. 10–16).
6. Misshaped dorsal spinous processes.[21]

Several authors have questioned the safety and accuracy of stressed (flexion, extension) radiographic studies. Many normal anesthetized dogs appear to have borderline vertebral body subluxation when the cervical spine is flexed.[21] In addition, it is possible to traumatize the spinal cord further when these procedures are performed.

Minor changes in spinal canal architecture, soft tissue compression, or disk protrusions are detected only by myelographic examination. Because multiple lesions usually are present, myelography is recommended, so that the exact site or cause of the spinal cord compression can be identified (Fig. 10–17). Extension of the neck during the taking of myelograms often demonstrates soft tissue compression. Based on the myelographic results, rational surgical therapy can be instituted. Myelographic stud-

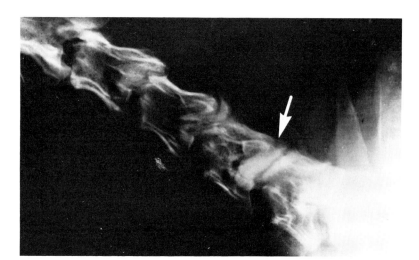

Figure 10–14. Myelogram of a 6-year-old Great Dane with tetraplegia. There is marked sclerosis and exostosis of the articular facets. The spinal canal is extremely narrowed at C5–C6 (*arrow*) by the changes in the bone. Euthanasia was performed.

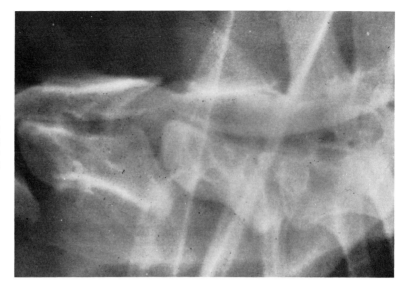

Figure 10–15. Myelogram of a 4-year-old Doberman pinscher with cervical spondylopathy. Note the subluxation of C6 and the stenosis of the vertebral canal at this level.

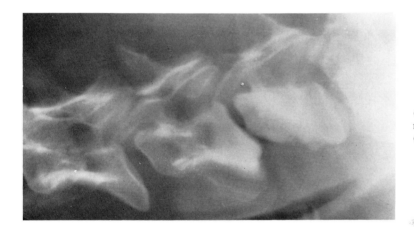

Figure 10–16. Misshaped C5 and C6 vertebrae in a 9-year-old Doberman pinscher with cervical spondylopathy.

Figure 10–17. Myelogram of the cervical area with the neck extended. Note the dorsal compression of the spinal cord from ligamentous proliferation in this area. Myelograms are needed in order to demonstrate compression by soft tissues in certain cases of cervical spondylopathy.

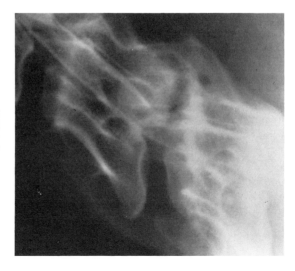

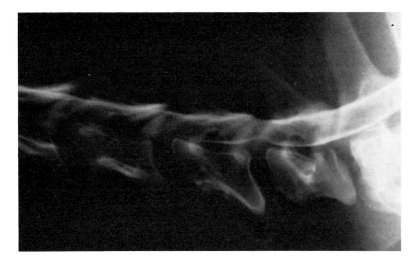

Figure 10–18. Myelogram of an adult Doberman pinscher with C5–C6 subluxation and disk protrusion at C6–C7.

ies are mandatory in the older Doberman pinscher in order to exclude disk disease as the primary cause of the neurologic signs (Fig. 10–18).

In the horse, cervical spondylopathy must be differentiated from degenerative myeloencephalopathy and protozoal myeloencephalitis. As in the dog, carefully performed cervical radiography can confirm the diagnosis in the horse. The radiographic techniques have been described adequately elsewhere.[29] Survey radiographs of the extended and hyperflexed cervical spine are taken. Metrizamide myelography then is performed. Several abnormalities may be detected:

1. a decrease in the minimum sagittal diameter of the cervical vertebral canal (less than 16 mm),[5,29]
2. a decrease in the minimum flexion diameter of the intervertebral spaces between adjacent vertebrae during flexion of the neck (less than 13 mm),[5,29]
3. a narrowing of the dorsal and ventral subarachnoid dye column with the cervical spine in the hyperflexed position (one of the most common radiographic lesions), usually at C3–C4,[29]
4. a remodeling of the caudal aspect of the cranial vertebrae at the affected sites,[29] and
5. proliferative lesions of the articular facets (usually C5–C6, C6–C7).[5,29]

Lesions in horses with cervical vertebral instability are demonstrated best with myelography of the hyperflexed neck. In general, compressive abnormalities are most apparent when the cervical spine is assessed myelographically.[29]

Therapy

Some dogs with mild neurologic signs improve with cage rest and corticosteroid therapy. The neurologic status usually deteriorates with resumption of normal activity. Therefore, the best long-term benefits are provided by surgical stabilization or decompression, or both. Several techniques have been described and are listed in Table 10–1. Some of these techniques require special orthopedic equipment, and the surgeon must decide which method best suits the patient's needs. Regardless of the procedure used, the surgical results largely depend upon the degree of spinal cord damage present at the time of surgery.

The medical therapy for equine cervical spondylopathy is similar to that for dogs. Since 1979, at least two surgical procedures to augment medical therapy have been described.[30] Ventral cervical fusion is indicated for those

Table 10–1. SURGICAL TECHNIQUES USED IN THE TREATMENT OF CERVICAL SPONDYLOPATHY

Procedure	References
Canine	
Plating of dorsal spines	13
Ventral vertebral body screws (with disk fenestration)	15,20,21,24
Dorsal laminectomy	19,20,21
Ventral decompression and fusion	19
Dorsal laminectomy—wire stabilization of articular facets	23
Equine	
Ventral cervical fusion	30
Subtotal dorsal decompression	30

horses with cord compression caused by cervical vertebral instability. In such cases, compression of the dorsal dye column does not occur when the neck is extended but is obvious when the neck is flexed. Subtotal dorsal decompression is used to treat stenotic lesions that cause cord compression irrespective of neck position (i.e., myelographic compression when the neck is extended). The results of surgery depend to some degree upon the severity, the distribution, and the duration of cervical cord compression.

Prognosis

In general, the prognosis for full recovery is poor, especially in tetraplegic dogs. Several factors contribute to the poor recovery rates, including (1) irreparable spinal cord damage, (2) failure to provide adequate decompression or stabilization, (3) development of compression at sites cranial to the initial lesions, and (4) postsurgical complications caused by failure to rehabilitate the recumbent large-breed dog. The prognosis is better in those cases in which the clinical signs result primarily from cervical disk protrusion or herniation. Most affected animals respond to ventral decompression with or without stabilization. Many dogs that initially benefited by surgery develop neurologic signs later in life because of compression at sites cranial to the initial lesion. Certain stabilization procedures actually may increase stress forces at intervertebral sites

Table 10–2. DIFFUSE LMN DISEASES

Acute progressive disorders
  Polyradiculoneuritis
  Tick paralysis
  Botulism
  Aminoglycoside paralysis
Chronic progressive disorders
  Motor neuronopathies
    Spinal muscle atrophy of Brittany spaniels
    Swedish Lapland dog paralysis
    Stockard's paralysis
  Polyneuritis (polyneuropathy)—see Table 10–4
  Muscle disorders
    Polymyositis
    Degenerative myopathy
    Myotonia
Episodic progressive disorders
  Myasthenic syndromes
  Metabolic (polysystemic) disorders (see Chapter 17)
    Hypoglycemia
    Hyperkalemia
    Hypercalcemia
    Hypocalcemia
    Hypomagnesemia
  Chronic relapsing polymyositis

cranial to the surgical sites. Owners should be warned that the surgery is difficult to perform and that the results may not be satisfactory.

In horses, the prognosis is poor without surgery. The results of ventral cervical fusion appear to be better than the results following subtotal dorsal decompression.

Diseases with Diffuse LMN Signs

Diseases that affect one or more components of the LMNs result in hyporeflexic or areflexic paresis or paralysis with little or no loss of pain perception. The various diseases listed in Table 10–2 can be classified as acute progressive, chronic progressive, or episodic. All are characterized by diffuse symmetric or asymmetric involvement of LMNs.

ACUTE PROGRESSIVE DISEASES

Polyradiculoneuritis (Coon-Hound Paralysis)

This acute neurologic syndrome has been recognized largely in hunting dogs that have been exposed to raccoons. It also has been observed in other dogs with no raccoon exposure. The disease is remarkably similar to acute polyneuritis in humans (Landry-Guillain-Barré syndrome).

Pathophysiology. The exact cause is not known, although an immunologic disturbance affecting myelin production has been suggested. Cummings suggests that raccoon bites or scratches provide the antigenic stimulation necessary for triggering the immune reaction.[31] The disease in human beings has been reported to have several causes, including respiratory infections and influenza vaccinations.

The disease attacks primarily the ventral roots and the spinal nerves. Characteristic microscopic lesions include segmental demyelination, degeneration of both myelin and axons, leukocyte infiltration, secondary degeneration of the ventral horn cells, and neurogenic muscle atrophy. Neurologic signs develop because motor signal transmission from the spinal cord to the muscle fibers is blocked. Pain perception is usually normal, because the dorsal root is only mildly affected in this disease. Diffuse hyperesthesia is occasionally seen.

Clinical Signs. Neurologic signs develop suddenly—in some cases, 7 to 14 days following raccoon exposure. Early clinical signs include pelvic limb paresis and hyporeflexia.

Ascending weakness or paralysis develops quickly. Affected dogs become tetraparetic 24 to 48 hours after the neurologic signs first develop. Spinal reflexes are severely depressed or absent. Passive flexion and extension of the limbs reveals severe hypotonus of affected muscles. Cerebral responses to painful stimuli are normal, or even exaggerated. Dogs with rapidly progressive disease may develop respiratory paralysis. Cranial nerve involvement is uncommon. The animal's voice is usually weak; the patient remains alert, responsive, and afebrile. The disease spares the sacral and coccygeal nerve roots. Defecation, urination, and tail mobility usually are normal. Muscle atrophy develops quickly and can be detected by direct palpation 10 to 14 days after the onset of paresis. Occasionally, the initial clinical signs are detected in the thoracic limbs and progress caudally to the pelvic limbs. The clinical course is usually 3 to 6 weeks. Improvement begins by the third week, and complete recovery may take 6 to 8 weeks. In patients that develop severe muscle atrophy, recovery may not be complete.

Diagnosis. The differential diagnosis should include tick paralysis and botulism, because these diseases have clinical signs that are essentially identical to those of the early stages of polyradiculoneuritis. Polyradiculoneuritis should be suspected when no ticks are found on physical examination and no exposure to botulism toxin is possible. Laboratory and radiographic studies are normal. A diagnosis of polyradiculoneuritis is supported by electromyographic (EMG) evidence of the diffuse denervation of affected muscles. These changes appear 5 to 7 days after the motor axon has been injured. EMG abnormalities include increased insertion activity, fibrillation potentials, and positive sharp waves. Evoked potentials are reduced in amplitude and may be polyphasic. Nerve conduction velocities may be normal or reduced. Table 10–3 compares the diagnostic features of polyradiculoneuritis, tick paralysis, and botulism.

Treatment. There is no specific treatment for polyradiculoneuritis. Despite its popularity, there is no evidence to support the use of glucocorticoid therapy, even though an immune reaction is suspected. In at least one human study, corticosteroids were associated with prolonged recovery times.[32] When corticosteroid therapy is employed, the agents are administered only during the first 48 to 72 hours of the illness. Their chronic use may foster urinary tract infection, muscle wasting, and delayed healing of decubital ulcers.

Supportive care consists of attentive nursing that (1) prevents decubital ulcers, (2) minimizes muscle atrophy and contractures, (3) prevents urinary tract infection, (4) prevents pneumonia, and (5) supports respiratory function. The animals should be bedded on deep straw or hay, air mattresses, sealed foam, or waterbeds. The patients should be turned frequently and kept clean. Voluntary micturition should be preserved; however, many dogs cannot produce a normal abdominal press and may fail to empty their bladders totally. Gentle

Table 10–3. DIAGNOSTIC COMPARISON OF ACUTE PROGRESSIVE LMN DISORDERS

	Polyradiculoneuritis	Tick Paralysis	Botulism
History	Single case; previous exposure to raccoon in some cases	Single case— engorged tick	Multiple cases are very suggestive; access to carrion
Pathophysiology	Nonsuppurative nerve inflammation and demyelination	Interference with action potential release of acetylcholine and action potential production	Block of neuromuscular transmission
Cranial nerve involvement	Rare	Rare	Usual
EMG	Fibrillation potentials and positive sharp waves	No denervation	Usually no denervation
Conduction velocity	Normal to decreased	Normal to slightly decreased	Normal
Evoked potentials	Reduced	Reduced	Reduced
Special tests	None	None	Toxin in feces, serum, and so forth
Treatment	Supportive	Tick removal	Polyvalent antitoxin, supportive
Recovery time	3 to 6 weeks	24 to 48 hours	2 to 3 weeks

manual expression of the bladder is helpful. Physical therapy, consisting of muscle massage and passive manipulation of the limbs, is important. Hydrotherapy is helpful for preventing muscle atrophy and contractures and for keeping the dog clean.

The prognosis for recovery is usually good. Recurrences have been observed. The course of the illness is 3 to 6 weeks. Recovery of neurologic function is usually in the reverse order of sign development.

Botulism

For many years, this disease was suspected in dogs but never documented. Carrion eaters and some carnivores, including dogs, were thought to be resistant to botulism toxin. In 1978, Barsanti and coworkers at the University of Georgia documented an outbreak of Type C botulism in foxhounds from northeastern South Carolina.[33] Previously, other workers from England and France had reported on outbreaks of this disease.[34,35] Before a detailed description of polyradiculoneuritis was published, many hunting dogs with acute progressive LMN disease were thought to have botulism or pseudobotulism. After Cummings' report on coon-hound paralysis, most dogs were thought to be affected with this disorder. Both conditions now are known to exist in dogs, and it can be difficult to make a differential diagnosis.

In large animals, botulism results from the ingestion of toxin or from the contamination of an ulcerated gastrointestinal tract with proliferating *Clostridium botulinum* spores. Outbreaks in cattle occur as a result of the ingestion of hay, ensilage, or water that has been contaminated by dead rodents. In horses, the disease is seen in foals 25 to 30 days old. Foals that are given highly nutritious feed develop gastrointestinal ulcers. These ulcers are colonized by *Cl. botulinum,* which then produces the offending toxin.

Pathophysiology. Clinical signs develop when the preformed toxin of *Clostridium botulinum* is ingested. Several different strains of exotoxin-producing organisms have been identified. Types A, B, and E are the strains most commonly associated with human disease. Types C and D, found in carrion, cause most cases of botulism in birds and mammals other than human beings. Botulinal toxin produces generalized neuromuscular blockade by inhibiting the release of acetylcholine from the terminals of cholinergic nerve fibers. The exact mechanism is unknown.

Clinical Signs. The incubation period is less than 6 days. The clinical signs are those of a progressive, symmetric, generalized LMN disorder. The severity of clinical signs varies with the amount of toxin ingested. Affected animals may develop only mild generalized weakness or tetraplegia with respiratory failure. Both cranial and spinal nerves are affected.[33] In dogs, the usual clinical course is less than 14 days.

Diagnosis. Botulism must be suspected in animals with acute progressive LMN disease. Botulism is especially likely to be present in cases of multiple animal involvement. Tick paralysis and polyradiculoneuritis are sporadic diseases involving individual animals. EMG studies can be used to differentiate botulism from polyradiculoneuritis by the lack of denervation in botulism. EMG findings in botulism include a small muscle action potential in response to a single supramaximal stimulus.[33] Nerve conduction velocities may be normal or slightly decreased.

Toxin identification in the food, the carrion, the serum, the feces, or the vomitus of an affected animal is necessary for the formulation of a conclusive diagnosis. The organism can be isolated from the viscera of clinically normal animals, and its isolation from feces therefore is insufficient for the formulation of a positive diagnosis.

Treatment. The treatment of botulism, like that of polyradiculoneuritis, is largely supportive. To be effective, the specific antitoxin must be administered before the botulinal toxin binds to receptors at the myoneural junction. It is rarely possible to achieve this timing, because the signs usually are present before the animal is treated. Polyvalent products that contain Type C antitoxin are recommended for dogs. The efficacy of antibiotic therapy has not been proved. The prognosis for recovery is generally good, unless the dog develops severe, rapidly progressive signs. Mildly affected animals recover without therapy.[33]

Tick Paralysis

This disease has been recognized worldwide for several years, but most in-depth reports have come from the United States and Australia. The clinical signs are similar to those of polyradiculoneuritis and botulism.

Pathophysiology. A neurotoxin secreted by engorged feeding female ticks either inhibits depolarization in the terminal portions of motor nerves or blocks the release of acetylcholine at the neuromuscular junction. The toxin may affect both motor and sensory nerve fibers by altering ionic fluxes that mediate action potential production.[36] In the United States, *Dermacentor andersoni* and *D. variabilis* are the primary ticks involved. In Australia, the disease is produced by *Ixodes holocyclus,* although *I. cornuatus* and *I. histi* are also incriminated.[37]

Clinical Signs. Clinical signs develop 7 to 9 days after attachment of the tick. The earliest clinical sign is marked ataxia with rapid progression to paresis, paralysis, areflexia, and hypotonus. In human beings, cases of primary ataxia and areflexia with little muscle weakness have been described.[38,39] Early tick paralysis in dogs may have similar signs. In the United States, cranial nerve involvement is rare. Nystagmus occasionally may be observed. Death can occur from respiratory failure if the ticks are not removed. Painful stimuli normally are perceived. In Australia, affected dogs or cats apparently develop more severe signs. Respiratory failure and retching occur with greater frequency in these animals than in those from the United States. In the Australian syndrome, clinical signs may worsen progressively, even though the ticks have been removed.[37] In the United States, dramatic improvement follows tick removal.

Diagnosis. Tick paralysis is diagnosed by the rapid improvement after tick removal. In unusual cases, EMGs can be used to differentiate this disease from acute polyradiculoneuritis.[40] EMG evidence of denervation is not found in tick paralysis. In tick paralysis, there is marked reduction in amplitude of evoked motor potentials. Nerve conduction velocities may be slightly slower than normal, and terminal conduction times may be prolonged.

Treatment. In the United States, removal of the tick results in marked improvement within 24 hours and complete recovery within 72 hours. Animals must be examined thoroughly for ticks. The areas evaluated should include the ear canals and the interdigital spaces. Ticks are removed carefully so that the head is not left embedded in the animal's skin. The toxin probably comes from the salivary glands of the tick. Failure to remove the head may result in a worsening of the clinical signs. Insecticide solutions should be sponged over the entire dog when ticks cannot be found and tick paralysis is suspected. In Australian tick paralysis, tick removal does not prevent further progression of the disease. The use of hyperimmune dog serum has been advocated to prevent death from respiratory failure.[37] In the United States, the prognosis for complete recovery is good.

Aminoglycoside Paralysis

The aminoglycoside antibiotics, when given parenterally, can cause neuromuscular blockade. Their effects are similar to those of curare. We have observed one animal that developed severe muscle weakness and hyporeflexia following 5 days of gentamycin therapy for deep pyoderma. The clinical signs resolved within 48 hours after the drug was discontinued.

CHRONIC PROGRESSIVE DISEASES

Motor Neuronopathies

These diseases are listed in Table 10–2. As a group, they are characterized by progressive degeneration of motor neurons in the gray matter of the spinal cord and the nuclei of the brain stem. Progressive denervation of muscle fibers results in paresis, paralysis, and severe muscle atrophy. The diseases in dogs resemble the inherited spinal muscular atrophies of human beings.

Brittany Spaniel Spinal Muscular Atrophy. This inherited disease was first reported in 1979 in a family of Brittany spaniel dogs in the southeastern United States.[41] The signs typically develop by the time the animal has reached 4 months of age. The characteristic signs include severe atrophy of the paraspinal and proximal pelvic girdle muscles. Affected animals walk with a crouched, waddling gait in the pelvic limbs. The involvement of the thoracic limbs is less severe. C.N. V, C.N. VII, and C.N. XII are involved in some dogs. The distal appendicular muscles tend to be spared. The disease progresses over several months to severe tetraparesis, respiratory failure, and death. A variant of the typical syndrome has been observed in puppies. These young dogs develop clinical signs at 4 to 6 weeks of age, and the disease rapidly progresses to severe paralysis within 4 to 6 months. Pathologic studies have established that degeneration of motor neurons produces the clinical signs. Breeding studies suggest a polygenic basis for the disease. The condition is nearly identical to juvenile spinal muscular atrophy of children. There is no effective known treatment.

Swedish Lapland Dog Paralysis. Dogs with this disorder develop paralysis at 5 to 7 weeks of age and within 2 weeks become tetraparetic.[42] There is no predilection for more severe involvement of the pelvic limbs, and weakness and atrophy are most conspicuous in the distal muscles. The disease shows little tendency to progress after the initial 2 weeks. The disease may be inherited as an autosomal recessive trait. There is no known effective treatment.

Stockard's Paralysis. This is a paraplegic syndrome that affects the offspring of Great Dane–bloodhound or Great Dane–Saint Bernard matings.[43] There is a predilection for pelvic limb involvement. Signs of pelvic limb paresis develop when the animal is 11 to 14 weeks of age and progressively worsen for a few days. Thereafter, the signs remain rather constant. There is preferential involvement of the distal muscles of the limbs.

Polyneuritis (Polyneuropathies)

These diseases are listed in Table 10–4.[46] They are well documented in human beings and occur sporadically in dogs. These diseases have an insidious onset and slowly progress over several months. Attacks of the disease may be disrupted by periods of spontaneous improvement. As Cummings and deLahunta have stated, "[C]hronic polyneuritis denotes a rather characteristic assemblage of clinical

Table 10–4. CAUSES OF POLYNEUROPATHY IN HUMAN BEINGS*

Polyneuropathy (Multiple Disorders)
Malnutrition and vitamin deficiency
Carcinoma and other malignancy
Collagen diseases
  Systemic lupus
  Rheumatoid arthritis
Diabetes mellitus†
Drugs or toxins
  Heavy metals
    Lead
    Mercury
    Thallium
    Copper, antimony, zinc
  Organophospate compounds
    (Triorthocresylphosphate)
  Industrial
    Trichloroethylene
    N-hexane
    Acrylamide
Hypothyroidism
Immune-mediated
  Acute polyneuritis†
  Chronic progressive or relapsing neuropathy†
  Hereditary neuropathy (neuronopathy)†

*Modified from Dyck, P. J.: Diseases of nerve roots, plexuses, and peripheral nerves. In Beeson, P. B., and McDermott, W.: Cecil and Loeb Textbook of Medicine. Philadelphia, W. B. Saunders Co., 1971.
†Existence is well-documented in dogs.

findings rather than a discrete disease entity."[44]

Idiopathic Polyneuritis. This disease affects mature dogs primarily. Signs of lameness, muscle atrophy, paresis, and, eventually, paralysis develop slowly over several months. Neurologic findings vary with the stage of the illness. Hopping responses and tendon reflexes are decreased. C.N. V and C.N. VII may be involved. Hypalgesia may occur later in the disease, when sensory nerves become involved. The clinical course varies from several months to years. This disease can resemble primary muscle disorders.

The diagnosis is made by biopsy of the muscles and the sensory nerves, EMG, and nerve conduction velocity studies. Evidence of peripheral nerve inflammation, denervation atrophy of muscle, and slow nerve conduction velocities and EMG evidence of denervation support the diagnosis. Pathologic studies of a few affected dogs suggest that nonsuppurative inflammation, perhaps with an immune basis, is responsible for the disease. Approximately 10 per cent of human patients with Landry-Guillain-Barré syndrome develop chronic relapsing or chronic progressive polyneuritis.[45] Some of these patients are benefited by corticosteroid therapy. At present, there appear to be no effective treatment strategies for the dog. Corticosteroid therapy should be evaluated once the diagnosis is confirmed.

Diffuse Muscle Disorders

Diseased muscles are usually weak. Muscle pain (myalgia), failure of muscles to relax (myotonia), and sudden muscle contraction (cramp) also suggest muscle disease. Myopathies include disorders characterized by weakness that does not have neurogenic causes. A myopathy may be a result of inflammation (myositis) or degeneration. Muscular dystrophies are progressive degenerative myopathies that are genetically determined. The signs of diffuse muscle disease are very similar to those of diffuse polyneuropathies. Because of the ambiguities in diagnosis, increasing attention has been given to three laboratory aids: serum enzyme levels, EMG and nerve conduction velocity (NCV) studies, and muscle biopsy. A classification of animal myopathies is presented in Table 10–5. These diseases will be discussed briefly in subsequent sections of this chapter.

Polymyositis. Polymyositis is classified as diffuse muscle inflammation of infectious or noninfectious origin (Table 10–5).[47] Inflamma-

Table 10–5. CAUSES OF
POLYMYOPATHY IN ANIMALS*

Inflammatory
  Infectious
    Toxoplasma gondii
    Leptospira icterohaemmorrhagiae
    Clostridium species
  Noninfectious
    Idiopathic polymyositis
    Systemic lupus erythematosus–polymyositis
    Eosinophilic myositis
Degenerative
  Inherited†
    Irish terrier myopathy
    Labrador retriever myopathy
    Chow myopathy
  Nutritional (white muscle disease)
    Vitamin E deficiency
    Selenium deficiency
  Endocrine
    Hyperadrenocorticism (steroid myopathy)†
    Hypothyroidism
  Exertional rhabdomyolysis

*Modified from Kornegay, J. N., Gorgacz, E. J., Dawe, D. L., Bowen, J. M., White, N. A., and De Buysscher, E. V.: Polymyositis in the dog. JAVMA 176:431, 1980.
†Diseases associated with myotonia.

tions of noninfectious origin appear to be immune-mediated. The most common clinical signs include muscle pain, weakness, a stilted gait, and fever. Less frequent signs include muscle atrophy, depression, anorexia, weight loss, and voice change.[47] Regurgitation may develop in dogs that have diseased esophageal muscles and megaesophagus. Signs may be episodic—characterized by acute attacks followed by periods of spontaneous remission. Other dogs have chronic progressive signs. The clinical signs resemble those of chronic polyneuritis or myasthenic syndromes. The acute, painful episodes must be differentiated from meningitis and skeletal diseases.

A definitive diagnosis of polymyositis is based upon (1) evidence of muscle pain or weakness, (2) elevations in the concentrations of serum muscle enzymes (CPK, LDH, SGOT), (3) EMG abnormalities, and (4) histopathologic evidence of muscle necrosis and inflammation.[47,48] A probable diagnosis can be made when three of these four findings are present. There appears to be little correlation between muscle enzyme concentrations and either the severity of clinical signs or the degree of muscle necrosis or inflammation on biopsy.[47] EMG changes include fibrillation potentials, polyphasic motor unit potentials, motor unit potentials of decreased duration, positive potentials, and increased insertional activity. The

fading of evoked motor unit potentials, reversed with neostigmine, has been reported.[47] Pathologic changes may include muscle fiber necrosis, muscle regeneration, and variable fiber size and hyaline fibers. Inflammatory cells include lymphocytes and some neutrophils. Eosinophilic inflammation has been reported.[49]

Idiopathic polymyositis should be treated with prednisone, 2.0 mg per kg per day, until remission is achieved. Alternate-day steroid therapy then is instituted in order to maintain remission. Dogs with megaesophagus may develop aspiration pneumonia. Management of these cases is difficult, and the prognosis is poor for regaining normal esophageal function.

Degenerative Myopathies. These disorders have been reported in the Irish terrier and Labrador retriever breeds. The myopathy of Irish terriers appears to be sex-linked and is characterized by a stiff gait and a weakness that develop after the animal has reached 8 weeks of age.[50] Dysphagia and muscle atrophy occur in most cases. Skeletal muscle changes include degeneration, calcification, and mild to moderate inflammatory cell infiltration. Prolonged high-frequency discharges have been found on EMG examination (see the section on myotonia). The myopathy affecting Labrador retrievers becomes clinically evident before the dogs have reached 6 months of age.[51] Affected dogs appear stiff and walk with a hopping gait. Muscle atrophy and weakness are noticeable. Myopathic changes include variably sized muscle fibers, an increase in muscle connective tissue, and a decreased number of Type II fibers. The disease is not progressive.

Nutritional Myopathies (White Muscle Disease). White muscle disease is a degenerative myopathy of calves and lambs, caused by a dietary deficiency of α-tocopherol or selenium.[52] Two forms of the disease exist in calves. An acute form is characterized by sudden death resulting from cardiac muscle degeneration during exertion or exercise. The second form is marked by a gradual onset of tetraparesis in calves 2 weeks of age or older. Lambs develop similar signs and are affected when they are 10 days to 2 months of age. Lambs may have a stiff gait and tetraparesis. Other diseases linked to a selenium deficiency include mulberry heart disease in baby pigs, white muscle disease in foals, the equine tying-up syndrome, and retained placenta in cattle.

The diagnosis is based on clinical signs, biopsy of affected muscles, quantitation of glutathione peroxidase levels, and the animal's response to therapy. In the skeletal form of the disease, muscle degeneration is characterized by symmetric grayish or white streaks in groups of skeletal muscle. Selenium–α-tocopherol preparations are very beneficial if the signs are severe. Diets should be corrected if selenium deficiencies are found. Selenium can be highly toxic if it is used at high concentrations.

Exertional Rhabdomyolysis. This disorder of racing greyhounds and horses develops from local muscle ischemia. The final event appears to be muscle swelling and necrosis. Gannon has categorized the clinical signs in dogs as hyperacute, acute, and subacute.[53] Factors that tend to lead to the syndrome include (1) a lack of physical fitness, (2) excitement prior to racing, (3) hot and humid conditions, and (4) excessive frequency of running. In the more acute forms of the disease, clinical signs are observed during the race. The most severe signs include generalized muscle pain, hyperpnea, and heavy myoglobinuria. Death may occur within 48 hours. In the milder (subacute) form of the disease, muscle pain is confined to the longissimus thoracis muscle and may not be apparent for 24 to 72 hours after the race. Myoglobinuria is rarely observed in subacute exertional rhabdomyolysis.

The hyperacute and acute forms of the disease are treated in a similar fashion. Intravenous fluids are given to treat or to prevent hypovolemic shock and to aid in the renal excretion of myoglobin. Sodium bicarbonate is added to the fluid to combat muscle acidosis and to help prevent the precipitation of myoglobin in rental tubules. The patient is cooled to help remove excess heat. Other treatments to be considered include anabolic steroids, oral sodium bicarbonate, B vitamins, and analgesics.

The prophylactic therapy that should be contemplated includes (1) installation of air conditioning in kennels, (2) reduction of the body temperature with cool-water baths before racing, (3) administration of oral bicarbonate-glucose solutions prior to kenneling for the race, (4) alkalinization of the urine with sodium bicarbonate or potassium citrate, (5) administration of oral potassium supplement, and (6) decreasing the frequency of racing.[53]

Myotonia. A contraction of muscle that persists after the cessation of voluntary effort or stimulation is called myotonia (if generalized) or a cramp (if localized). Myotonia occurs in a number of canine muscle disorders. Affected animals have difficulty in rising and walk with a stiff gait. There is an inability to flex the stifle joints, and a bunny hop or a shuffling gait may develop. Muscle hypertrophy may be present on palpation. Percussion of the muscles may elicit a dimple. The limbs may be hyperextended and are difficult to flex.

A form of myotonia has been reported in the chow chow. Myopathic changes are variable but include hypertrophy of the fibers from the proximal muscles, variability in muscle fiber size, fiber degeneration and regeneration, hyaline fibers, and an increase in muscle connective tissue. The disease usually is manifested when the animal is 2 to 3 months of age, and there is evidence that it represents an inherited progressive degenerative myopathy similar to human myotonia congenita.[54] Both insertional and spontaneous high-frequency discharges are found on EMG examinations. These typical myotonic discharges increase and decrease in both frequency and amplitude. There is no definitive therapy for the myopathy; however, both procainamide and phenytoin are useful for the management of human myotonia congenita. These drugs usually are not effective in chow chows.[54]

Steroid-Induced Myopathy. This muscle disease is caused by exogenous or endogenous glucocorticoids. It is observed in both spontaneous and iatrogenic Cushing's disease. Dogs with steroid-induced myopathy develop muscle atrophy and weakness. Some develop an associated myotonia-like syndrome. Bizarre high-frequency discharges that do not wax and wane are typical EMG findings. The exact biochemical cause of steroid-induced myopathy is not known. Disturbances of calcium metabolism have been suggested. Myopathic changes include fiber atrophy, necrosis, regeneration, and increased muscle fat and connective tissue. Withdrawal of exogenous steroids or suppression of endogenous steroids may benefit many dogs greatly. Dogs with severe disease may not improve even after plasma steroid levels are decreased. Even in dogs that improve with appropriate therapy, bizarre high-frequency discharges can be detected in muscles several years after remission has been achieved.[55]

EPISODIC PROGRESSIVE DISEASES

Diseases in which episodes of weakness are interspersed with periods of normality are perplexing, because many different body systems may be envolved. Episodic weakness

Table 10–6. EPISODIC PROGRESSIVE DISEASES

Diseases	Diagnostic Tests
Metabolic disorders (see Chapter 17)	
Hyperkalemia	Serum potassium levels, electrocardiogram (EKG)
Adrenal insufficiency	Plasma cortisol levels
Severe acidosis	Blood gases and pH
Severe renal failure	Blood urea nitrogen (BUN) levels, urinalysis
Hypokalemia	Serum potassium levels
Hypocalcemia	Serum calcium and phosphorus levels
Hypoparathyroidism	Serum parathyroid hormone (PTH) assay
Hypercalcemia	Serum calcium levels
Primary hyperparathyroidism	Serum PTH assay, parathyroid mass
Pseudohyperparathyroidism	Evidence of lymphosarcoma
Hypoglycemia	Fasting blood glucose levels
Functional beta cell carcinoma	Amended glucose insulin ratio
Glycogen storage disease	Glucagon response test, tissue biopsy
Adrenal insufficiency	Plasma cortisol levels
Cardiovascular disorders	
Arrhythmias	EKG
Conduction disturbances	EKG
Congestive heart failure	EKG, thoracic radiographs
Dirofilariasis	Thoracic radiographs, modified Knott test
Neuromuscular Disorders	
Myasthenia gravis	Repetitive nerve stimulation, anticholinesterase testing
Polymyositis	Serum muscle enzyme levels, muscle biopsy, EMG

usually results from cardiovascular, metabolic, or neuromuscular diseases (Table 10–6). The primary neuromuscular disorder is myasthenia gravis, which will be discussed in this section. The endocrine-metabolic causes will be discussed in Chapter 17.

Myasthenia Gravis

Pathophysiology. Myasthenia gravis is a disease involving the motor end-plate that results in progressive loss of muscle strength with exercise. The basic defect is a reduction of available acetycholine receptors at neuromuscular junctions, which is caused by autoimmune attack.[56] Human myasthenic muscles have a 70 to 90 per cent reduction in the number of acetylcholine receptors per motor end-plate. The decreased number of available receptors reduces the probability that acetylcholine molecules will react with muscle receptor sites. The safety margin of neuromuscular transmission is greatly reduced in myasthenia gravis. With repeated nerve stimulations of the motor end-plate, severe muscle weakness results.

In human beings, myasthenia gravis has been associated with several thymic disorders and other autoimmune diseases. Recent studies have demonstrated that antimuscle membrane antibodies are present in the serum of myasthenic patients. A reaction of these antibodies with acetylcholine receptors results in the muscle weakness that is characteristic of myasthenia gravis. Myasthenic syndromes have been well documented in the dog; however, studies confirming that the canine disease has a pathogenesis similar to that of true myasthenia gravis have not been completed.

Clinical Signs. With exercise, muscle weakness becomes progressively worse. This phenomenon is most apparent in the appendicular muscles. Animals become fatigued, develop a shortened stride, and then lie down to rest. Strength improves with rest. Ptosis of the upper eyelids and drooping of the lips occur in some dogs with weak facial muscles. Sialosis, regurgitation of food, and dysphagia develop in a high percentage of cases. Megaesophagus is common, because the esophagus of the dog contains a considerable amount of striated muscle. Aspiration pneumonia occurs in many dogs with megaesophagus.

Diagnosis. The formulation of the diagnosis is aided by the exclusion of cardiovascular and metabolic diseases with appropriate laboratory or electrophysiologic tests. The examiner makes a definite diagnosis of myasthenia gravis by finding a decremental response in the amplitude of motor unit potentials induced by repetitive nerve stimulation at a rate of 30 stimuli per second. After the initial nerve stimulation studies, anticholinesterase drugs, such as edrophonium chloride (Tensilon) or neostigmine, are given. Repetitive nerve stimulation studies then are performed again. The anticholinesterase drugs should prevent the decremental response in the amplitude of motor unit potentials.

In field testing, the diagnosis of myasthenia gravis has been supported by the administration of edrophonium or neostigmine. The patient is exercised until weakness develops. Edrophonium or neostigmine is given by parenteral injection. The patient is then exercised again and is watched for evidence of increased strength and endurance. Care must be exercised both in the performance and in the interpretation of the test results. The anticholinesterase drugs may cause excessive muscle depolarization (cholinergic crisis), vomiting, salivation, and defecation. In addition, these drugs may improve the strength of dogs that are affected with primary muscle disease (polymyositis). A definitive diagnosis must be based on electrodiagnostic techniques.

Treatment. Once the diagnosis has been confirmed, initial therapy consists of the administration of anticholinesterase agents. Neostigmine bromide, 0.5 mg per kg per os, or pyridostigmine bromide, 2.0 mg per kg per os, is given as needed to control the clinical signs. If the results are not satisfactory, one should consider the addition of glucocorticoids, such as prednisone, at a dosage of 0.50

to 1.0 mg per kg per day. This dosage can be increased to 1.0 to 2.0 mg per kg per day after a few days. Once remission is achieved, the patient is continued on alternate-day steroid therapy at a dosage of 2.0 mg per kg. The dosage of anticholinesterase drugs is gradually decreased and, if possible, eliminated. Drastic changes in the therapy should not occur. Thymectomy should be considered for those dogs that respond poorly to medical therapy.

Some dogs with myasthenia-like syndromes spontaneously improve, or the condition resolves after several weeks. In human patients, in contrast, the disease tends to get progressively worse with time. The prognosis is poor for dogs with megaesophagus. The eosphageal dilatation is permanent in many dogs, although this abnormality has been reported to resolve with anticholinesterase therapy.

CASE HISTORIES

Case History 10A

Signalment

Canine, mixed breed, male, 6 months old.

History

An acute onset of tetraparesis progressed rapidly to total hypotonic paralysis. The dog has been paralyzed for 24 hours.

Physical Examination

Negative except for the neurologic problem.

Neurologic Examination *

A. Observation
  1. Mental status: Alert.
  2. Posture: Recumbent.
  3. Gait: The dog cannot support weight or maintain sternal recumbency. Tetraplegia. The dog can wag his tail.

B. Palpation
  The limbs are very hypotonic.

C. Postural Reactions

Left	Reactions	Right
0	Proprioceptive positioning PL	0
0	TL	0
0	Wheelbarrowing	0
0	Hopping, PL	0
0	Hopping, TL	0
0	Extensor postural thrust	0
0	Hemistand-hemiwalk	0
0	Tonic neck	0
0	Placing, tactile PL	0
0	TL	0
0	Placing, visual TL	0

Key: 0 = absent, +1 = decreased, +2 = normal, +3 = exaggerated, +4 = very exaggerated or clonus, PL = pelvic limb, TL = thoracic limb.

D. Spinal Reflexes

Left	Reflex Spinal Segment	Right
0	Quadriceps L4−L6	0
+1	Extensor carpi radialis C7−T1	+1
+1	Triceps C7−T1	+1
0 to +1	Flexion, PL L5−S1	0 to +1
0 to +1	Flexion, TL C6−T1	0 to +1
0	Crossed extensor	0
+2	Perineal S1−S2	+2

E. Cranial Nerves

Left	Nerve + Function	Right
+2	C.N. II vision menace	+2
Nor.	C.N. II + C.N. III pupil size	Nor.
+2	Stim. left eye	+2
+2	Stim. right eye	+2
Nor.	C.N. II fundus	Nor.
0	C.N. III, C.N. IV, C.N. VI Strabismus	0
0	Nystagmus	0
+2	C.N. V sensation	+2
Nor.	C.N. V mastication	Nor.
Nor.	C.N. VII facial muscles	Nor.
+2	Palpebral	+2
+2	C.N. IX, C.N. X swallowing	+2
Nor.	C.N. XII tongue	Nor.

F. Sensation: Location
  Hyperesthesia _____ None _____
  Superficial pain _____ +2 _____
  Deep pain _____ +2 _____

Complete sections G and H before reviewing Case Summary.

G. Assessment (Anatomic diagnosis and estimation of prognosis)

H. Plan (Diagnostic)
  Rule-outs   Procedure
  1.
  2.
  3.
  4.

Case History 10B

Signalment

Canine, miniature schnauzer, male, 6 years old.

History

The dog had a sudden onset of falling to the right with weakness of both pelvic limbs and paralysis of the right thoracic limb. No previous trauma. The signs began 7 days ago.

Physical Examination

Negative except for the neurologic problem.

Neurologic Examination *

A. Observation
1. Mental status: Alert.
2. Posture: Lateral recumbency.
3. Gait: The dog can stand if assisted for a short period of time. He knuckles severely on the right limbs.

B. Palpation
Atrophy of the right supraspinatus, deltoid, and triceps muscles.

C. Postural Reactions

Left	Reactions	Right
+2	Proprioceptive positioning PL	0
+2	TL	+1
+2	Wheelbarrowing	+1
+2	Hopping, PL	0
+2	Hopping, TL	+1
+2	Extensor postural thrust	0
+2	Hemistand-hemiwalk	0
+2	Tonic neck	+1
+2	Placing, tactile PL	0
+2	TL	+1
+2	Placing, visual TL	+1

D. Spinal Reflexes

Left	Reflex / Spinal Segment	Right
+2	Quadriceps L4−L6	+3
+2	Extensor carpi radialis C7−T1	+1
+2	Triceps C7−T1	+1
+2	Flexion, PL L5−S1	+2
+2	Flexion, TL C6−T1	+1
0	Crossed extensor	Present
+2	Perineal S1−S2	+2

E. Cranial Nerves

Left	Nerve + Function	Right
+2	C.N. II vision menace	+2
Nor.	C.N. II + C.N. III pupil size	Nor.
+2	Stim. left eye	+2
+2	Stim. right eye	+2
Nor.	C.N. II fundus	Nor.
0	C.N. III, C.N. IV, C.N. VI Strabismus	0
0	Nystagmus	0
Nor.	C.N. V sensation	Nor.
+2	C.N. V mastication	+2
Nor.	C.N. VII facial muscles	Nor.
+2	Palpebral	+2
Nor.	C.N. IX, C.N. X swallowing	Nor.
+2	C.N. XII tongue	+2

F. Sensation: Location
Hyperesthesia _____ None _____
Superficial pain _____ +2 _____
Deep pain _____ +2 _____

Complete sections G and H before reviewing Case Summary.

G. Assessment (Anatomic diagnosis and estimation of prognosis)

H. Plan (Diagnostic)
Rule-outs   Procedure
1.
2.
3.
4.

*Key: 0 = absent, +1 = decreased, +2 = normal, +3 = exaggerated, +4 = very exaggerated or clonus, PL = pelvic limb, TL = thoracic limb.

Case History 10C

Signalment

Canine, miniature poodle, male, 11 years old.

History

One month ago, lameness developed in the left thoracic limb followed by progression to both thoracic limbs within 7 days. Two weeks later, the dog developed ataxia of both pelvic limbs and one week ago, he developed severe paresis of both pelvic limbs. The dog does not wag his tail.

Physical Examination

Grade IV/VI holosystolic mitral murmur. Fluid lung sounds. Severe periodontal disease.

Neurologic Examination *

A. Observation
  1. Mental status: Alert.
  2. Posture: Recumbent (sternal).
  3. Gait: Tetraparesis.

B. Palpation
  Extensor rigidity of thoracic limbs. Hypertonus of pelvic limbs.

C. Postural Reactions

Left	Reactions	Right
	Proprioceptive positioning PL	
0		0
0	TL	0
0	Wheelbarrowing	0
0	Hopping, PL	0 to +1
0	Hopping, TL	0 to +1
0	Extensor postural thrust	0
0	Hemistand-hemiwalk	0
0	Tonic neck	0
0	Placing, tactile PL	0
0	TL	0
0	Placing, visual TL	0

*Key: 0 = absent, +1 = decreased, +2 = normal, +3 = exaggerated, +4 = very exaggerated or clonus, PL = pelvic limb, TL = thoracic limb.

D. Spinal Reflexes

Left	Reflex Spinal Segment	Right
+2	Quadriceps L4−L6	+3
+2	Extensor carpi radialis C7−T1	+3
+2	Triceps C7−T1	+3
+2	Flexion, PL L5−S1	+2
+2	Flexion, TL C6−T1	+2
0	Crossed extensor	0
+2	Perineal S1−S2	+2

E. Cranial Nerves

Left	Nerve + Function	Right
+2	C.N. II vision menace	+2
Nor.	C.N. II + C.N. III pupil size	Nor.
+2	Stim. left eye	+2
+2	Stim. right eye	+2
Nor.	C.N. II fundus	Nor.
0	C.N. III, C.N. IV, C.N. VI Strabismus	0
0	Nystagmus	0
Nor.	C.N. V sensation	Nor.
Nor.	C.N. V mastication	Nor.
Nor.	C.N. VII facial muscles	Nor.
+2	Palpebral	+2
Nor.	C.N. IX, C.N. X swallowing	Nor.
Nor.	C.N. XII tongue	Nor.

F. Sensation: Location
  Hyperesthesia   Mild in cervical area
  Superficial pain   Good
  Deep pain   Good

Complete sections G and H before reviewing Case Summary.

G. Assessment (Anatomic diagnosis and estimation of prognosis)

H. Plan (Diagnostic)
  Rule-outs   Procedure
  1.
  2.
  3.
  4.

Case History 10D

Signalment

Canine, poodle, male, 1 year old.

History

Five weeks ago the dog experienced severe pain and could not walk up or down stairs. The head was slightly flexed, and the neck was stiff. One week ago, the dog bumped his head, cried out in pain, fell down, and became stiff. He cries out when the head is moved.

Physical Examination

Negative except for 5 per cent dehydration and the neurologic problem.

Neurologic Examination *

A. Observation
  1. Mental status: Alert; cries out if manipulated.
  2. Posture: Lateral recumbency; neck is flexed and rigid.
  3. Gait: Severe tetraparesis.

B. Palpation
  The thoracic limbs are in extensor rigidity. Open fontanelle.

C. Postural Reactions

Left	Reactions	Right
	Proprioceptive positioning	
+1	PL	+1
+1 to +2	TL	+1 to +2
+1	Wheelbarrowing	+1
+1	Hopping, PL	+1
+1	Hopping, TL	+1
+1	Extensor postural thrust	+1
+1	Hemistand-hemiwalk	+1
Not present	Tonic neck	Not present
	Placing, tactile	
0	PL	0
+1	TL	+1
	Placing, visual	
+1	TL	+1

*Key: 0 = absent, +1 = decreased, +2 = normal, +3 = exaggerated, +4 = very exaggerated or clonus, PL = pelvic limb, TL = thoracic limb.

D. Spinal Reflexes

Left	Reflex Spinal Segment	Right
	Quadriceps	
+3	L4–L6	+3
	Extensor carpi radialis	
+3	C7–T1	+3
	Triceps	
+3	C7–T1	+3
	Flexion, PL	
+2	L5–S1	+2
	Flexion, TL	
+2	C6–T1	+2
0	Crossed extensor	0
	Perineal	
+2	S1–S2	+2

E. Cranial Nerves

Left	Nerve + Function	Right
	C.N. II vision	
+2	menace	+2
Nor.	C.N. II + C.N. III pupil size	Nor.
+2	Stim. left eye	+2
+2	Stim. right eye	+2
Nor.	C.N. II fundus	Nor.
	C.N. III, C.N. IV, C.N. VI	
0	Strabismus	0
0	Nystagmus	0
Nor.	C.N. V sensation	Nor.
Nor.	C.N. V mastication	Nor.
Nor.	C.N. VII facial muscles	Nor.
+2	Palpebral	+2
Nor.	C.N. IX, C.N. X swallowing	Nor.
Nor.	C.N. XII tongue	Nor.

F. Sensation: Location
  Hyperesthesia _____Cervical_____
  Superficial pain _____Good_____
  Deep pain _____Good_____

Complete sections G and H before reviewing Case Summary.

G. Assessment (Anatomic diagnosis and estimation of prognosis)

H. Plan (Diagnostic)
  Rule-outs   Procedure
  1.
  2.
  3.
  4.

Case History 10E

Signalment

Canine, Doberman pinscher, male, 2 years old.

History

For several months, the dog has had knuckling, ataxia, and paresis in the pelvic limbs. He occasionally knuckles on the thoracic limbs. He has been treated with intramuscular injections of corticosteroids that gave temporary improvement. He recently developed paralysis of the right pelvic limb.

Physical Examination

Negative except for the neurologic signs described in the next section.

Neurologic Examination *

A. Observation
   1. Mental status: Alert.
   2. Posture: Ambulatory.
   3. Gait: Paraparesis and ataxia. Occasionally knuckles on the thoracic limbs.

B. Palpation
   Stiff neck. Muscle atrophy is severe in the right pelvic limb below the stifle. Abrasions are present on the dorsal surface of the right pelvic foot.

C. Postural Reactions

Left	Reactions	Right
	Proprioceptive positioning	
0	PL	0
+2	TL	+2
Knuckles	Wheelbarrowing	Knuckles
+1	Hopping, PL	0
+2	Hopping, TL	+2
+1	Extensor postural thrust	+1
+1	Hemistand-hemiwalk	+1
Knuckling	Tonic neck	Knuckling
	Placing, tactile	
+1	PL	0
+2	TL	+2
	Placing, visual	
+2	TL	+2

Key: 0 = absent, +1 = decreased, +2 = normal, +3 = exaggerated, +4 = very exaggerated or clonus, PL = pelvic limb, TL = thoracic limb.

D. Spinal Reflexes

Left	Reflex Spinal Segment	Right
	Quadriceps	
+3	L4−L6	+3
	Extensor carpi radialis	
+3	C7−T1	+3
	Triceps	
+2	C7−T1	+2
	Flexion, PL	Flexes
+2	L5−S1	0: at hip
	Flexion, TL	
+2	C6−T1	+2
0	Crossed extensor	0
	Perineal	
+2	S1−S2	+2

E. Cranial Nerves

Left	Nerve + Function	Right
	C.N. II vision	
+2	menace	+2
Nor.	C.N. II + C.N. III pupil size	Nor.
+2	Stim. left eye	+2
+2	Stim. right eye	+2
Nor.	C.N. II fundus	Nor.
	C.N. III, C.N. IV, C.N. VI	
0	Strabismus	0
0	Nystagmus	0
Nor.	C.N. V sensation	Nor.
Nor.	C.N. V mastication	Nor.
Nor.	C.N. VII facial muscles	Nor.
+2	Palpebral	+2
Nor.	C.N. IX, C.N. X swallowing	Nor.
Nor.	C.N. XII tongue	Nor.

F. Sensation: Location
   Hyperesthesia   Mild in midcervical area
   Superficial pain   Good but absent on right
   Deep pain   Pelvic foot

Complete sections G and H before reviewing Case Summary.

G. Assessment (Anatomic diagnosis and estimation of prognosis)

H. Plan (Diagnostic)
   Rule-outs   Procedure
   1.
   2.
   3.
   4.

Case History 10F

Signalment

Canine, Weimaraner, male, 4½ years old.

History

Sudden onset of fever, diarrhea, depression, and weakness. The dog will not walk and collapses if forced to stand.

Physical Examination

Temperature: 104.5 degrees F. The dog experiences pain when handled.

Neurologic Examination*

A. Observation
1. Mental status: Alert.
2. Posture: Sternal recumbency.
3. Gait: The dog will not stand and falls when forced to stand. Tetraparesis is present.

B. Palpation
Pain in long bones.

C. Postural Reactions

Left	Reactions	Right
	Proprioceptive positioning	
+2	PL	+2
+2	TL	+2
0	Wheelbarrowing	0
+1	Hopping, PL	+1
+1	Hopping, TL	+1
+2	Extensor postural thrust	+2
+1	Hemistand-hemiwalk	+1
+1	Tonic neck	+1
	Placing, tactile	
+2	PL	+2
+2	TL	+2
	Placing, visual	
+2	TL	+2

D. Spinal Reflexes

Left	Reflex Spinal Segment	Right
	Quadriceps	
+2	L4−L6	+2
	Extensor carpi radialis	
+2	C7−T1	+2
	Triceps	
+2	C7−T1	+2
	Flexion, PL	
+2	L5−S1	+2
	Flexion, TL	
+2	C6−T1	+2
0	Crossed extensor	0
	Perineal	
+2	S1−S2	+2

E. Cranial Nerves

Left	Nerve + Function	Right
	C.N. II vision	
+2	menace	+2
Nor.	C.N. II + C.N. III pupil size	Nor.
+2	Stim. left eye	+2
+2	Stim. right eye	+2
Nor.	C.N. II fundus	Nor.
	C.N. III, C.N. IV, C.N. VI	
0	Strabismus	0
0	Nystagmus	0
Nor.	C.N. V sensation	Nor.
Nor.	C.N. V mastication	Nor.
Nor.	C.N. VII facial muscles	Nor.
+2	Palpebral	+2
Nor.	C.N. IX, C.N. X swallowing	Nor.
Nor.	C.N. XII tongue	Nor.

F. Sensation: Location
Hyperesthesia _____ Long bones _____
Superficial pain _____ Normal _____
Deep pain _____ Normal _____
Complete sections G and H before reviewing Case Summary.
G. Assessment (Anatomic diagnosis and estimation of prognosis)

H. Plan (Diagnostic)
Rule-outs   Procedure
1.
2.
3.
4.

---

*Key: 0 = absent, +1 = decreased, +2 = normal, +3 = exaggerated, +4 = very exaggerated or clonus, PL = pelvic limb, TL = thoracic limb.

ASSESSMENT 10A

Anatomic diagnosis: Generalized LMN signs are present, and pain perception is preserved. Generalized neuropathy or motor end-plate disease should be suspected.

Diagnostic plan (Rule-outs):
1. Tick paralysis—examine for ticks (present).
2. Botulism—history, EMGs, toxin analysis.
3. Polyradiculoneuritis—EMGs.
Therapeutic plan:
1. Remove ticks.
2. Support the dog with attentive nursing care.
Client education: The prognosis is good.
Case summary: Tick paralysis was diagnosed. The ticks were removed, and the dog improved within 24 hours and was normal in 36 hours. This is a typical recovery for tick paralysis.

ASSESSMENT 10B

Anatomic diagnosis: This dog has a right hemiparesis with a normal left thoracic limb and a nearly normal left pelvic limb. The right hemiparesis is characterized by LMN signs in the thoracic limb and UMN signs in the pelvic limb. The lesion is most likely C6—T2.

Diagnostic plan (Rule-outs):
1. Trauma—history, cervical radiography (negative).
2. Cervical disk disease—myelography (negative).
3. Myelitis—CSF examination (negative).
4. Cervical spinal cord infarction—supported by negative diagnostic tests.
Therapeutic plan:
1. Prescribe cage rest, prevent decubital sores, perform hydrotherapy.
2. Corticosteroid therapy is of questionable value at this stage of the spinal cord infarction.
Client education: The prognosis is poor.
Case summary: A severe hemorrhagic vascular lesion on the right (C7−C8, C8−T1) was diagnosed. The dog did not improve, and euthanasia was performed. Necropsy confirmed the presence of the lesion. The cause of the infarction was not found.

ASSESSMENT 10C

Anatomic diagnosis: The dog has UMN tetraparesis with no evidence of brain stem disease. This finding localizes the lesion to the segment C1−C5.

Diagnostic plan (Rule-outs):
1. Cervical disk disease—radiology (disk herniation at C2−C3).
2. Cervical neoplasia—myelography (not performed).
3. Cervical myelitis—CSF analysis (not performed).
Therapeutic plan: Because of the age of the animal, the heart condition, and client concern, the dog should be managed with cage rest and corticosteroids.
Client education: The prognosis is fair to poor. Surgery would give better results; however, the anesthetic risk precludes surgery.
Case summary: Cervical disk disease was diagnosed. The dog improved with corticosteroid therapy; however, a relapse did occur. Most cases of this severity require surgery because of protruded disk material in the vertebral canal.

ASSESSMENT 10D

Anatomic diagnosis: Severe tetraparesis is present with UMN signs in all four limbs. Cervical pain plus the absence of brain stem signs localize the lesion to the segment C1−C5.

Diagnostic plan (Rule-outs):
1. Atlantoaxial subluxation—cervical radiography (atlantoaxial subluxation is present).
2. Cervical disk—myelography (not performed).
3. Meningomyelitis—CSF examination (not performed).
Therapeutic plan: Surgical stabilization.
Client education: The prognosis is fair to good.
Case summary: Atlantoaxial subluxation was diagnosed. Following surgery, the patient recovered.

ASSESSMENT 10E

Anatomic diagnosis: Two lesions must be present in order for the clinical findings in this case to be explained. LMN disease and hypalgesia are present in the right pelvic limb, suggesting a selective sciatic nerve injury (probably a needle injury from intramuscular injections). The other neurologic signs suggest a midcervical lesion.

Diagnostic plan (Rule-outs):
1. Cervical spondylopathy—cervical radiography and myelography (instability of C5−C6).
2. Cervical disk—see Diagnostic Plan Number 1.
3. Cervical myelitis—CSF analysis (normal).
4. Injection neuritis—EMG (denervation potentials in the flexors of the stifle and all muscles below the stifle).
Therapeutic plan:
1. Ventral stabilization of C5−C6 with lag screw compression and fenestration.
2. Physical therapy and a boot for the right pelvic limb.
Client education: The prognosis is very guarded.
Case summary: Cervical spondylopathy and sciatic neuritis were diagnosed. The dog improved for 4 months. Cervical signs returned from compression at C4−C5. Euthanasia was performed. The right pelvic limb improved over 50 per cent during the 4 months following surgery.

ASSESSMENT 10F

Anatomic diagnosis: The generalized weakness with normal reflexes and normal pain perception tends to discount primary neurologic disease. The pain helps in the localization of the disease to the musculoskeletal system.

Diagnostic plan (Rule-outs):
1. Metabolic bone disease—skeletal radiography (hypertrophic osteodystrophy).
2. Primary myopathy or myositis—EMG (negative) and muscle enzyme analysis (normal).

Therapeutic plan:
1. cage rest,
2. aspirin, and
3. mild calcium supplementation.
   Client education: The prognosis is guarded.
   Case summary: Hypertrophic osteodystrophy was diagnosed. The dog recovered in 7 days with no recurrence of the condition. This case illustrates the point that primary musculoskeletal diseases may closely resemble primary neurologic disorders.

REFERENCES

1. Hoerlein, B. F.: Intervertebral disks. *In* Hoerlein, B. F.: Canine Neurology: Diagnosis and Treatment, 3rd ed. Philadelphia, W. B. Saunders Co., 1978.
2. Gage, E. D.: Incidence of clinical disk disease in the dog. JAAHA 11:135, 1975.
3. Goggins, J. E., Li, A. S., and Franti, C. E.: Canine intervertebral disk diseases: characterized by age, sex, breed, and anatomical site of involvement. Am. J. Vet. Res. 9:1687, 1980.
4. Mayhew, I. G., deLahunta, A., Whitlock, R. H., and Geary, J. C.: Equine degenerative myeloencephalopathy. JAVMA 170:195–201, 1977.
5. Mayhew, I. G., deLahunta, A., Whitlock, R. H., Krook, L., and Tasker, J. B.: Spinal cord disease in the horse. Cornell Vet. 68 (Suppl. 6): 1–207, 1978.
6. Geary, J. C., Oliver, J. E., Jr., and Hoerlein, B. F.: Atlantoaxial subluxation in the canine. J. Small Anim. Pract. 8:577–582, 1967.
7. Oliver, J. E., Jr., and Lewis, R. E.: Lesions of the atlas and axis in dogs. JAAHA 9:304, 1973.
8. Geary, J. C.: Canine spinal lesions not involving discs. JAVMA 155:2038–2044, 1969.
9. Gage, E. D., and Smallwood, J. E.: Surgical repair of atlanto-axial subluxation in a dog. VM/SAC 65:583–592, 1970.
10. Gage, E. D.: Atlanto-axial subluxation. *In* Bojrab, M. J.: Current Techniques in Small Animal Surgery I. Philadelphia, Lea & Febiger, 1975.
11. Chambers, J. N., Betts, C. W., and Oliver, J. E., Jr.: The use of nonmetallic suture material for stabilization of atlantoaxial subluxation. JAAHA 13:602, 1977.
12. Palmer, A. C., and Wallace, M. E.: Deformation of cervical vertebrae in Basset hounds. Vet. Rec. 80:430–433, 1967.
13. Gage, E. D., and Hall, C. L.: Surgical repair of caudal cervical subluxation in a dog. JAVMA 160:424–426, 1972.
14. Wright, F., Rest, J. R., and Palmer, A. C.: Ataxia of the Great Dane caused by stenosis of the cervical vertebral canal: Comparison with similar conditions in the Basset Hound, Doberman Pinscher, Ridgeback and the thoroughbred horse. Vet. Rec. 92:1–6, 1973.
15. Gage, E. D., and Hoerlein, B. F.: Surgical repair of cervical subluxation and spondylolisthesis in the dog. JAAHA 9:385, 1973.
16. Parker, A. J., Park, R.D., Cusick, P. K., Small, E., and Jeffers, C. B.: Cervical vertebral instability in the dog. JAVMA 163:71–74, 1973.
17. Parker, A. J., Park, R. D., and Henry, J. D.: Cervical vertebral instability associated with cervical disk disease in the dog. JAVMA 163:1369–1371, 1973.
18. Selcer, R. R., and Oliver, J. E., Jr.: Cervical spondylopathy—wobbler syndrome in dogs. JAAHA 11:175, 1975.
19. Trotter, E. J., deLahunta, A., Geary, J. C., and Brasmer, T. H.: Caudal cervical vertebral malformation-malarticulation in Great Danes and Doberman Pinschers. JAVMA 168:917–930, 1976.
20. Denny, H. R., Gibbs, C., and Gaskell, C. J.: Cervical spondylopathy in the dog—a review of thirty-five cases. J. Small Anim. Pract. 18:117–132, 1977.
21. Chambers, J. N., nd Betts, C. W.: Caudal cervical spondylopathy in the dog: A review of 20 clinical cases and the literature. JAAHA 13:571, 1977.
22. Raffe, M. R., and Knecht, C. D.: Cervical vertebral malformation in bull mastiffs. JAAHA 14:593, 1978.
23. Hurov, L. I.: Treatment of cervical vertebral instability in the dog. JAVMA 175:278, 1979.
24. Mason, T. A.: Cervical vertebral instability (wobbler syndrome) in the dog. Vet. Rec. 104:142–145, 1979.
25. Wright, J. A.: A study of the radiographic anatomy of the cervical spine in the dog. J. Small Anim. Pract. 18:341–357, 1977.
26. Wright, J. A.: The use of sagittal diameter measurements in the diagnosis of cervical spinal stenosis. J. Small Anim. Pract. 20:331, 1979.
27. Hedhammar, A., Wu, F. M., and Krook, L.: Overnutrition and skeletal disease. An experimental study in growing Great Dane dogs. Cornell Vet. 64 (Suppl. 5):115–127, 1974.
28. Reed, S. M., et al.: Ataxia and paresis in horses. Part I. Differential diagnosis. Comp. Cont. Ed. 3:S88, 1981.
29. Rantanen, N. W., et al.: Ataxia and paresis in horses. Part II. Radiographic and myelographic examination of the cervical vertebral column. Comp. Cont. Ed. 3:S161, 1981.
30. Wagner, P. C., Grant, B. D., and Gallina, A.: Ataxia and paresis in horses. Part III. Surgical treatment of cervical spinal cord compression. Comp. Cont. Ed. 3:S192, 1981.
31. Cummings, J. F., and Haas, D. C.: Coonhound paralysis. An acute idiopathic polyradiculoneuritis in dogs resembling the Landry-Guillain-Barré syndrome. J. Neurol. Sci. 4:51–81, 1967.
32. Goodall, J. A. D., Kosmidis, J. C., and Geddes, A. M.: Effect of corticosteroids on course of Guillain-Barré syndrome. Lancet 1:524–526, 1974.
33. Barsanti, J. A., Walser, M., Hatheway, C. L., Bowen, J. M., and Crowell, W.: Type C botulism in American Foxhounds. JAVMA 172:809–813, 1978.
34. Darke, P. G. G., Roberts, T. A., Smart, J. L., and Bradshaw, P. R.: Suspected botulism in foxhounds. Vet. Rec. 99:98–99, 1976.
35. Pilet, C., Cazabat, H., and Ardonceau, R.: Line nouvelle enzotic de botulisme chez le chien de meute. Bull. Acad. Vet. Fr. 32:297, 1959.
36. Swift, T. R., and Ignacio, O. J.: Tick paralysis: Electrophysiologic studies. Neurology 25:1130–1133, 1975.
37. Ilkiw, J. E.: Tick paralysis in Australia. *In* Kirk, R. W.: Current Veterinary Therapy VII. Philadelphia, W. B. Saunders Co., 1980.
38. Lagos, J. C., and Thies, R. E.: Tick paralysis without muscle weakness. Arch. Neurol. 21:471–474, 1969.
39. Haller, J. S., and Fabara, J. A.: Tick paralysis. Case report with emphasis on neurological toxicity. Am. J. Dis. Child 124:915–917, 1972.
40. Chrisman, L. L.: Differentiation of tick paralysis and acute idiopathic polyradiculoneuritis in the dog using electromyography. JAAHA 11:455, 1975.
41. Lorenz, M. D., Cork, L. C., Griffin, J. W., Adams, R. J., and Price, D. L.: Hereditary spinal muscular atrophy in Brittany spaniels: Clinical manifestations. JAVMA 175:833, 1979.

42. Sandefeldt, E., Cummings, J. F., deLahunta, A., Bjorck, G., and Krook, L.: Hereditary neuronal abiotrophy in the Swedish Lapland dog. Cornell Vet. 63 (Suppl. 3):1–71, 1973.
43. Stockard, L. R.: An hereditary lethal for localized motor and preganglionic neurones with a resulting paralysis in the dog. Am. J. Anat. 59:1–53, 1936.
44. Cummings, J. F., and deLahunta, A.: Canine polyneuritis. In Kirk, R. W.: Current Veterinary Therapy VI. Philadelphia, W. B. Saunders Co., 1977.
45. Sibley, W. A.: Polyneuritis. Med. Clin. North Am. 56:1299–1319, 1972.
46. Dyck, P. J.: Diseases of nerve roots, plexuses, and peripheral nerves. In Beeson, P. B., and McDermott, W.: Cecil and Loeb Textbook of Medicine. Philadelphia, W. B. Saunders Co., 1971.
47. Kornegay, J. N., Gorgacz, E. J., Dawe, D. L., Bowen, J. M., White, N. A., and DeBuysscher, E. V.: Polymyositis in the dog. JAVMA 176:431, 1980.
48. Duncan, I. D., and Griffiths, I. R.: Inflammatory muscle disease in the dog. In Kirk, R. W.: Current Veterinary Therapy VII. Philadelphia, W. B. Saunders Co., 1980.
49. Scott, D. W., and deLahunta, A.: Eosinophilic polymyositis in a dog. Cornell Vet. 64:47–56, 1974.
50. Wentink, G. H., van der Linde-Sipman, J. S., Keijer, A. E. F. H., Kamphuisen, H. A. C., van Vorstenbosch, C. J. A. H. V., Hartman, W., and Hendricks, H. J.: Myopathy with a possible recessive x-linked inheritance in a litter of Irish terriers. Vet. Pathol. 9:328, 1972.
51. Kramer, J. W., Hegreberg, G. A., Bryan, G. M., Meyers, K., and Ott, R. L.: A muscle disorder of Labrador retrievers characterized by deficiency of type II muscle fibers. JAVMA 169:817–820, 1976.
52. Muth, O. H., et al.: White muscle disease (myopathy) in lambs and calves. VI. Effects of selenium and vitamin E on lambs. Am. J. Vet. Res. 20:231, 1959.
53. Gannon, J. R.: Exertional rhabdomyolysis (myoglobinuria) in the racing greyhound. In Kirk, R. W.: Current Veterinary Therapy VII. Philadelphia, W. B. Saunders Co., 1980.
54. Duncan, I. D.: Myotonia in the dog. In Kirk, R. W.: Current Veterinary Therapy VII. Philadelphia, W. B. Saunders Co., 1980.
55. Greene, C. E., Lorenz, M. D., Munnell, J., Prasse, K. W., White, N. A., and Bowen, J. M.: Myopathy associated with hyperadrenocorticism in the dog. JAVMA 174:1310, 1979.
56. Drachman, D. B.: Myasthenia gravis (first of two parts). N. Eng. J. Med. 298:136–142, 1978.

Ataxia is a lack of coordination that may be present without spasticity, paresis, or involuntary movements. It is characterized by a broad-based stance and uncoordinated movements of the head, the trunk, or the limbs. Lesion localization of ataxic animals has been discussed in Chapter 4 and is summarized in Figure 11–1. A brief review is presented in this chapter.

11

ATAXIA OF THE HEAD AND THE LIMBS

LESION LOCALIZATION

Ataxia is a sign of specific sensory dysfunction. For clinical purposes, it can be classified in three major categories: sensory, vestibular, and cerebellar. Clinical signs result when a disease interferes with the recognition or coordination of position changes involving the head, the trunk, or the limbs. Key neurologic signs that are useful for localizing the lesion may be observed. Figure 11–2 is an algorithm that is clinically beneficial for the formulation of a differential diagnosis of ataxia. This algorithm is largely based on a few key differential signs. For example, abnormal movements of the head or the eyes indicate that the lesion is not in the spinal cord but rather in the vestibular system, the brain stem, or the cerebellum.

Sensory Ataxia

Loss of proprioceptive signals from the limbs and, in some cases, the trunk produces sensory ataxia. For the purpose of localization, abnormalities of proprioception in the limbs are interpreted in exactly the same way as motor dysfunction (see Chapters 4, 9, and 10). For example, loss of proprioception in the pelvic limbs with normal thoracic limbs indicates a lesion caudal to T3 involving sensory long tracts, spinal nerves, or peripheral nerves. Further localization is achieved by an examination of spinal reflexes and segmental pain responses. Sensory ataxia is frequently associated with motor dysfunction (paresis).

Vestibular Ataxia

The vestibular system detects linear acceleration and rotational movements of the head. This system does not originate motor activity; however, its sensory input is used to modify and coordinate movement. The vestibular system primarily controls the muscles that are involved in maintaining equilibrium, position-

ing the head, and regulating eye movements. Sensory receptors are located in the inner ear in the vestibular labyrinth. Two kinds of receptors are present: maculae in the utriculi and sacculi and cristae in the semicircular canals. The maculae are arranged approximately at right angles to each other. They function to detect head position with respect to gravity and linear acceleration and help to maintain equilibrium. The cristae in the semicircular canals detect the onset of angular or rotational acceleration. These receptors predict loss of balance and cause the appropriate adjustments to be made in order for equilibrium to be maintained. Input to the brain is by way of C.N. VIII (vestibular division). The vestibular nerve terminates in one of four vestibular nuclei or in the cerebellum. Pathways from the vestibular nuclei project to other brain stem centers, to the cerebellum, to the cerebral cortex, and to the spinal cord (Fig. 11–3). Projections to the nuclei of nerves controlling eye movements travel by way of the medial longitudinal fasciculus (MLF).

This system controls normal physiologic nystagmus, and one can demonstrate it in the normal animal by moving the animal's head from side to side or up and down. When this control mechanism is disrupted, nystagmus occurs independently of head movement (pathologic nystagmus). Projections to the emetic center in the brain stem are important in the development of motion sickness (visual-vestibular sensory dissociation). The vestibular apparatus works in close association with the cerebellum to maintain balance and coordination. Pathways project from the ves-

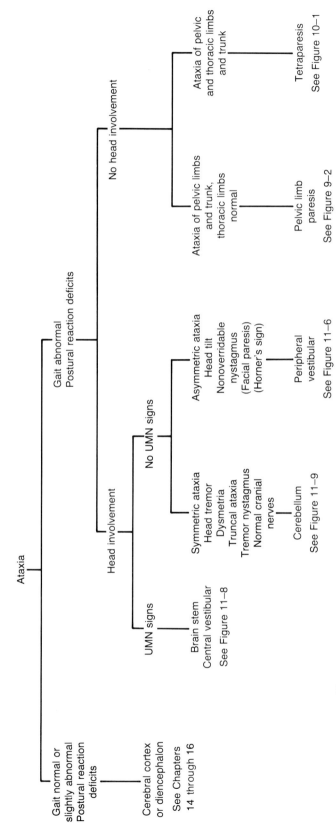

Figure 11-1. Algorithm for the diagnosis of ataxia based on gait, head involvement, and motor function of the limbs.

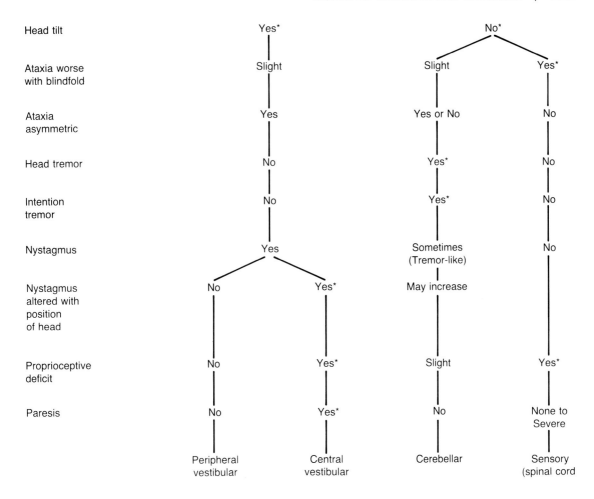

Head tilt	Yes*		No*	
Ataxia worse with blindfold	Slight		Slight	Yes*
Ataxia asymmetric	Yes		Yes or No	No
Head tremor	No		Yes*	No
Intention tremor	No		Yes*	No
Nystagmus	Yes		Sometimes (Tremor-like)	No
Nystagmus altered with position of head	No	Yes*	May increase	
Proprioceptive deficit	No	Yes*	Slight	Yes*
Paresis	No	Yes*	No	None to Severe
	Peripheral vestibular	Central vestibular	Cerebellar	Sensory (spinal cord

*Key differential signs. Lesions in the brain stem can cause central vestibular, cerebellar, and sensory signs.

Figure 11–2. Algorithm for the differential diagnosis of ataxia resulting from vestibular, cerebellar, or spinal cord disease.

tibular nuclei through the cerebellar peduncles to several cerebellar centers (see Fig. 11–3). Vestibular impulses reach the cerebral cortex and inform the animal of its position during movement. Projections to the spinal cord travel by way of the vestibulospinal tracts. These pathways are important for the regulation of the antigravity muscles of the limbs and

Figure 11–3. Neuronal pathways of the vestibular system. (From Hoerlein, B. F.: Canine Neurology, 3rd ed. Philadelphia, W. B. Saunders Co., 1978. Used by permission.)

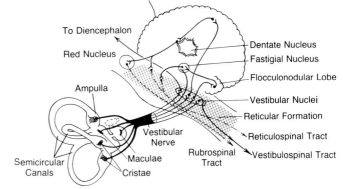

the trunk. Most importantly, the vestibulo-spinal tracts stimulate the ipsilateral extensor muscles. Unilateral vestibular lesions cause animals to fall toward the side of the lesion. Animals actually are forced to fall in this direction, because extensor tone on the contralateral side is not antagonized by extensor muscle tone on the ipsilateral side. (Extensor tone is lost because of the lesion.)

On the basis of a neurologic examination, vestibular ataxia can be localized to peripheral vestibular disease or central vestibular (brain stem) disease. A head tilt indicates vestibular system disease. In most cases, the head will be tilted toward the side of the lesion. The ataxia is often asymmeteric unless bilateral lesions are present. The animal usually falls or drifts toward the side of the lesion. Turning in tight circles is usually a vestibular sign, although exceptions have been observed. The movement is usually toward the side of the lesion, but movement in the opposite direction has been observed with central vestibular lesions. Signs of paresis or proprioceptive deficit associated with a head tilt indicate central vestibular disease. Paresis in central vestibular disease is caused by injury of the motor tracts that project through the brain stem. *Thus, a major way of differentiating central and peripheral vestibular disease is to evaluate the animal critically for evidence of motor dysfunction or sensory ataxia.*

Nystagmus may be present in central or peripheral vestibular disease. In peripheral vestibular disease, the nystagmus may be horizontal or rotatory, with the quick phase directed away from the side of the lesion. With a central vestibular lesion, the nystagmus may be similar to that described for peripheral lesions; however, nystagmus that frequently changes direction with alterations in head position or that is vertical in direction strongly suggests a central vestibular lesion. Facial and sympathetic nerve function may be impaired in cases of peripheral vestibular diseases.

Dysfunction of other cranial nerves associated with head tilt indicates a central vestibular lesion with extension to other areas of the brain stem. Physiologic nystagmus may be depressed or absent with vestibular lesions. Caloric tests and assessment of postrotatory nystagmus are usually not needed in the evaluation of vestibular disease in small animals.

Paradoxical vestibular disease is evidenced by one or more vestibular signs (e.g., head tilt, nystagmus) that are in the direction opposite the other localizing signs. These signs generally are caused by lesions near the cerebellar peduncles.

Cerebellar Ataxia

The cerebellum functions as a major coordinator of motor activity. It compares the intent of motor activity with the performance required to complete the activity. The cerebellum receives its sensory input through three paired peduncles (Fig. 11–4). The caudal cerebellar peduncles carry sensory fibers from the vestibular system, the basal nuclei, and the spinal cord. The middle cerebellar peduncle carries information from the cerebral cortex by way of brain stem centers. Cerebellar output to the cerebral cortex, the brain stem, and the spinal cord travels through the rostral and caudal cerebellar peduncles (Fig. 11–5). A disease of the cerebellum or its peduncles results in characteristic clinical signs. The cerebellum performs below the level of consciousness to control muscle movements accurately, to assist in maintaining equilibrium, and to control posture.

Because the cerebellum does not initiate motor activity, paresis is not a sign of cerebellar dysfunction. Symmetric ataxia characterized by a hypermetric gait, truncal ataxia, a head tremor, and an intention tremor is very suggestive of cerebellar disease. Unlike vestibular disorders, cerebellar dysfunction rarely

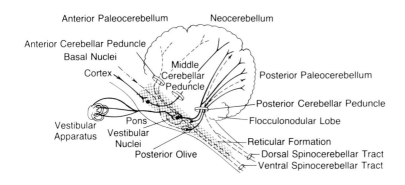

Figure 11–4. Sensory pathways from the cerebellum. (From Hoerlein, B. F.: Canine Neurology, 3rd ed. Philadelphia, W. B. Saunders Co., 1978. Used by permission.)

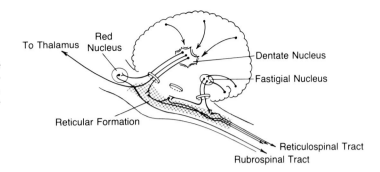

Figure 11–5. Motor pathways from the cerebellum. (From Hoerlein, B. F.: Canine Neurology, 3rd ed. Philadelphia, W. B. Saunders Co., 1978. Used by permission.)

produces head tilt or circling. Nystagmus, when present, is tremor-like (rapid eye flutter). A deficient menace response has been observed in animals with diffuse cerebellar disease.

Diseases that involve the caudal brain stem may cause a combination of signs suggesting both central vestibular and cerebellar dysfunction. These signs develop because of the close anatomic location of cerebellar pathways to the brain stem in the area of the pons.

DISEASES

The diseases discussed in this chapter include those that commonly affect the brain stem, the cerebellum, and the peripheral vestibular system. The disorders that produce sensory ataxia have been presented in Chapters 9 and 10 and will not be repeated here. As in previous chapters, this section is organized according to the anatomic location of the lesion and the course of the disease (acute versus chronic, progressive versus nonprogressive).

Peripheral Vestibular Diseases

A diagnostic approach to peripheral vestibular disorders is outlined in Figure 11–6. Using otoscopic and radiographic examinations of the ear canal and the osseous bulla, the cli-

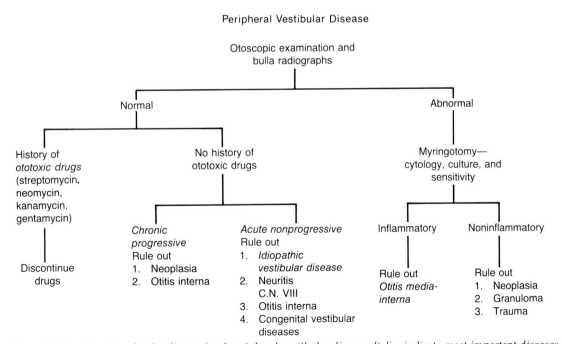

Figure 11–6. Algorithm for the diagnosis of peripheral vestibular disease. *Italics* indicate most important diseases clinically.

nician must decide if abnormalities exist. If no lesions are detected, a search is made for evidence of ototoxic drugs. If these agents have not been administered, the patient's history is used to place the condition in one of two categories: chronic progressive or acute nonprogressive disorders. If the initial otoscopic or radiographic examination is positive, the disorder is classified as inflammatory or noninflammatory, based on myringotomy, cytology, and culture and sensitivity testing. Certain inflammatory and neoplastic diseases can fall in either broad category, depending upon the propensity of the disease to produce grossly visible or radiographically detectable lesions.

OTITIS MEDIA-INTERNA

The most common cause of peripheral vestibular disease in the dog and the cat is an inner ear infection that has progressed from the middle ear. Otitis externa caused by bacteria is the most common cause of otitis media. Occasionally, otitis media-interna develops in animals with no historical or physical evidence of otitis externa. In these cases, retrograde infection through the auditory tube from the pharynx or hematogenous infection is suspected. In most cases, the infection is caused by bacteria, although yeast and fungal organisms occasionally are encountered. The causative bacteria include staphylococci, the *Proteus* species, the *Pseudomonas* species, and *Escherichia coli*. The last three organisms are usually secondary invaders. Breeds that are predisposed to chronic otitis externa (cocker spaniels, poodles, German shepherds, and so forth) or animals with chronic *Otodectes* are at increased risk for the development of otitis media-interna. Occasionally, otic foreign bodies (such as grass awns) are found as the underlying etiology. In areas where foxtail awns or spear grass is endemic, otic foreign bodies are a significant cause of otitis externa with progression to otitis media-interna. Recurrent episodes are not uncommon. In horses, streptococcal bacteria are the common pathogens. Pigs may develop otitis media-interna following outbreaks of *Hemophilus suis* (swine influenza). In cattle, most middle ear infections are caused by streptococcal or staphylococcal bacteria.

Clinical Signs

The clinical signs of otitis media-interna have been described previously at the beginning of this chapter. It is important to recognize that several of these clinical signs (head tilt, head shaking, aural pain, inflammatory discharge) also are associated with primary otitis externa. Torticollis, circling, ataxia, and nystagmus are specific neurologic signs that are suggestive of otitis interna if the patient has no demonstrable paresis. Unilateral facial nerve paralysis is common, because the inflammatory process often extends to the facial nerve as it passes through the petrous temporal bone. A complete or partial Horner's sign also can be seen on the affected side if there is involvement of the sympathetic nerve in the middle ear.

Otitis media is recognized by direct otoscopic examination of the tympanic membrane. If purulent otitis externa is present, the external ear is cultured for bacteria and the ear then is cleaned gently but thoroughly. Deep sedation or anesthesia aids in critical otoscopic examination. The tympanic membrane must be examined carefully for hyperemia, edema, hemorrhage, and erosion. Fluid in the middle ear makes the tympanic membrane appear opaque and produces bulging of the membrane into the external auditory canal.

Diagnosis

The diagnosis of otitis media-interna is confirmed by otoscopic examination and skull radiography. If the tympanic membrane is ruptured or eroded, fluid is aspirated gently from the middle ear for cytologic and bacteriologic examination. If the tympanic membrane is intact but abnormal, myringotomy is performed. In our opinion, this procedure should be done with the animal under general anesthesia and only after the external ear canal has been cleaned and dried thoroughly. Myringotomy can be performed with a 3-inch, 18G spinal needle or with a sterile myringotomy knife. The middle ear is flushed gently with sterile saline solution, and the fluid is examined for cells and bacteria.

Radiographic examination of the skull is a valuable aid in the diagnosis and prognosis of chronic otitis media-interna. Radiographic projections include lateral, dorsoventral, open-mouth, and oblique views of each tympanic bulla. Positive findings include fluid density in the bulla and exostosis, sclerosis, or erosion of the bulla (Fig. 11–7).

Treatment

The medical treatment of otitis media-interna consists of long-term systemic antibiotics chosen from positive culture and sensitivity examinations. Penicillinase-resistant

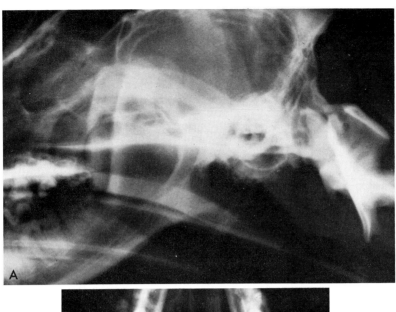

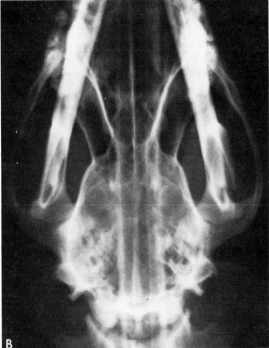

Figure 11–7. *A.* Lateral skull radiograph of a dog with severe otitis media-interna. Note the proliferative bony reaction of the osseous bulla. *B.* Ventrodorsal skull radiograph of the same dog. Note the opacity of the right tympanic bulla. A bulla osteotomy was performed to curette the diseased bone and to establish drainage from the middle ear.

penicillins, cephalosporins, and chloramphenicol are good initial antibiotics. Long-term chloramphenicol therapy is used with caution in cats because of its propensity to cause anorexia, depression, weight loss, and occasional blood dyscrasia. We prefer to use long-term bactericidal antibiotic therapy. In chronic cases, therapy for 6 to 8 weeks is recommended. Therapy with systemic aminoglycosides must be performed with caution, because ototoxic signs are masked by the existing disease. Topical therapy with antibiotics and corticosteroids instilled in the external ear canal, although beneficial for cases of otitis externa, rarely reaches the middle ear and therefore is seldom useful for resolving the inner ear infection.

In chronic disease involving the middle ear and the bulla, surgical debridement and drainage often are needed in order to resolve the infection. Various techniques have been described; however, we prefer the ventral bulla osteotomy because it affords the best visibility and exposure for biopsy, debridement, and drainage. Following surgery, drains are left in place for 10 days, and medical therapy is followed as described previously.

Therapy for otitis media-interna must resolve the infection and prevent its extension into the brain stem. The prognosis for recovery depends upon several factors: (1) the resistance of the organism, (2) the chronicity of disease, (3) the extent of the bone involvement, and (4) the reversibility of the neurologic damage. In chronic otitis interna, neurologic deficits may be permanent; however, most animals soon compensate for their vestibular deficits. Facial paralysis is usually permanent, and the resulting keratoconjunctivitis sicca requires long-term therapy with artificial tears.

IDIOPATHIC VESTIBULAR DISEASES

Feline Vestibular Syndrome

An acute nonprogressive vestibular disturbance has been recognized in cats. The cause is unknown. The disease occurs sporadically and is not associated with other infectious feline diseases. At one time, some clinicians believed the incidence to be higher during the late summer or fall following epizootics of upper respiratory viral diseases. These observations have not been substantiated. In the southern United States, the syndrome has been termed *lizard poisoning* and is believed to be related to the ingestion of blue-tailed lizards. These speculations also are unsubstantiated. No lesions in the vestibular system have been found at necropsy in limited studies.[1]

Clinical Signs. Clinical signs develop acutely and are usually unilateral, although bilateral involvement has been observed. Signs of otitis externa are lacking, and affected cats are usually healthy in all other respects. There appears to be no sex, breed, or age predilection. Cats with unilateral disease develop severe head tilt, disorientation, falling, rolling, and nystagmus. In bilateral disease, affected cats have little head tilt but are unable to move because of severe disorientation. The head may

swing in wide excursions from side to side. The cat usually remains in a crouched posture with the limbs widely abducted. It may cry out as if extremely frightened. Nystagmus may not be present; however, vestibular eye movements are depressed bilaterally.

Diagnosis. The diagnosis is based on the clinical signs and the absence of evidence supporting a diagnosis of bacterial otitis externa, otitis media, or otitis interna.

Treatment. No specific therapy is available. Affected cats spontaneously improve within 72 hours and are usually normal in 2 to 3 weeks. Antimotion drugs do not benefit the vestibular signs. Sedation may be necessary during the acute phase of the disease in order to suppress crying or thrashing about. Although bacteria are not incriminated in the pathogenesis of this disease, antibiotics should be considered in those cases in which differentiation from acute bacterial otitis media-interna is difficult. The prognosis for recovery is excellent. Residual vestibular dysfunction is uncommon.

Canine Vestibular Syndrome

Idiopathic acute vestibular syndromes are recognized in older dogs. The disease is not associated with any known infectious agent. The syndrome has been diagnosed erroneously as a stroke, even though the signs are those of a peripheral vestibular disturbance.

Clinical Signs. Signs develop acutely and on occasion may be preceded by vomiting and nausea. The signs are similar to those described in the section on the feline syndrome.

Diagnosis. The diagnosis is based on the clinical signs and the absence of evidence supporting a disgnosis of bacterial otitis media-interna.

Treatment. No specific therapy is available. Dogs spontaneously improve in 72 hours and are usually normal in 7 to 10 days. Head tilt may persist in some cases but usually does not interfere with function.

CONGENITAL VESTIBULAR SYNDROMES

These syndromes occur sporadically in litters of purebred dogs and cats. They have been reported in beagle, German shepherd, and Doberman pinscher dogs. Affected Siamese and Burmese cats also have been identified. Vestibular signs develop from the time of birth until the animal is several weeks of age. Deafness may accompany the vestibular disease and may be unilateral or bilateral. The pathogenesis of the lesion is unknown. Some animals gradually improve, whereas others have persistent head tilt and are deaf. No effective therapy is known.

NEOPLASTIC DISEASES

Primary neurologic tumors initially may cause peripheral vestibular dysfunction if the tumor originates from or compresses the vestibular nerve. Neurofibromas rarely develop in this nerve; however, when present, a slowly progressive course of vestibular disease evolves over several months. Eventually, this tumor grows into the brain stem, and central vestibular signs become apparent. Tumors of the osseous bullae or the labyrinth (fibrosarcomas, chondrosarcomas, osteosarcomas) may destroy structures in the inner ear. Unlike neurofibromas, these tumors are recognized easily with skull radiography.

OTOTOXICITY

In addition to renal toxicity, the aminoglycoside antibiotics can produce degeneration within the vestibular and auditory nerves. The

Etiologic Category	Brain Stem		
	Acute		***Chronic***
	Progressive	*Nonprogressive*	
Degenerative		Vascular disorders (See also *Cerebral cortex*) Hemorrhage, embolism	1. *Hypoglycemia* 2. *Hepatic encephalopathy* 3. *Storage diseases* 4. *Demyelinating diseases* 5. Neuronopathies
Anomalous			1. Congenital malformation of the foramen magnum 2. *Hydrocephalus* (see *Cerebral cortex*)
Metabolic	1. Hypoglycemia 2. Hepatic encephalopathy		See *Chronic degenerative*
Neoplastic	Metastatic—in patients with vascular thrombosis		1. *Primary* a. Meningioma b. Gliomas c. Neurofibroma of the cranial nerve 2. Metastatic 3. Skull origin (osteogenic sarcoma, etc.) 4. Lymphosarcoma
Inflammatory Infectious	1. Viral a. *Distemper* b. *Rabies* c. Pseudorabies d. Infectious hepatitis 2. Bacterial meningoencephalitis 3. Salmon poisoning (rickettsial)		1. Viral a. *Distemper* Old dog encephalitis b. *Atypical (noneffusion) feline infectious peritonitis)* 2. Bacterial a. Abscess b. Meningoencephalitis 3. *Mycotic* a. Blastomycosis b. Cryptococcosis c. Histoplasmosis d. Coccidioidomycosis e. Nocardiosis 4. *Toxoplasmosis* 5. Other a. Algae: Prototheosis b. Primary CNS reticulosis
Traumatic	Tentorial herniation	Head injury (hemorrhage, hematoma)	
Toxic	1. *Lead* 2. *Hexachlorophene* 3. Tetanus ?? See *Seizures,* Tables 15–2 and 15–3		1. Lead, other heavy metals 2. Hexachlorophene

Figure 11–8. Algorithm for the diagnosis of brain stem (central vestibular) disease. *Italics* indicate most important diseases clinically.

signs may be unilateral or bilateral. High doses of these drugs, prolonged therapy (over 14 days), or use in patients with impaired renal function are factors that contribute to ototoxicity. These drugs cause degeneration within receptors in the inner ear and in the fastigial and flocculonodular lobes of the cerebellum.

Patients receiving these drugs are monitored closely for signs of renal toxicity and ototoxicity. Dosages are reduced or replaced by other nontoxic antibiotics in patients with decreased renal function. Vestibular signs usually improve once the offending antibiotics are discontinued; however, deafness may be permanent.

Central Vestibular Diseases

A diagnostic approach to central vestibular (brain stem) disorders is outlined in Figure 11–8. Of the various categories listed, the chronic degenerative and inflammatory conditions are most important. These disorders produce multifocal neurologic lesions and systemic signs. They will be discussed as a group in Chapter 17. The localization of lesions to the caudal brain stem has been discussed previously.

Cerebellar Diseases

A diagnostic approach to cerebellar disorders is outlined in Figure 11–9. Of the categories listed, the chronic degenerative and inflammatory conditions are most important. Those diseases likely to produce multifocal neurologic lesions will be discussed in Chapter 17. Disorders that are confined to the cerebellum will be discussed in the following sections. These conditions are largely congenital, in which the abnormality occurs during gestation or prior to normal ambulation. In a review of congenital cerebellar diseases, deLahunta grouped these disorders in three categories: (1) in utero or neonatal viral infections (2) malformations of genetic or unknown causes, and (3) degenerative diseases, referred to as *abiotrophies*.[2] Tables 11–1 and 11–2 list the congenital disorders occurring in animals.

NEONATAL SYNDROMES

Clinical signs are present at birth or in the early postnatal period prior to normal ambulation. These syndromes are characterized by symmetric signs and a nonprogressive course.

Table 11–1. CONGENITAL CEREBELLAR DISEASES IN DOGS AND CATS*

Neonatal Syndromes
Viral infections
  Feline panleukopenia, feline cerebellar hypoplasia
  Canine herpesvirus
Malformations
  Cerebellar hypoplasia (dysplasia) with lissencephaly
    Wire-haired fox terriers
    Irish setters
  Cerebellar hypoplasia
    Chow chows
Abiotrophies
  Beagles
  Samoyeds
  Irish setters
  Cats—olivopontocerebellar atrophy
Postnatal Syndromes—Abiotrophies
Dogs
  Kerry blue terriers
  Rough-coated collies
  Gordon setters
  Airedale terriers
  Finnish terriers
  Bern running dogs

*Modified from deLahunta, A.: Comparative cerebellar disease in domestic animals. Comp. Cont. Ed. 2:8, 1980.

Viral Infection

Feline Parvovirus. The parvovirus responsible for feline infectious enteritis (panleukopenia) can produce a variety of cerebellar malformations, including cerebellar hypoplasia. In utero or perinatal infection of the brain adversely affects the development of the cerebellum. Destruction of the external germinal layer produces hypoplasia of the granular cell layer. Growing Purkinje neurons also may be destroyed. The destruction may be so severe that the size of the cerebellar cortex is grossly reduced (hence the term *cerebellar hypoplasia*) (Fig. 11–10). The resulting lesions are permanent.

Symmetric nonprogressive cerebellar signs are present in affected kittens at the time of ambulation. There are no systemic signs of panleukopenia. Kittens that are infected with the virus after 2 weeks of age rarely develop neurologic signs, even though the systemic signs may be severe. In addition to the virulent virus, a modified live vaccine virus also may produce this syndrome. Pregnant queens and kittens less than 3 weeks of age therefore should not be given MLV vaccines. Killed virus vaccines are used in these situations. There is no effective therapy for this disease. Some kittens can function as pets; however, many

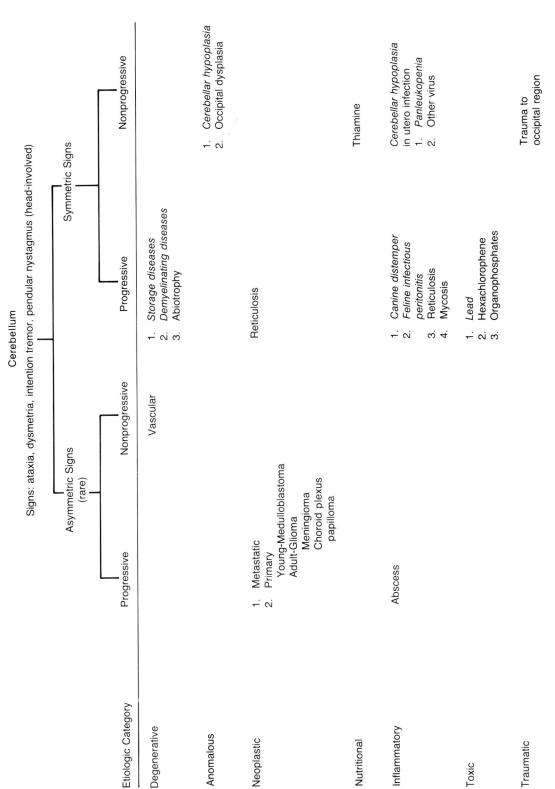

Figure 11–9. Algorithm for the diagnosis of cerebellar disease. *Italics* indicate most important diseases clinically.

Table 11–2. CONGENITAL CEREBELLAR
DISEASES IN LARGE ANIMALS*

Neonatal Syndromes
Viral infections
  Cattle
    Bovine virus diarrhea
    Akabane virus
    Bluetongue virus
  Sheep
    Akabane virus
    Bluetongue virus
  Swine
    Hog cholera virus
Malformations
  Cattle
    Cerebellar hypoplasia (dysplasia) with polymicrogyria—Herefords (autosomal recessive)
    Cerebellar hypoplasia—Shorthorns (autosomal recessive)
Abiotrophies
  Cattle
    Hereford cattle—suspected inheritance
  Sheep
    Welsh Mountain—autosomal recessive
    Corriedale—autosomal recessive

Postnatal Syndromes—Abiotrophies
Horses
  Arabian—presumed recessive
  Gotland ponies—autosomal recessive
Cattle
  Holstein Friesian—presumed recessive
Swine
  Yorkshire—presumed recessive

*Modified from deLahunta, A.: Comparative cerebellar disease in domestic animals, Comp. Cont. Ed. 2:8, 1980.

have incapacitating disease, and euthanasia should be performed in these instances.

Canine Herpesvirus. This viral agent affects puppies less than 2 weeks of age. The disease is characterized by generalized systemic signs, including sudden death. Rarely, puppies survive the systemic effects of the virus and develop a residual cerebellar ataxia. This form of cerebellar disease should be suspected in puppies that survive systemic herpes infection. The cerebellar signs are nonprogressive.

Bovine Virus Diarrhea (BVD). Fetal calves infected with this virus between 100 and 200 days of gestation develop severe cerebellar degeneration and atrophy. Ocular lesions include retinal atrophy, optic neuritis, cataracts, and microphthalmia with retinal dysplasia. Affected calves have symmetric nonprogressive cerebellar signs at birth. The clinical signs usually remain constant, although a few calves may show an improved ability to ambulate as they compensate for the cerebellar disease. No treatment is known. The disease can be prevented by vaccinating heifers at 4 months of age with BVD vaccine.

Akabane Virus. This virus produces severe destruction of germinal cells in the brains of fetal lambs and calves. It has been observed in Australia, Japan, and Israel. The clinical

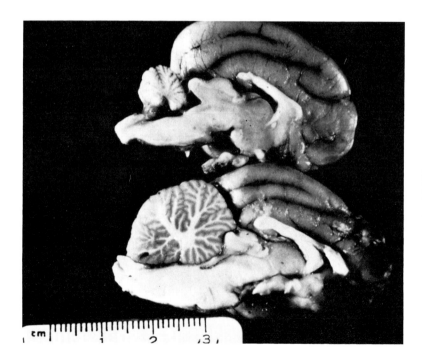

Figure 11–10. Cerebellar hypoplasia in a kitten affected in utero with panleukopenia virus. Note the small cerebellum compared with that of a normal cat.

signs are related to the cerebral and cerebellar lesions.

Bluetongue Virus. This virus produces severe destruction of germinal cells in the brains of fetal lambs and calves. Hydranencephaly and cerebellar atrophy are the usual lesions. Lambs develop the most severe lesions when infected at 50 to 58 days of gestation.

Hog Cholera Virus. Hog cholera vaccine virus, when administered to susceptible pregnant sows, produces numerous lesions in fetal pigs, including lesions in the cerebellum. The clinical signs are those of a diffuse whole body tremor (see the section on myoclonia congenita).

Malformation

Dysplasia of the cerebrum and the cerebellum has been reported in wire-haired fox terriers and Irish setters.[3] The clinical signs are nonprogressive. Generalized seizures developed in one dog after 1 year of age and were associated with lissencephaly. The cerebellum is symmetrically small as a result of abnormal development of the cerebellar cortex. The cause is unknown, but a genetic mode is suspected.

A microscopic cerebellar hypoplasia has been reported in chow chow puppies.[4] Cerebellar ataxia was present at birth and persisted as the puppies developed. The clinical signs resulted from a depletion of Purkinje neurons and granular cells. An autosomal recessive mode of inheritance was suspected. This syndrome should not be confused with a similar syndrome in chow chow puppies that results from dysmyelinogenesis. The latter syndrome tends to improve as the age of the dog increases.

Abiotrophies

These neonatal syndromes are characterized by degenerative changes that affect Purkinje neurons primarily and result in clinical signs at the time of ambulation. The disease has been studied most extensively in the beagle and Samoyed breeds.[2,3] Microscopic lesions include swelling and diffuse absence of Purkinje neurons.

POSTNATAL SYNDROMES: ABIOTROPHIES

The term *abiotrophy* denotes premature death of neurons, presumably from abnormal metabolic processes within the cell. The term implies a lack of the intrinsic biologic activity that is necessary for cell vitality and function.[2] After a variable period of normal neurologic function, cerebellar signs develop and may progress slowly or acutely. Microscopic lesions are most profound in the Purkinje neurons. Occasionally, lesions are found in granular cells, cerebellar medullary nuclei, and brain stem nuclei.[3] These diseases have been studied most extensively in Kerry blue terriers and Gordon setters in the United States and in rough-coated collies in Australia.

Kerry Blue Terrier Abiotrophy

This syndrome has been observed since 1968 in a study involving nine dogs from New York and California.[5] The puppies developed a progressive cerebellar disorder at 9 to 16 weeks of age. The earliest signs included stiffness of the pelvic limbs and a mild head tremor. These signs progressed to severe dysmetria (hypermetria). Most animals are unable to stand by 10 to 12 months of age. Progressive cerebellar cortical degeneration with loss of Purkinje cells has been demonstrated. Degenerative lesions also have been observed in the olivary nuclei, the substantia nigra, and the caudate nucleus. An autosomal recessive inheritance has been proposed.

Gordon Setter Abiotrophy

This syndrome has been studied in dogs from New York, Virginia, North Carolina, and California.[6] The clinical sign is a slowly progressive cerebellar ataxia that develops when the dog is 6 to 24 months of age. The ataxia may become severe but does not prevent the dog from standing. Early signs include mild thoracic limb stiffness, hypermetria, and stumbling. The signs progress slowly and at times even appear static. Necropsy studies have established a diffuse degeneration of neurons in the cerebellar cortex. The accumulated evidence suggests an autosomal recessive mode of inheritance.

Rough-Coated Collie Abiotrophy

This autosomal recessive inherited disease has been documented in rough-coated collies in Australia.[7] The signs develop when the animal is 4 to 12 weeks of age and progress fairly rapidly for 1 to 4 weeks. In addition to cerebellar cortical degeneration, lesions also occur in cerebellar and brain stem nuclei.

Arabian Horse Abiotrophy

Signs of cerebellar ataxia may develop from the time of birth until the animal is a few months of age. The signs may progress rapidly and then stabilize, or they may progress slowly. Most affected foals can walk but have a symmetric spasticity of all four limbs. Foals tend to fall over backward when the head is elevated. Nystagmus and opisthotonos are absent. An hereditary basis is suspected. A similar syndrome has been described in Gotland ponies.

Holstein-Friesian Cattle Abiotrophy

Acute cerebellar ataxia has been noted in Holstein cattle, beginning when the animals are 3 to 9 months of age. The signs initially are rapidly progressive and then become static or slowly progressive. The neck is extended with the ears retracted. Dorsomedial strabismus and nystagmus may be present. A recessive inheritance is suspected.

Yorkshire Swine Abiotrophy

Acute pelvic limb stiffness and cerebellar ataxia have been observed in Yorkshire pigs that are from 1 to 5 weeks of age. The clinical signs are progressive over a few days. A recessive inheritance is suspected.

OCCIPITAL DYSPLASIA

This syndrome somewhat resembles the Arnold-Chiari malformation in human beings. It occurs primarily in toy-breed dogs and results in an enlargement of the foramen magnum and congenital shortening of C1. Concomitant hydrocephalus has been observed. In severe cases, the cerebellum and the brain stem are exposed, making these structures vulnerable to compression. The clinical signs include cranial neck pain, personality change, and cerebellar ataxia. Many dogs remain asymptomatic. Often, the clinical signs are more related to the hydrocephalus. The diagnosis is confirmed by radiographs of the skull and the cervical vertebrae. No surgical treatment has been reported.

Miscellaneous Ataxias and Tremors

CONGENITAL TREMOR (MYOCLONIA CONGENITA)

Congenital tremor is a disease of neonatal swine that is characterized by rapid, repeated contractions of one or more skeletal muscle groups. There is evidence that suggests that congenital tremor is a boar-transmitted viral disease that produces mild spinal hypomyelinization.[8] In many respects, the clinical signs resemble a hypomyelinization syndrome that has been observed in chow chow puppies.

Clinical Signs

Clonic muscle contractions develop in the neck, the legs, or the trunk within a few hours of birth. The myoclonus may cease within 2 to 8 weeks but may persist longer (even in adult swine). The severity of the clinical signs varies from slight muscular tremors to violent jerking. The tremors are exacerbated by exercise and improve or cease when the pigs are asleep or at rest. All or only a portion of the litter may be affected. Violent head shaking may interfere with nursing, and severely affected pigs may starve to death.

Treatment

No specific treatment is known. Since many pigs will improve with time, attentive nursing care may salvage many affected pigs. Hog cholera vaccine virus also may induce a similar syndrome in pigs when it is administered to susceptible sows. A method of identification of carrier boars has not been reported; however, in certain herds with multiple occurrences, breeding programs should be altered so that boars that are suspected of being carriers are eliminated.

PERIODIC SPASTICITY OF CATTLE

This chronic progressive disease occurs primarily in cattle that are kept in barns or stalls. It occurs in both sexes and in many breeds but is seen most frequently in Holstein and Guernsey cattle. The etiology is unknown. The disease probably results from a combination of environmental and hereditary factors.

Clinical Signs

Intermittent attacks of muscle spasm or cramps characterize this disease. The examiner may initiate the sign by moving the animal sideways or backward. There is spasm of the muscles of the pelvic limbs and the back. The spasms may extend forward and may involve the neck, the head, and the thoracic limbs. The attacks may last for several minutes and may disappear when the animal lies down. Affected animals lose weight because they have difficulty eating while standing. The signs apparently are most severe during the winter and the early spring. Periodic spasticity must be differentiated from spastic paresis and hypomagnesemic tetany.

Treatment

There is no known therapy except for symptomatic care. Affected animals should not be used for breeding. The overall prognosis is poor.

PLANT-INDUCED ATAXIAS

Ergotism (Dallis Grass Staggers)

This is an acute disorder of the nervous system that is seen in cattle (and, rarely, in horses) that ingest Dallis grass or rye infected with the fungus *Claviceps paspali*. The sclerotium of this fungus develops in the seed head of Dallis grass and is present in highest concentrations during wet summers. Toxic fungal alkaloids, found primarily in the mature sclerotia, produce the neurologic signs. A very similar syndrome has been described in cattle grazing in Bermuda grass pastures in Louisiana.

Affected animals demonstrate an uncoordinated gait when stimulated. Tremors, twitching, and dysmetria are apparent. Affected animals are bright and alert and gradually recover when removed from toxic pastures. Severely affected animals may develop extensor rigidity, opisthotonos, and clonic convulsions. The treatment consists of removing cattle from affected pastures. Control of the disorder is achieved by grazing cattle on pastures before the seed heads develop or by mowing affected pastures to remove the seed heads.

Bermuda Grass Staggers

This syndrome is nearly identical to nervous ergotism, except that the toxic material has not been identified. Cattle grazing in toxic Bermuda grass pastures develop signs within 36 hours. The stems, leaves, and hay of affected pastures are toxic. The signs cease within 2 to 12 days following removal of the toxic feed.

Ryegrass Staggers

The exact etiology of ryegrass toxicity is not known. Ryegrass staggers affects primarily sheep but also occurs in cattle and horses. The syndrome is nearly identical to nervous ergotism and Bermuda grass staggers.

CASE HISTORIES

Case History 11A

Signalment

Canine, spitz, female, 3 years old.

History

Severe lack of coordination and loss of balance since the dog was 6 weeks of age. The signs have been non-progressive.

Physical Examination

Negative except for the neurologic problem

Neurologic Examination *

A. Observation
  1. Mental status: Alert.
  2. Posture: Severe symmetric trunkal ataxia. Head tremors. No head tilt or circling.
  3. Gait: Severe hypermetria and ataxia. Wide-based stance. Intention tremors of the head and the body.

B. Palpation

C. Postural Reactions

Left	Reactions	Right
	Proprioceptive positioning	
+2	PL	+2
+2	TL	+2
Dysmetric	Wheelbarrowing	Dysmetric
+2	Hopping, PL	+2
+2	Hopping, TL	+2
+2	Extensor postural thrust	+2
+1 to +2	Hemistand-hemiwalk	+1 to +2
Hypermetric	Tonic neck	Hypermetric
	Placing, tactile	
Hypermetric	PL	Hypermetric
Hypermetric	TL	Hypermetric
	Placing, visual	
Hypermetric	TL	Hypermetric

D. Spinal Reflexes

Left	Reflex Spinal Segment	Right
	Quadriceps	
+2 to +3	L4–L6	+2 to +3
	Extensor carpi radialis	
+2	C7–T1	+2
	Triceps	
+2	C7–T1	+2
	Flexion, PL	
+2	L5–S1	+2
	Flexion, TL	
+2	C6–T1	+2
0	Crossed extensor	0
	Perineal	
+2	S1–S2	+2

E. Cranial Nerves

Left	Nerve + Function	Right
	C.N. II vision	
+2	menace	+2
Nor.	C.N. II + C.N. III pupil size	Nor.
+2	Stim. left eye	+2
+2	Stim. right eye	+2
Nor.	C.N. II fundus	Nor.
	C.N. III, C.N. IV, C.N. VI	
0	Strabismus	0
0	Nystagmus	0
Nor.	C.N. V sensation	Nor.
Nor.	C.N. V mastication	Nor.
Nor.	C.N. VII facial muscles	Nor.
+2	Palpebral	+2
Nor.	C.N. IX, C.N. X swallowing	Nor.
Nor.	C.N. XII tongue	Nor.

F. Sensation: Location
  Hyperesthesia _____ None _____
  Superficial pain _____ Normal _____
  Deep pain _____ Normal _____

Complete sections G and H before reviewing Case Summary.

G. Assessment (Anatomic diagnosis and estimation of prognosis)

H. Plan (Diagnostic)
  Rule-outs   Procedure
  1.
  2.
  3.
  4.

Case History 11B

Signalment

Canine, Pekingese, male, 2 years old.

History

Progressive lack of coordination and falling from side to side during the past 72 hours. The head swings from side to side and bobs up and down. No history of trauma or other clinical signs.

Physical Examination

See neurologic findings.

Neurologic Examination *

A. Observation
   1. Mental status: Alert, hyperventilating.
   2. Posture: Sternal recumbency, rolls to right, extreme head tilt to right.
   3. Gait: Cannot stand. Moderate truncal and severe head ataxia. Head drop is present. Severe dysmetria of limbs.

B. Palpation
   Negative.

C. Postural Reactions

Left	Reactions	Right
	Proprioceptive positioning	
+1 to +2	PL	0 to +1
0 to +1	TL	+1
+2	Wheelbarrowing	+1
+1	Hopping, PL	0
+1 to +2	Hopping, TL	+1
+1	Extensor postural thrust	0
0	Hemistand-hemiwalk	0
+2	Tonic neck	+1
	Placing, tactile	
0	PL	0
+1	TL	0 to +1
	Placing, visual	
+1	TL	0 to +1

D. Spinal Reflexes

Left	Reflex Spinal Segment	Right
	Quadriceps	
+3	L4−L6	+4
	Extensor carpi radialis	
+3	C7−T1	+3
	Triceps	
+3	C7−T1	+3
	Flexion, PL	
+3	L5−S1	+3
	Flexion, TL	
+2	C6−T1	+2
0	Crossed extensor	Present
	Perineal	
+2	S1−S2	+2

E. Cranial Nerves

Left	Nerve + Function	Right
	C.N. II vision	
+2	menace	+2
Nor.	C.N. II + C.N. III pupil size	Nor.
+2	Stim. left eye	+2
+2	Stim. right eye	+2
Nor.	C.N. II fundus	Nor.
	C.N. III, C.N. IV, C.N. VI	
0	Strabismus	0
Positional-Left	Nystagmus	Positional-Left
Nor.	C.N. V sensation	Nor.
Nor.	C.N. V mastication	Nor.
Nor.	C.N. VII facial muscles	Nor.
+2	Palpebral	+2
Nor.	C.N. IX, C.N. X swallowing	Nor.
Nor.	C.N. XII tongue	Nor.

F. Sensation: Location
   Hyperesthesia _____ None _____
   Superficial pain _____ Good _____
   Deep pain _____ Good _____

Complete sections G and H before reviewing Case Summary.

G. Assessment (Anatomic diagnosis and estimation of prognosis)

H. Plan (Diagnostic)
   Rule-outs   Procedure
   1.
   2.
   3.
   4.

---

*Key: 0 = absent, +1 = decreased, +2 = normal, +3 = exaggerated, +4 = very exaggerated or clonus, PL = pelvic limb, TL = thoracic limb.

Case History 11C

Signalment

Feline, domestic, male, 6 months old.

History

The cat has been ill for 10 days. He is depressed, confused, and ataxic and sleeps most of the time. He has gotten progressively worse.

Physical Examination

The cat is dehydrated, thin, and extremely depressed. Temperature: 102.5 degrees F.

Neurologic Examination *

A. Observation
1. Mental status: Depressed, stuporous, grinds teeth when aroused.
2. Posture: Recumbent, slight head tilt.
3. Gait: Tetraparesis. Falls to left and right when forced to stand. Front legs are extended.

B. Palpation
Hypertonus of thoracic limbs.

C. Postural Reactions

Left	Reactions	Right
	Proprioceptive positioning	
+1	PL	+1
0 to +1	TL	0 to +1
+1	Wheelbarrowing	+1
+1	Hopping, PL	+1
+1	Hopping, TL	+1
+1	Extensor postural thrust	+1
0	Hemistand-hemiwalk	0
+1	Tonic neck	+1
	Placing, tactile	
+1 to +2	PL	+1 to +2
+1	TL	+1
	Placing, visual	
+1	TL	+1

D. Spinal Reflexes

Left	Reflex Spinal Segment	Right
	Quadriceps	
+3	L4−L6	+3
	Extensor carpi radialis	
+2	C7−T1	+2
	Triceps	
+2	C7−T1	+2
	Flexion, PL	
+3	L5−S1	+3
	Flexion, TL	
+3	C6−T1	+3
Present	Crossed extensor	
	Perineal	
+2	S1−S2	

E. Cranial Nerves

Left	Nerve + Function	Right
	C.N. II vision	
+2	menace	
Nor.	C.N. II + C.N. III pupil size	Nor.
+2	Stim. left eye	+2
+2	Stim. right eye	+2
Nor.	C.N. II fundus	Nor.
	C.N. III, C.N. IV, C.N. VI	
0	Strabismus	0
Rotatory	Nystagmus	Rotatory
Nor.	C.N. V sensation	Nor.
Nor.	C.N. V mastication	Nor.
Nor.	C.N. VII facial muscles	Nor.
+2	Palpebral	+2
Nor.	C.N. IX, C.N. X swallowing	Nor.
Nor.	C.N. XII tongue	Nor.

F. Sensation: Location
Hyperesthesia _____ None _____
Superficial pain _____ Good _____
Deep pain _____ Good _____

Complete sections G and H before reviewing Case Summary.

G. Assessment (Anatomic diagnosis and estimation of prognosis)

H. Plan (Diagnostic)
   Rule-outs   Procedure
   1.
   2.
   3.
   4.

---

*Key: 0 = absent, +1 = decreased, +2 = normal, +3 = exaggerated, +4 = very exaggerated or clonus, PL = pelvic limb, TL = thoracic limb.

Case History 11D

Signalment

Feline, domestic, female, 2 years old.

History

The cat developed acute ataxia and lack of coordination. The head tilts to the right and the cat circles right. Appetite is good. No history of previous ear infection.

Physical Examination

Otic examination is negative.

Neurologic Examination *

A. Observation
   1. Mental status: Alert.
   2. Posture: Circles to right, head tilt to right, falls to right.
   3. Gait: Asymmetric ataxia. The cat drifts and falls to right.

B. Palpation

C. Postural Reactions

Left	Reactions	Right
	Proprioceptive positioning PL	
+2		+2
+2	TL	+2
+2	Wheelbarrowing	Dysmetria
+2	Hopping, PL	+2
+2	Hopping, TL	+2
+2	Extensor postural thrust	+2
Ataxia	Hemistand-hemiwalk	Ataxia
Ataxia	Tonic neck	Severe ataxia
+2	Placing, tactile PL	+2
+2	TL	+2
+2	Placing, visual TL	+2

D. Spinal Reflexes

Left	Reflex Spinal Segment	Right
+2	Quadriceps L4–L6	+2
+2	Extensor carpi radialis C7–T1	+2
+2	Triceps C7–T1	+2
+2	Flexion, PL L5–S1	+2
+2	Flexion, TL C6–T1	+2
0	Crossed extensor	0
+2	Perineal S1–S2	+2

E. Cranial Nerves

Left	Nerve + Function	Right
+2	C.N. II vision menace	+2
Nor.	C.N. II + C.N. III pupil size	Nor.
+2	Stim. left eye	+2
+2	Stim. right eye	+2
Nor.	C.N. II fundus	Nor.
0	C.N. III, C.N. IV, C.N. VI Strabismus	Ventrolateral when head is extended
Horizontal—left	Nystagmus	Horizontal—left
Nor.	C.N. V sensation	Nor.
Nor.	C.N. V mastication	Nor.
Nor.	C.N. VII facial muscles	Nor.
+2	Palpebral	+2
Nor.	C.N. IX, C.N. X swallowing	Nor.
Nor.	C.N. XII tongue	Nor.

F. Sensation: Location
   Hyperesthesia _____ None _____
   Superficial pain _____ Normal _____
   Deep pain _____ Normal _____

Complete sections G and H before reviewing Case Summary.

G. Assessment (Anatomic diagnosis and estimation of prognosis)

H. Plan (Diagnostic)

Rule-outs	Procedure
1.	
2.	
3.	
4.	

---

*Key: 0 = absent, +1 = decreased, +2 = normal, +3 = exaggerated, +4 = very exaggerated or clonus, PL = pelvic limb, TL = thoracic limb.

ASSESSMENT 11A

Anatomic diagnosis: The dog has generalized symmetric ataxia associated with head tremor and intention tremor. No paresis, cranial nerve dysfunction, or vestibular signs are present. The signs are related to generalized cerebellar disease. A congenital or early postnatal syndrome is suspected, because the signs began at an early age. The signs have been nonprogressive, which tends to rule out abiotrophies, storage diseases, and inflammation. A good choice for the diagnosis would be cerebellar hypoplasia.

Diagnostic plan (Rule-outs):
1. Cerebellar hypoplasia—there is no noninvasive method available (histopathology).
2. Cerebellar abiotrophy—history, histopathology.
3. Inflammation—CSF analysis (if early in course). This method probably is not useful at this time.

Therapeutic plan: None. The disease is untreatable.

Client education: The dog will not improve but can function as a pet in her current condition. The dog should not be bred, because the disease may be hereditary in this breed.

Case summary: The presumptive diagnosis was cerebellar hypoplasia. A follow-up was not recorded.

ASSESSMENT 11B

Anatomic diagnosis: Both cerebellar (head drop, head ataxia, truncal ataxia) and vestibular (head tilt, rolling, nystagmus) signs are present. Because the dog has motor deficits associated with the vestibular signs, central vestibular (brain stem) disease probably is present. A lesion or a disease involving the cerebellar-medullary junction could cause both cerebellar and central vestibular signs. The progressive course suggests inflammation, neoplasia, or degeneration.

Diagnostic plan: (Rule-outs):
1. Encephalitis—CSF examination (white blood cells 380, 88 per cent lymphocytes, 12 per cent neutrophils, protein 120 mg/dl), CSF culture (negative), conjunctival smear—fluorescent antibody titer for distemper (negative).
2. Neoplasia—skull radiography (negative).
3. Degeneration—Check complete blood count (CBC) and profile (normal) for evidence of polysystemic disease.

Therapeutic plan: Chloramphenicol, 50 mg per kg tid.

Client education: The prognosis is guarded, since it is most likely that a viral infection is present. Distemper encephalitis is still a strong possibility.

Case summary: The diagnosis was nonsuppurative encephalitis of unknown etiology. The dog recovered in 6 weeks.

ASSESSMENT 11C

Anatomic diagnosis: The predominant signs are those of central vestibular disease (brain stem disease). The head ataxia may be from cerebellar disease. The severe depression and altered mental attitude could be of cerebral or brain stem origin. The multifocal progressive features suggest inflammation or degeneration.

Diagnostic plan: (Rule-outs):
1. Nervous form of feline infectious peritonitis (FIP)—CSF analysis (white blood cells 200, 90 per cent segmented neutrophils, 10 per cent lymphocytes, protein 120 mg/dl), fundus examination (negative).
2. Lead poisoning—CBC (normal), blood lead levels (0.02 parts per million).
3. Thiamine deficiency—response to thiamine therapy.
4. Rabies—history, necropsy.

Therapeutic plan:
1. Intramuscular thiamine.
2. Chloramphenicol, 30 mg per kg tid.

Client education: The prognosis is poor.

Case summary: Noneffusive FIP was diagnosed. The diagnosis was confirmed by necropsy study.

ASSESSMENT 11D

Anatomic diagnosis: The circling, head tilt, asymmetric ataxia, and spontaneous nystagmus with the quick left phase suggest a right vestibular lesion. The positional strabismus in the right eye also suggests a right vestibular lesion. The absence of paresis localizes the lesion to the right peripheral vestibular apparatus.

Diagnostic plan: (Rule-outs):
1. Acute bacterial otitis media-interna—otoscopic examination (negative), skull radiographs (negative).
2. Trauma—History, physical examination, and radiographs.
3. Feline vestibular syndrome—exclude Diagnostic Plan Numbers 1 and 2.

Therapeutic plan: Although otitis media-interna is unlikely, one still could choose to treat the cat with the appropriate antibiotics just to be safe. In this case, the cat was treated with chloramphenicol for 10 days.

Client education: Feline vestibular syndrome is a disease of unknown cause and no specific therapy is known. Recovery usually takes 3 to 6 weeks.

Case summary: The cat recovered in 3 weeks. The presumptive diagnosis was feline vestibular syndrome.

REFERENCES

1. Chrisman, C. L.: Disorders of the vestibular system. Comp. Cont. Ed. 1:744, 1979.
2. deLahunta, A.: Comparative cerebellar disease in domestic animals. Comp. Cont. Ed. 2:8, 1980.
3. deLahunta, A.: Veterinary Neuroanatomy and Clinical Neurology. Philadelphia, W. B. Saunders Co., 1977.
4. Knecht, C. D., Larmar, C. H., Schaible, R., and Pflum, K.: Cerebellar hypoplasia in Chow Chows. JAAHA 15:51, 1979.
5. deLahunta, A., and Averill, D. R.: Hereditary cerebellar cortical and extrapyramidal nuclear abiotrophy in Kerry Blue Terriers. JAVMA 168:1119–1124, 1976.
6. deLahunta, A., Fenner, W. R., Indrieri, R. J., Mellick, P. W., Gardner, S., and Bell, J. S.: Hereditary cerebellar cortical abiotrophy in the Gordon Setter. JAVMA, 177:538–541, 1980.
7. Hartley, W. J., Barker, J. S. F., et al.: Inherited cerebellar degeneration in the rough coated Collie. Aust. Vet. Pract. 8:79–85, 1978.
8. Gustafson, D. P., and Kanitz, C. L.: Experimental transmission of congenital tremors in swine. Proc. 78th Meet. U.S.A.H.A., 338–345, 1974.

LESION LOCALIZATION

The problems described in this chapter result from dysfunction of C.N. V, C.N. VII, C.N. IX, C.N. X, and C.N. XII. Disorders of the other cranial nerves will be discussed in Chapter 13. The localization of cranial nerve lesions was presented in Chapter 4 and will be reviewed briefly in this chapter (see Table 4–8).

Once the clinician has identified cranial nerve dysfunction, he or she must decide if the injury involves the peripheral cranial nerve (nerve fibers) or the neuron cell bodies that are located in the brain stem. This differentiation is based on the results of a careful neurologic examination. Peripheral cranial nerve disorders are characterized by involvement of specific cranial muscles with no evidence of appendicular paresis.

Cranial nerve dysfunction resulting from brain stem lesions is characterized by multiple cranial nerve involvement and, more importantly, specific brain stem signs (paresis, central vestibular disease, depression, and so forth). Occasionally, the generalized lower motor neuron (LMN) diseases produce cranial nerve signs. These diseases are easily recognized because of the obvious LMN signs in the limbs.

C.N. V (Trigeminal Nerve)

ANATOMY

The motor neurons of C.N. V are located in the pons near the rostral cerebellar peduncles

12

CHAPTER

DISORDERS OF THE FACE, TONGUE, AND LARYNX

(Fig. 12–1). The motor fibers are distributed to the muscles of mastication by the mandibular branch of C.N. V. Sensation to the surface of the head is supplied by C.N. V through its divisions. The ophthalmic nerve innervates the eyelids and the cornea, and the maxillary division provides sensation to the face and the nasal area. The ophthalmic nerve is the sensory arc of the corneal reflex. The ophthalmic and maxillary nerves are the sensory arcs of the commonly performed palpebral reflex. The mandibular nerve provides sensation to the lower jaw. The cell bodies of these sensory

Figure 12–1. *A.* Midbrain structures. *B.* Pons and medulla, showing vital centers and nuclei of cranial nerves. (From Hoerlein, B. F.: Canine Neurology, 3rd ed. Philadelphia, W. B. Saunders Co., 1978. Used by permission.)

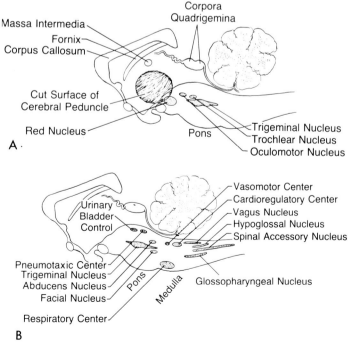

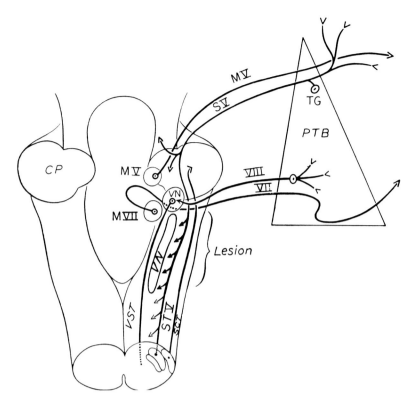

Figure 12-2. Diagram of the brain stem (pons and medulla) and the cranial cervical cord, showing the anatomy of the trigeminal nerve and its relationship to the facial and vestibulocochlear nerves. (From deLahunta, A.: Veterinary Neuroanatomy and Clinical Neurology. Philadelphia, W. B. Saunders Co., 1977. Used by permission.)

neurons are located in the trigeminal ganglia. The trigeminal nerve enters the pons just rostral to the origin of the facial and vestibulocochlear nerves. The sensory axons of the trigeminal nerve course caudally through the medulla in the spinal tract of the trigeminal nerve (Fig. 12-2). This tract continues caudally into the first cervical segment. Nerve fibers within this tract synapse upon neurons that are located in nuclei distributed along its course.

The anatomic distribution of pain fibers in C.N. V is of considerable importance in the location of lesions involving the trigeminal nerve. Lesions in the medulla involving the spinal tract of C.N. V result in ipsilateral loss of facial sensation but no impairment of the masticatory muscles. Loss of both sensory and motor function of the trigeminal nerve usually results from pontine lesions or extramedullary disorders that affect both motor and sensory neurons or fibers. Loss of motor function with no sensory impairment is associated with discrete lesions in the trigeminal motor nucleus located in the pons.

CLINICAL SIGNS

For the reasons just described, sensation may be lost ipsilaterally to the lesion. In addition, diminished corneal and palpebral reflexes may be observed as a result of interfer-

ence with the sensory arcs of these reflexes. Bilateral involvement of motor nerves results in a dropped jaw that cannot be closed voluntarily (mandibular paralysis). The jaw muscles are atonic and become atrophic if the paralysis persists for longer than 7 days. Unilateral motor lesions are difficult to detect until specific muscle atrophy develops.

C.N. VII (Facial Nerve)

ANATOMY

The facial nerve innervates the muscles of facial expression. The neurons are located in the facial nuclei of the rostral medulla (see Fig. 12-1). Nerve fibers leave the facial nuclei and course dorsomedially and around the abducent nucleus. The fibers leave the ventral surface of the medulla near C.N. VIII. The facial nerve courses through the petrosal bone en route to the face. It is separated from the tympanic bulla by a thin sheet of connective tissue. A disease involving the middle ear may extend to the facial nerve, resulting in an ipsilateral facial palsy. The facial nerve is the main motor pathway for the corneal and palpebral reflexes.

CLINICAL SIGNS

Lesions of C.N. VII result in ipsilateral facial paresis or paralysis. The lip may droop on the

244

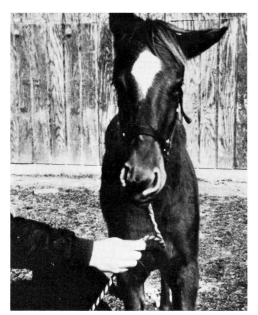

Figure 12–3. A horse with left facial nerve paralysis. Note the drooped ear and the deviation of the nose to the right.

affected side, and food or saliva may fall from that side of the mouth. The nasal philtrum may be deviated to the normal side. Drooping of the ear may be observed in animals with erect ears (Fig. 12–3). The palpebral fissure may be wider than normal and may fail to close upon elicitation of the palpebral or the corneal reflex. Exposure keratitis is a common sequela of facial nerve injury in the dog. It is especially prevalent in breeds that tend to have ectropion or exophthalmic globes.

Vestibular signs associated with facial paresis or paralysis are very commonly observed. These clinical findings are explained by the close anatomic relationship of the facial nerve to the vestibular nerve at the brain stem and in the course of these nerves into the petrosal bone. It is extremely important to differentiate these two locations because of the difference in prognosis and therapy. Lesions at the brainstem result in central vestibular disease, whereas lesions in the petrosal bone cause peripheral vestibular disease. See Chapter 11 for a discussion of these disorders.

C.N. IX (Glossopharyngeal Nerve), C.N. X (Vagus Nerve), and C.N. XI (Spinal Accessory Nerve)

Anatomy

These cranial nerves will be discussed as a group, because their nerve fibers originate from the same medullary nuclei and because they interact to control pharyngeal and laryngeal motor activity. These nerves originate in the nucleus ambiguus, located in the medulla (see Fig. 12–1). The rostral two thirds of the nucleus ambiguus is involved in swallowing by means of motor impulses through the glossopharyngeal and vagus nerves. The caudal nucleus ambiguus controls the laryngeal muscles through the accessory and vagus nerves and its branches (recurrent laryngeal nerves).

Clinical Signs

Dysphagia is the primary clinical sign of lesions involving the rostral nucleus ambiguus or its nerves (glossopharyngeal, vagus). The gag reflex is absent or depressed. Inspiratory dyspnea from laryngeal paralysis is the primary clinical sign of lesions involving the caudal nucleus ambiguus or its nerves (vagus, recurrent laryngeal).

C.N. XII (Hypoglossal Nerve)

Anatomy

This nerve originates from cell bodies located in the medulla (see Fig. 12–1). The hypoglossal nerve exits the medulla at a site just caudal to the spinal accessory nerve. It innervates the muscles of the tongue.

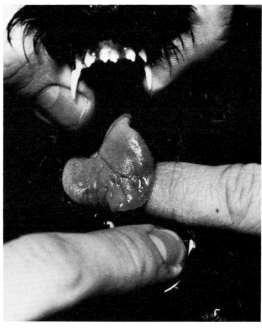

Figure 12–4. Unilateral hypoglossal paralysis resulting from trauma to the brain stem in an adult terrier dog. Note the right lateral deviation of the tongue and the atrophy of the tongue on the right side.

CLINICAL SIGNS

Paresis or paralysis of the tongue is the main clinical sign of bilateral lesions (usually in the medulla). Affected animals cannot prehend food or water. With unilateral lesions, the tongue, when protruded, tends to deviate toward the side of the lesion (Fig. 12–4).[1] Atrophy of the tongue may be severe.

DISEASES

Mandibular Paralysis

An idiopathic trigeminal neuritis that results in bilateral paralysis of the masticatory muscles has been observed in dogs. The disease apparently produces demyelination and some axonal degeneration of all portions of the trigeminal nerve and the ganglion.[1] Brain stem lesions have not been observed in the few cases that have been examined at necropsy.[1]

CLINICAL SIGNS

The onset of clinical signs is acute or subacute. The jaw hangs open, and the mouth cannot be closed voluntarily. The dog cannot prehend food and has difficulty drinking water. Mild dysphagia may be present. Dehydration and drooling saliva are associated signs. Affected dogs are alert and responsive and have no other detectable neurologic deficits. The clinical signs are suggestive of bulbar paralysis, which is observed with rabies. Clinicians should be extremely cautious in examining these dogs until accumulating sufficient evidence to rule out rabies. A diagnosis is based on the clinical signs and the absence of other brain stem signs. The disease should not be confused with masticatory myositis. In the latter disease, the mouth is closed, and the animal resents having its jaw moved or manipulated. Pain may be associated with muscle palpation. Sensation is usually normal in idiopathic mandibular paralysis.

TREATMENT

There is no definitive treatment. Affected animals are supported with fluid therapy and gastric gavage with food made into a gruel. Pharyngostomy tubes may be beneficial. The clinician should exercise caution to avoid aspiration pneumonia, especially in dysphagic animals. Performing frequent physical therapy by opening and closing the mouth helps to delay muscle atrophy. The recovery is usu-ally complete in 2 to 3 weeks. Multiple episodes may occur in the same dog. The prognosis is good.

Facial Paralysis

As was stated previously, the most common disease producing facial nerve injury is otitis media-interna (see Chapter 11). In this section, two other diseases involving the facial nerve will be described.

IDIOPATHIC FACIAL PARALYSIS

This disease occurs in the absence of otitis media-interna. The cause is unknown; however, the clinical signs are similar to those of human facial neuritis (Bell's palsy). Studies of human beings suggest that one etiology of facial paralysis is herpes simplex virus.[2] In 25 per cent of human patients, hypesthesia of the trigeminal nerve has been observed. In addition, evidence of a subclinical neuropathy has been observed on the unaffected side.[2] These findings suggest that the apparent mononeuritis of the facial nerve is a primary manifestation of a more generalized polyneuritis.[2] In this regard, the facial paralysis is similar to the cranial polyneuritis induced by herpes zoster virus. Although it has not been confirmed in dogs, a more generalized polyneuropathy may exist in idiopathic facial paralysis.

Clinical Signs

The onset of facial paralysis is sudden and the distribution is usually unilateral. There is no clinical evidence of vestibular disease or otitis media-interna. Affected animals are nonfebrile and have no polysystemic signs. The course is variable; however, the clinical signs are maximal in 7 days. The recovery takes 3 to 6 weeks. Exposure keratitis is a common problem that results from improper lubrication of the cornea.

Treatment

No specific treatment is known. The treatment of human Bell's palsy is controversial. Controlled studies conducted by Wolfe and associates have suggested that corticosteroid therapy offers some benefit, although the results are less impressive than earlier reports would indicate.[3] The administration of steroids in moderate or severe cases of Bell's palsy when there are no illnesses that might be exacerbated by their use is recommended. The

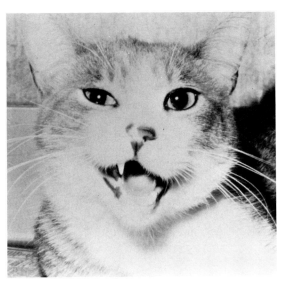

Figure 12–5.   A cat with right hemifacial spasm. Note the deviation of the nose and the wrinkling of the right upper lip. There is squinting of the right eyelids.

prognosis for recovery with or without therapy is good.

HEMIFACIAL SPASM

This syndrome is rarely observed in dogs or cats and is thought to occur secondarily to hypersensitivity of the facial nerve. The signs include blepharospasm, elevation of the ear, deviation of the nose to the affected side, and wrinkling or displacement of the upper lip (Fig. 12–5). Ipsilateral Horner's syndrome has been reported.[4] Facial neuritis resulting from trauma or from inflammation in the middle ear is thought to be the cause of the syndrome. It may precede signs of facial paralysis.

Hemifacial spasm also may occur as an upper motor neuron (UMN) sign involving the facial nerve. Lesions that isolate the facial nuclear motor neurons from UMN control could result in hemifacial spasm caused by the loss of inhibitory interneuronal activity. The palpebral reflex may be hyperactive, in that spasm of the eyelids may be observed when the reflex is elicited. This form of hemifacial spasm is associated with other brain stem neurologic signs.

The diagnosis and treatment are the same as those described for facial nerve paralysis.

Laryngeal Paralysis

Unilateral and bilateral paresis or paralysis of the laryngeal muscles have been reported in dogs and horses. Unilateral paralysis results in moderate inspiratory dyspnea and inspiratory noise. Bilateral paralysis results in episodes of gagging, cyanosis, severe inspiratory dyspnea, and collapse. The intrinsic muscles of the larynx are innervated by the recurrent laryngeal nerves that are branches of the vagus nerve. An injury to these nerve fibers or their cell bodies, which are located in the caudal nucleus ambiguus, results in the clinical signs. Laryngeal paralysis has been associated with chronic polyneuritis, injury to the vagus nerve during neck surgery, or retropharyngeal infection. A hereditary laryngeal paralysis occurs in the Bouvier des Flandres and will be discussed in the next section as the prototype of other forms of laryngeal paralysis in the dog.

HEREDITARY LARYNGEAL PARALYSIS IN THE BOUVIER DES FLANDRES

Laryngeal paralysis in Bouviers des Flandres is inherited as an autosomal dominant trait and results in bilateral partial destruction of the innervation of the larynx. The disease results from progressive degeneration of neurons within the nucleus ambiguus with subsequent wallerian degeneration throughout the length of the laryngeal nerves. In a few dogs, bilateral cranial tibial muscle denervation is observed.[5]

Clinical Signs

The onset of recognizable clinical signs is 4 to 6 months of age. The chief signs include decreasing endurance and noisy breathing. Severe respiratory distress associated with cyanosis or regurgitation occurs in more severely affected dogs. The signs are progressive. Laryngeal stridor, pharyngitis, and tonsillitis are consistent physical findings.

Diagnosis

Laryngoscopy usually reveals unilateral or bilateral immobility of the vocal folds. In a study of 105 affected Bouviers de Flandres, 28 dogs had bilateral immobility, 71 had immobility of the left vocal fold and moderate abduction of the right on inspiration, 3 had slight motion of both vocal folds, and 3 had abduction of both vocal folds on inspiration.[5]

An electromyographic (EMG) examination reveals a varying pattern of denervation of the abductor muscles on both sides. The EMG findings are usually in agreement with the laryngoscopic findings. Normal motor unit potentials frequently are found in muscles with denervation activity. A histologic examination of the affected muscles reveals changes that are characteristic of denervation atrophy.

Three dogs had bilateral cranial tibial muscle denervation, which resulted in a dropped foot.

In experimental studies, evidence of laryngeal dysfunction can be established when the animal is as young as 12 weeks of age with laryngoscopy or, more specifically, with electromyography. Normal abduction or adduction, or both, can be observed, even though EMG findings clearly indicate the presence of denervation.

Treatment

There is no effective cure. Since the disease is inherited as an autosomal dominant trait, it should be able to be eradicated through selective breeding programs.

Hypoglossal Paralysis

Paralysis of the tongue usually results from diseases affecting the medulla. It has been observed with neoplastic, granulomatous, viral, and bacterial inflammations of the caudal brain stem. It is a common sign in bulbar paralysis from rabies. Specific inflammatory disease of the hypoglossal nerve has not been reported.

Pharyngeal Paralysis

Pharyngeal paralysis is usually accompanied by signs of focal or diffuse brain stem disease. It also may accompany severe cerebral disease without specific lesions in the nucleus ambiguus or the swallowing center. Cerebral lesions destroy the neurons that influence the activity of the medullary nuclei (e.g., UMN pharyngeal paralysis, pseudobulbar palsy).[1]

Generalized LMN Diseases

Diseases that produce generalized LMN dysfunction may produce cranial nerve signs. Botulism and canine myasthenic syndromes more frequently produce cranial nerve involvement. Rarely, cranial nerve signs are observed with polyradiculoneuritis, tick paralysis, or chronic polyneuritis. Polymyositis occasionally may involve facial muscle, suggesting cranial nerve disease; however, this disease frequently involves the esophagus and

produces clinical signs similar to those of vagal nerve dysfunction. These diseases have been described in Chapter 10.

Facial Hypesthesia

Partial loss of pain sensation is termed *hypesthesia*. Facial hypesthesia without mandibular paresis or paralysis is caused by lesions involving the ipsilateral spinal tract of C.N. V in the medulla or the contralateral sensory cortex. Lesions involving the medulla are associated with decreased corneal or palpebral reflexes. In hypesthesia of cortical origin, reflex activity is usually normal.

Nigropallidal Encephalomalacia

This disease is characterized by the sudden onset of functional impairment of the muscles that are supplied by motor fibers of C.N. V, C.N. VII, and C.N. XII. It was first described in horses from northern California and southern Oregon that were grazed on pastures containing large quantities of yellow star thistle.[6] Because of the typical clinical signs and the association with yellow star thistle, the disease also is called "chewing disease" and yellow star thistle poisoning. The disease also has been reported in horses from Colorado and Utah that were grazed on pastures containing abundant Russian knapweed, a plant related to yellow star thistle.[7] Although the specific factor or toxin has not been identified, necrosis and malacia develop in the brain stem in the region of the globus pallidus and the substantia nigra. The disease occurs in the western United States, where the offending plants are endemic.

CLINICAL SIGNS

Affected horses range in age from 4 months to 10 years. In general, younger horses are affected more often. Foals that are nursed by clinically normal mares have been affected. Conversely, affected mares have continued to nurse normal foals. A prominent feature of this disease is the sudden onset of the inability to eat and drink. The ability to prehend food or water is partially or totally lost. The mouth is held partially open, the lips are retracted, and rhythmic tongue movements and purposeless chewing motions are apparent. Affected horses assume a drowsy pose and a fixed facial expression. The facial muscles are hypertonic.

Flaccidity of facial muscles and gait impairment do not develop. Food or water that is placed in the posterior pharynx can be swallowed. The clinical signs suggest specific UMN dysfunction of C.N. V, C.N. VII, and C.N. XII. Complete recovery has not been reported, although some horses may improve with time. The cause of death in most horses has been starvation or aspiration pneumonia.

DIAGNOSIS

Since no specific tests are available, the diagnosis is based on the history and the clinical signs. The disease must be differentiated from rabies, equine encephalomyelitis, brain stem abscess, and hematoma. The facial hypertonicity and the lack of ataxia or paresis differentiate nigropallidal encephalomalacia from these diseases.

TREATMENT

No specific treatment is known. Feeding affected horses by tube will prolong life while one waits to see if improvement will occur. The prognosis is poor. Horses should not be allowed to graze on pastures in which the offending plants are abundant.

CASE HISTORIES

Case History 12A

Signalment

Canine, poodle, male, 8 years old.

History

Right head tilt of 10 days' duration. The dog fell down stairs 1 week prior to developing signs. Severe ocular discharge in right eye.

Physical Examination

Exposure keratitis of the right eye.

Neurologic Examination *

A. Observation
  1. Mental status: Alert.
  2. Posture: Right head tilt.
  3. Gait: The dog drifts to the right and falls if he turns quickly.

B. Palpation
  Negative.

C. Postural Reactions

Left	Reactions	Right
	Proprioceptive positioning	
+2	PL	+2
+2	TL	+2
+2	Wheelbarrowing	
+2	Hopping, PL	+2
+2	Hopping, TL	+2
+2	Extensor postural thrust	+2
+2	Hemistand-hemiwalk	+2
Nor.	Tonic neck	Nor.
	Placing, tactile	
+2	PL	+2
+2	TL	+2
	Placing, visual	
+2	TL	+2
	Rear	

D. Spinal Reflexes

Left	Reflex / Spinal Segment	Right
	Quadriceps	
+2	L4–L6	+2
	Extensor carpi radialis	
+2	C7–T1	+2
	Triceps	
+2	C7–T1	+2
	Flexion, PL	
+2	L5–S1	+2
	Flexion, TL	
+2	C6–T1	+2
0	Crossed extensor	0
	Perineal	
+2	S1–S2	+2

E. Cranial Nerves

Left	Nerve + Function	Right
	C.N. II vision	
+2	menace	+2
Nor.	C.N. II + C.N. III pupil size	Nor.
+2	Stim. left eye	+2
+2	Stim. right eye	+2
Nor.	C.N. II fundus	Nor.
	C.N. III, C.N. IV, C.N. VI	
0	Strabismus	Vestibular
Present	Nystagmus	Present
+2	C.N. V sensation	+2
+2	C.N. V mastication	+2
	C.N. VII facial	
Nor.	muscles	Paralyzed
+2	Palpebral	0
Nor.	C.N. IX, C.N. X swallowing	Nor.
Nor.	C.N. XII tongue	Nor.

F. Sensation: Location
  Hyperesthesia _____ None _____
  Superficial pain _____ Good _____
  Deep pain _____ Good _____

Complete sections G and H before reviewing Case Summary.

G. Assessment (Anatomic diagnosis and estimation of prognosis)

H. Plan (Diagnostic)
  Rule-outs   Procedure
  1.
  2.
  3.
  4.

Key: 0 = absent, +1 = decreased, +2 = normal, +3 = exaggerated, +4 = very exaggerated or clonus, PL = pelvic limb, TL = thoracic limb.

Case History 12B

Signalment

Canine, English setter, female, 5 years old.

History

Long history of chronic otitis externa, which last was treated 5 months ago. Signs of head tilt have waxed and waned since that time. During the past few weeks, muscle atrophy has developed in the right temporal area.

Physical Examination

The dog is very thin and mildly dehydrated.

Neurologic Examination*

A. Observation
   1. Mental status: Alert.
   2. Posture: Circles to the right.
   3. Gait: Falls to the right, drifts to the right.

B. Palpation
   Negative.

C. Postural Reactions

Left	Reactions	Right
	Proprioceptive positioning	
+2	PL	+2
+2	TL	+2
+2	Wheelbarrowing	+2
+2	Hopping, PL	+2
+2	Hopping, TL	+2
+2	Extensor postural thrust	+2
+2	Hemistand-hemiwalk	+2
+2	Tonic neck	+2
	Placing, tactile	
+2	PL	+2
+2	TL	+2
	Placing, visual	
+2	TL	+2
	Rear	

D. Spinal Reflexes

Left	Reflex Spinal Segment	Right
	Quadriceps	
+2	L4–L6	+2
	Extensor carpi radialis	
+2	C7–T1	+2
	Triceps	
+2	C7–T1	+2
	Flexion, PL	
+2	L5–S1	+2
	Flexion, TL	
+2	C6–T1	+2
0	Crossed extensor	0
	Perineal	
+2	S1–S2	+2

E. Cranial Nerves

Left	Nerve + Function	Right
	C.N. II vision	
+2	menace	0
Nor.	C.N. II + C.N. III pupil size	Nor.
+2	Stim. left eye	+2
+2	Stim. right eye	+2
Nor.	C.N. II fundus	Nor.
	C.N. III, C.N. IV, C.N. VI	
0	Strabismus	0
Horizontal left	Nystagmus	Horizontal left
+2	C.N. V sensation	+2
+2	C.N. V mastication	+2
+2	C.N. VII facial muscles	+2
+2	Palpebral	0
+2	C.N. IX, C.N. X swallowing	+2
+2	C.N. XII tongue	+2

F. Sensation: Location
   Hyperesthesia _____ None _____
   Superficial pain _____ Good _____
   Deep pain _____ Good _____

Complete sections G and H before reviewing Case Summary.

G. Assessment (Anatomic diagnosis and estimation of prognosis)

H. Plan (Diagnostic)
   Rule-outs   Procedure
   1.
   2.
   3.
   4.

*Key: 0 = absent, +1 = decreased, +2 = normal, +3 = exaggerated, +4 = very exaggerated or clonus, PL = pelvic limb, TL = thoracic limb.

Case History 12C

Signalment

Canine, poodle, male, 6 years old.

History

Sudden onset of an inability to close the mouth. The jaw hangs open. The dog cannot prehend food but can lap water. No other signs have been observed.

Physical Examination

Negative except for the neurologic signs.

Neurologic Examination *

A. Observation
   1. Mental status: Alert.
   2. Posture: Normal.
   3. Gait: Normal.

B. Palpation
   Lower jaw hangs open. Hypotonus of masticatory muscles.

C. Postural Reactions

Left	Reactions	Right
	Proprioceptive positioning	
Normal	PL	Normal
Normal	TL	Normal
Normal	Wheelbarrowing	Normal
Normal	Hopping, PL	Normal
Normal	Hopping, TL	Normal
Normal	Extensor postural thrust	Normal
Normal	Hemistand-hemiwalk	Normal
Normal	Tonic neck	Normal
	Placing, tactile	
Normal	PL	Normal
Normal	TL	Normal
	Placing, visual	
Normal	TL	Normal
	Rear	

D. Spinal Reflexes

Left	Reflex Spinal Segment	Right
	Quadriceps	
Normal	L4–L6	Normal
	Extensor carpi radialis	
Normal	C7–T1	Normal
	Triceps	
Normal	C7–T1	Normal
	Flexion, PL	
Normal	L5–S1	Normal
	Flexion, TL	
Normal	C6–T1	Normal
Normal	Crossed extensor	Normal
	Perineal	
Normal	S1–S2	Normal

E. Cranial Nerves

Left	Nerve + Function	Right
	C.N. II vision	
+2	menace	+2
Normal	C.N. II + C.N. III pupil size	Normal
+2	Stim. left eye	+2
+2	Stim. right eye	+2
Normal	C.N. II fundus	Normal
	C.N. III, C.N. IV, C.N. VI	
0	Strabismus	0
0	Nystagmus	0
Normal	C.N. V sensation	Normal
Paralysis	C.N. V mastication	Paralysis
Normal	C.N. VII facial muscles	Normal
+2	Palpebral	+2
+2	C.N. IX, C.N. X swallowing	+2
Normal	C.N. XII tongue	Normal

F. Sensation: Location
   Hyperesthesia _____ None _____
   Superficial pain _____ Good _____
   Deep pain _____ Good _____

Complete sections G and H before reviewing Case Summary.

G. Assessment (Anatomic diagnosis and estimation of prognosis)

H. Plan (Diagnostic)
   Rule-outs   Procedure
   1.
   2.
   3.
   4.

Key: 0 = absent, +1 = decreased, +2 = normal, +3 = exaggerated, +4 = very exaggerated or clonus, PL = pelvic limb, TL = thoracic limb.

ASSESSMENT 12A

Anatomic diagnosis: Two major findings are important in the localization of this lesion. Vestibular signs with no paresis strongly suggest a right peripheral vestibular disease. Facial paralysis on the right side probably has occurred secondarily to the peripheral vestibular disorder.

Diagnostic plan (Rule-outs):
1. Otitis media-interna—otoscopic examination (negative), skull radiography (negative).
2. Geriatric vestibular syndrome—exclusion diagnosis.
3. Facial nerve paralysis—EMG.

Therapeutic plan:
1. Treat the exposure keratitis of the right eye.
2. Chloramphenicol, 50 mg per kg tid for 10 days.

Client education: The prognosis is good.

Case Summary: Otitis media-interna with facial paralysis was suspected. The dog recovered following therapy. The facial paralysis persisted.

ASSESSMENT 12B

Anatomic diagnosis: There is a right-sided peripheral vestibular disorder associated with a partial right facial paralysis. The muscle atrophy in the right temporal area suggests partial involvement of the right mandibular nerve. A lesion in the right inner ear extending along the floor of the brain stem or peripherally could injure the mandibular nerve branches supplying the temporal muscles.

Diagnostic plan (Rule-outs):
1. Neoplasia—skull radiography (erosive lesion of the right petrous temporal bone).
2. Inflammation—otoscopic examination (the ear canal is filled with ulcerated tissue), CSF analysis (negative).

Therapeutic plan: None is available.

Client education: The prognosis is very poor. The tumor is inoperable.

Case summary: A squamous cell carcinoma was diagnosed. Euthanasia was performed.

ASSESSMENT 12C

Anatomic diagnosis: The neurologic findings localize the lesion to bilateral involvement of the motor division of C.N. V. (Normal facial sensation and palpebral reflex suggest clinically normal function of the sensory fibers of C.N. V.) Since the lesion is rather specific for motor neurons and is bilateral, involvement of the peripheral nerves is unlikely. (The peripheral nerves have both motor and sensory fibers.) The lesion therefore most likely affects both motor nuclei of C.N. V. One disease that causes these lesions is clinically recognized; idiopathic mandibular paralysis.

Diagnostic plan (Rule-outs):
1. Mandibular nerve paralysis—EMG of masticatory muscles (diffuse evidence of denervation 7 days after the onset of the signs).
2. Temporal, masseter myositis—history and physical examination (negative for pain, the jaw is open rather than closed, and the muscles are hypotonic rather than firm), muscle biopsy (not done in this case).
3. Rabies—clinical history and course of the disease. Rabies always is considered when bulbar signs are present.
4. Trauma—skull radiographs (negative).

Therapeutic plan: Support hydration and nutrition with tube feedings.

Client education: The disease is of unknown etiology. Recovery takes 3 to 6 weeks and is usually complete. No specific therapy is known.

Case summary: A uneventful recovery occurred in 4 weeks. A second episode was recorded 6 months later. A complete recovery again occurred in 4 weeks.

REFERENCES

1. deLahunta, A.: Veterinary Neuroanatomy and Clinical Neurology. Philadelphia, W. B. Saunders Co., 1977.
2. Adour, K. K., Bell, D. N., and Hilsinger, R. L., Jr.: Herpes simplex virus in idiopathic facial paralysis (Bell palsy). JAMA 233:527–530, 1975.
3. Wolfe, S. M., et al.: Treatment of Bell's palsy with prednisone: A prospective, randomized study. Neurology 28:158, 1978.
4. Roberts, S. R., and Vainisi, S. J.: Hemifacial spasm in dogs. JAVMA 150:381–385, 1967.
5. Venker-van Haagen, A. J., Hartman, W., and Goedegebuure, S. A.: Spontaneous laryngeal paralysis in young Bouviers: A study in 105 affected Bouviers. JAAHA 14:714–720, 1978.
6. Fowler, M. E.: Nigropallidal encephalomalacia in the horse. JAVMA 147:607–616, 1965.
7. Young, S., Brown, W. W. and Klinger, B.: Nigropallidal encephalomalacia in horses caused by the ingestion of weeds of the genus Centaurea. JAVMA 157:1602–1605, 1970.

13

CHAPTER

BLINDNESS, ANISOCORIA, AND ABNORMAL EYE MOVEMENTS

Problems related to abnormalities of the eyes and the visual pathways are especially useful in the formulation of a neurologic diagnosis.[1] The retina and the optic nerve are the only sensory receptors and the only nerve that can be examined directly. The sensory and motor pathways of vision and eye movements traverse the brain from the orbit to the occipital region of the cerebral cortex and the medulla oblongata, so diseases affecting the brain are likely to affect some portion of the visual system. The retina is often affected by systemic diseases.

ANATOMIC DIAGNOSIS: LOCALIZATION

The visual system will be considered in three parts: (1) vision, (2) pupillary light reflexes, and (3) eye movements. Combinations of abnormal signs should lead to an anatomic diagnosis.

Vision

The visual pathways are presented in Figures 13–1 and 13–2 and Table 13–1. Methods of testing vision were discussed in Chapter 3. Lesions of the lateral geniculate nucleus of the thalamus, the optic radiation (fiber tracts), or the occipital cortex cause a loss of sight without affecting pupillary reflexes. Many of these lesions are unilateral, resulting in a loss of vision in the contralateral field. Bilateral lesions due to encephalitis or hydrocephalus cause complete blindness. Lesions of the retina, the optic nerve, the optic chiasm, or the optic tracts will cause blindness *and* pupillary abnormalities (see Fig. 13–1). Optic chiasm lesions almost always cause bilateral blindness. Retinal and optic nerve lesions are frequently bilateral (e.g., retinal atrophy, optic neuritis) but may be unilateral (e.g., trauma, neoplasia). Optic tract lesions are rare.

The degree of decussation of optic nerve fibers at the optic chiasm varies in different species. In primates, essentially all of the fibers from the nasal half of the retina cross, whereas all of the fibers from the temporal half of the retina remain ipsilateral. In carnivores, approximately one half of the fibers of the temporal retina cross, and all of the nasal retinal fibers cross. Most of the herbivores have 80 per cent or more of the fibers crossing. Therefore, visual field testing may be of importance for lesion localization in dogs and cats, but each eye can be considered to have an independent pathway in other domestic animals.

Assessment of the visual field is difficult. The usual methods of the menace and visual plac-

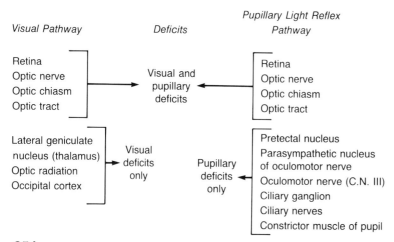

Figure 13–1. Deficits from lesions of the visual and pupillary light reflex pathways.

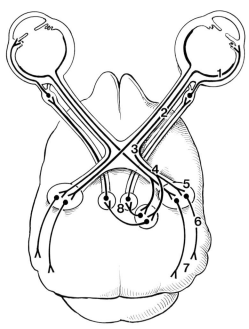

Figure 13–2. Pathways for vision and the pupillary light reflex. The numbers correspond to those in Table 13–1.

ing reactions test the lateral field and the crossing fibers. Deficits in these responses that are central to the optic chiasm are usually on the contralateral side of the brain.

Caution must be exercised in the interpre-tation of visual deficits. Because the examiner must rely on motor or behavioral reactions, he or she should use several tests to confirm an impression that the animal does not see. See Chapter 3 for details.

Pupillary Light Reflexes

The pathway for pupillary light reflexes is outlined and illustrated in Figures 13–1 to 13–3 and in Table 13–1. The methods of testing pupillary reflexes have been described in Chapter 3.

Lesions of C.N. III (the oculomotor nerve, including the ciliary ganglion and the short ciliary nerves) or of the constrictor muscle of the pupil cause loss of pupillary constriction in response to light on the affected side with-out affecting vision. Bilateral lesions are un-usual. Lesions of the pretectal nucleus or the parasympathetic nucleus of C.N. III cause loss of pupillary constriction. Usually, both eyes are affected, because the nuclei are anatomically close together in the brain stem. Lesions of the retina, the optic nerve, or the optic chiasm cause loss of constriction of the pupil on the affected side in response to direct stimulation, but the pupil reacts to light shined in the op-posite eye. Vision is impaired in the affected eye (see Table 13–1).

Table 13–1. SIGNS OF LESIONS IN THE VISUAL PATHWAYS

Complete Lesion on *Right Side* *	Vision		Resting Pupil		Pupillary Light Reflex	
	OD †	OS ‡	OD	OS	Light OD	Light OS
1. Retina or optic nerve	Absent	Normal	Slight dilatation	Normal	No response	Both constrict
2. Orbit (C.N. II and C.N. III)	Absent	Normal	Dilated	Normal	No response	OS constricts
3. Optic chiasm	Absent	Absent	Dilated	Dilated	No response	No response
4. Optic tract	Normal	Poor§	Normal	Slightly dilated	Both constrict	Both constrict
5. Lateral geniculate nucleus	Normal	Poor§	Normal	Normal	Both constrict	Both constrict
6. Optic radiation	Normal	Poor§	Normal	Normal	Both constrict	Both constrict
7. Occipital cortex	Normal	Poor§	Normal	Normal	Both constrict	Both constrict
8. Parasympathetic nucleus of C.N. III *bilateral*	Normal	Normal	Dilated	Dilated	No response	No response
9. Oculomotor nerve	Normal	Normal	Dilated	Normal	OS constricts	OS constricts

*Numbers identify structures in Figure 13–2.
†OD = Right eye.
‡OS = Left eye.
§Loss of sight in the left visual field with partial sparing in the right visual field.

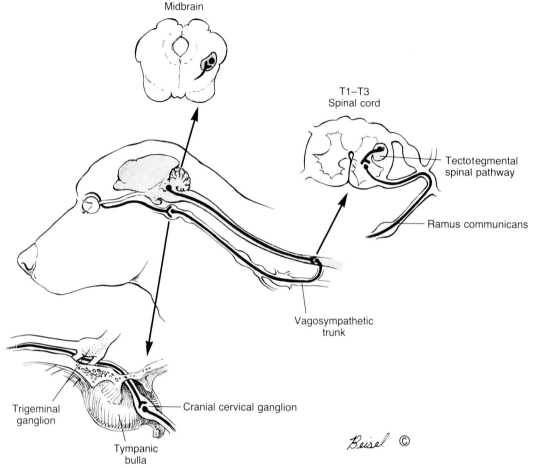

Figure 13–3. Pathway of sympathetic innervation to the eye. (From Greene, C. E., and Oliver, J. E., Jr.: Neurologic examination. *In* Ettinger, S. E.: Textbook of Veterinary Internal Medicine, 2nd ed. Philadelphia, W. B. Saunders Co., 1982. Used by permission.)

The sympathetic control of the dilator muscle of the pupil is illustrated in Figure 13–3. Sympathetic activation is produced by emotional reactions, such as fear and rage. The sympathetic nerves also innervate smooth muscle in the periorbital fascia and the eyelids, including the third eyelid. Lesions of this pathway cause a constricted pupil (miosis), a slight retraction of the globe because of loss of tone in the periorbita (enophthalmos), a narrowing of the palpebral fissure (ptosis), and extrusion of the third eyelid. This cluster of signs is called Horner's syndrome. Horner's syndrome usually is not associated with visual deficits. Localization is dependent on associated clinical signs. For example, avulsion of the brachial plexus may cause a monoparesis and Horner's syndrome on the same side. T1–T3 spinal cord lesions cause upper motor neuron (UMN) signs in the pelvic limb, lower motor neuron (LMN) signs in the thoracic limb, and Horner's syndrome.

Differentiation of pre- and postganglionic lesions can be determined in the first few weeks of Horner's syndrome. Instillation of 0.1 ml of 0.001 per cent epinephrine hydrochloride causes rapid dilatation of the pupil in postganglionic lesions. The response takes 35 to 40 minutes in preganglionic lesions. This response is unreliable after 1 to 2 weeks and is only moderately reliable at best.[2]

Eye Movements

The extraocular eye muscles are innervated by C.N. III (oculomotor), C.N. IV (trochlear), and C.N. VI (abducent) (Fig. 13–4). Eye movements are controlled by UMNs from the cerebral cortex and through brain stem vestibular

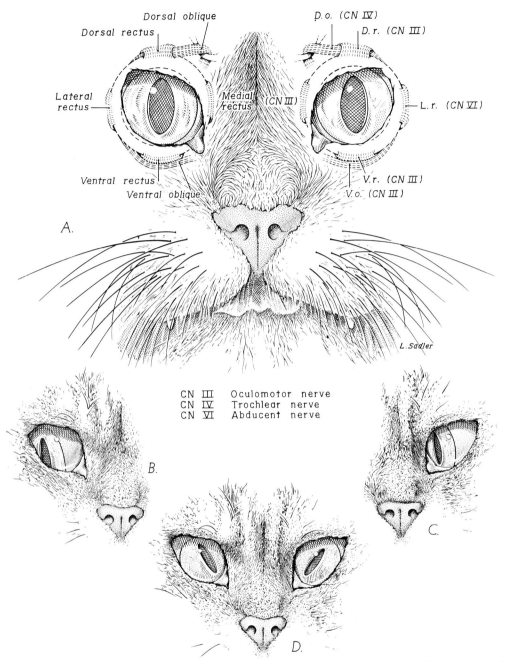

Figure 13–4. Functional anatomy of the extraocular muscles (A). Direction of strabismus following paralysis of the oculomotor (B), abducent (C), and trochlear (D) neurons. (From deLahunta, A.: Veterinary Neuroanatomy and Clinical Neurology. Philadelphia, W. B. Saunders Co., 1977. Used by permission.)

reflexes. The eye muscles normally act in a synergistic or antagonistic manner to provide coordinated conjugate movements. The testing of eye movements has been discussed in Chapter 3. Abnormalities of eye movements include paralysis of gaze in a direction related to a muscle or a group of muscles; strabismus,

or deviation, of the globe; loss of conjugate movements; and nystagmus.

When the globe is fixed, regardless of head position, a lesion of C.N. III, C.N. IV, or C.N. VI is suspected. Lesions of the trochlear nerve (C.N. IV) may cause a slight rotation of the globe, which is difficult to evaluate in animals that have a round pupil (Fig. 13–4).[3] Lesions of C.N. III cause a ventrolateral strabismus, and lesions of C.N. VI cause a medial strabismus. Several weeks after an injury the globe may return to its normal midposition, but there is loss of movement dorsally, medially, and ventrally with a lesion of C.N. III and laterally with a lesion of C.N. VI (Fig. 13–4). Positional strabismus (dysconjugate deviation of the eye in certain head positions) is characteristic of lesions of the vestibular system. In this case, eye movements can be elicited in all directions by appropriate movements of the head, demonstrating that all extraocular muscles are functional (see Chapter 11). Medial strabismus without deficits in eye movements is seen in some animals, especially Siamese cats. These animals have an abnormal arrangement of the visual pathways rather than an abnormality of C.N. VI.[4]

The function of the extraocular muscles has not been established in large animals. It is assumed that the movements and the physiologic deficits produced after lesions of the cranial nerves are similar to those that occur in other species.

Conjugate eye movements require coordination of the three cranial nerves and their muscles. The pathway responsible for this coordination is the medial longitudinal fasciculus (MLF), which runs in the center of the brain stem from the vestibular nuclei to the nuclei of C.N. III, C.N. IV, and C.N. VI. Lesions of the MLF may cause dysconjugate movements or, more commonly, a lack of motion in response to moving the head. The phenomenon of the eyes' remaining fixed in the orbit as the head is moved is called the "doll's-eye" syndrome and is seen most commonly after an acute head

injury that produces hemorrhage in the center of the brain stem (see Chapter 14).

Nystagmus is involuntary rhythmic movement of the eyes. Normal nystagmus may be visual in origin (for example, watching telephone poles go by from a moving car) or it may be vestibular in origin (for example, turning the head rapidly). The visual and vestibular types are called jerk nystagmus, because there is a slow phase to one side followed by a rapid recovery movement (jerk). The direction of the nystagmus is classified according to the fast component. Nystagmus also is categorized by the direction of the movement (horizontal, vertical, or rotatory) and according to whether it changes direction with varying head positions (overridable or nonoverridable). Jerk nystagmus that is horizontal or rotatory and nonoverridable is indicative of peripheral vestibular disease. All other forms of jerk nystagmus are associated with central vestibular brain stem lesions (including lesions of the flocculonodular lobe of the cerebellum) (Fig. 13–5; see also Chapter 11).

A less frequently seen form, called pendular nystagmus, consists of small oscillations of the eye that do not have fast and slow components. Pendular nystagmus usually is seen with cerebellar disease and is most pronounced during fixation of the gaze. It also may be seen in animals with visual deficits.

Except for lesions of the globe and the orbit, most diseases affecting the visual system produce other clinical signs that are related to abnormal function of surrounding structures. For example, masses affecting the optic chiasm or the optic tracts usually affect hypothalamic function. Lesions of C.N. III, C.N. IV, or C.N. VI cause other brain stem signs (see Chapters

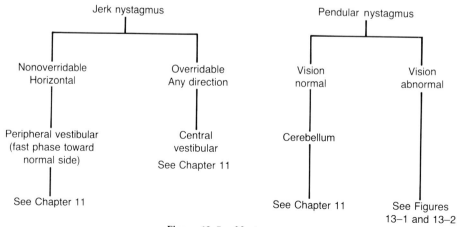

Figure 13–5. Nystagmus.

| Etiologic Category | Acute | | Chronic |
	Progressive	Nonprogressive	Progressive
Degenerative			Storage diseases
Anomalous		1. Retinal dysplasia	Retinal abiotrophies
		2. Collie eye syndrome	
		3. Coloboma (Charolais	
		and albinotic Hereford)	
Metabolic			Diabetes mellitus
Neoplastic	1. Lymphosarcomas		
	2. Malignant melanoma		
Nutritional			1. Hypovitaminosis A
			2. Taurine-deficient
			diets (cats)
Inflammatory	1. Canine distemper		1. FIP
	2. Feline infectious		2. Toxoplasmosis
	peritonitis (FIP)		3. Systemic mycoses
	3. Toxoplasmosis		
	4. Thromboembolic		
	meningoencephalitis		
	(bovine)		
	5. Bovine virus diarrhea		
Traumatic		1. Retinal detachment	
		2. Retinal hemorrhage	

Figure 13–6. Etiology of retinal diseases.

10 through 12). Lesions of the occipital cortex affect other cerebral functions (see Chapters 14 and 15). The combination of signs defines the location of the lesion.

ETIOLOGIC DIAGNOSIS

The most common diseases causing clinical signs in various parts of the visual system are mentioned in Figures 13–6 through 13–12. The history and the physical and neurologic ex-

aminations should provide the clinician with a list of the most probable diseases to be considered. Most of the diseases presented in the figures are discussed in other chapters. Only those that are related primarily to the visual system are discussed here.

Degenerative Diseases

An abnormality of the intracellular enzyme systems causes an accumulation of the prod-

| Etiologic Category | Acute | | Chronic |
	Progressive	Nonprogressive	Progressive
Degenerative			Demyelinating diseases
Anomalous		1. Hypoplasia	
		2. Coloboma	
Neoplastic			1. Primary
			a. Neurofibroma
			b. Pituitary adenoma
			c. Meningioma
			d. Glioma
			2. Metastatic
			3. Lymphoreticular
Nutritional			Hypovitaminosis A
Inflammatory	1. Canine distemper		See *Acute Progressive*
	2. Feline infectious		1. Feline infectious peritonitis
	peritonitis		2. Toxoplasmosis
	3. Systemic mycoses		3. Systemic mycoses
	4. Systemic bacterial infection		
	5. Bovine virus diarrhea		
Traumatic		1. Avulsion	
		2. Hematoma	
		3. Laceration	

Figure 13–7. Etiology of optic neuropathy.

| Etiologic Category | Acute | | Chronic |
	Progressive	Nonprogressive	Progressive
Degenerative			

Neoplastic			Demyelinating diseases
			1. Primary
			  a. Pituitary adenoma
			  b. Meningioma
			  c. Neurofibroma
			  d. Glioma
			2. Metastatic
			3. Lymphoreticular

Inflammatory	1. Canine distemper 2. Feline infectious peritonitis 3. Systemic mycoses 4. Systemic bacterial infection		See *Acute Progressive* 1. Feline infectious peritonitis 2. Toxoplasmosis 3. Systemic mycoses 4. Abscess

Figure 13–8. Etiology of optic chiasm disorders.

ucts of metabolism in the neurons. Affected neurons function abnormally and eventually die. This group of diseases is listed in Figures 13–6 through 13–12 as storage diseases (see Chapter 17). Because neurons are affected, the retina, the lateral geniculate nucleus, and the occipital cortex are the most obvious targets in the visual system. Cranial nerve nuclei usually are not affected until late in the disease. The diseases are hereditary, progressive and, invariably, fatal. The formulation of an antemortem diagnosis is difficult except by assessment of the history, knowledge of the breed selectivity, and exclusion of other diagnoses. A brain biopsy can confirm a diagnosis. A biopsy of other tissues can provide a diagnosis in some of the systemic forms of these diseases.

Demyelinating diseases also are considered degenerative diseases; for example, one type, globoid cell leukodystrophy, is caused by an abnormal enzyme system similar to that of the neuronal storage diseases. The signs of cerebellar and spinal cord tract involvement (UMN signs, proprioception deficits) are characteristic of the clinical syndrome. Visual pathways (optic nerve, optic tract, optic radiation) may be affected. Demyelination also may occur secondarily to inflammatory diseases, especially canine distemper. The visual pathways are often affected, but other signs predominate.

Anomalies

Hydrocephalus, which may be the result of a congenital anomaly or may be secondary to mass lesions or inflammation, affects primarily the optic radiations and the occipital cortex through enlargement of the lateral ventricles. Hydrocephalus always should be considered

| Etiologic Category | Acute | | Chronic |
	Progressive	Nonprogressive	Progressive
Degenerative			

Neoplastic			Demyelinating diseases
			1. Primary
			  a. Meningioma
			  b. Glioma
			  c. Pituitary adenoma
			2. Metastatic
			3. Lymphoreticular

Inflammatory	1. Canine distemper 2. Feline infectious peritonitis 3. Systemic mycoses 4. Bacterial infection		See *Acute Progressive* 1. Feline infectious peritonitis 2. Toxoplasmosis 3. Systemic mycoses

Traumatic		1. Compression
		  a. Fracture
		  b. Hematoma	

Figure 13–9. Etiology of optic tract disorders.

Etiologic Category	Acute Progressive	Acute Nonprogressive	Chronic Progressive
Degenerative		1. Vascular disorders a. Infarcts b. Hemorrhage	Demyelinating diseases
Anomalous Neoplastic			Hydrocephalus 1. Primary a. Glioma b. Ependymoma c. Choroid plexus papilloma 2. Metastatic 3. Lymphoreticular See *Acute Progressive*
Inflammatory	1. Canine distemper 2. Feline infectious peritonitis 3. Systemic mycoses		

Figure 13–10. Etiology of optic radiation disorders.

in a blind animal that has intact pupillary light reflexes. A diagnosis of hydrocephalus requires a ventricular tap, penumoventriculography, or electroencephalography (see Chapter 14).

Primary retinal anomalies and abiotrophies are relatively common in the dog. The types of anomaly and the breeds affected are listed in Table 13–2. These diseases cause blindness without other clinical signs. Several books on

Etiologic Category	Acute Progressive	Acute Nonprogressive	Chronic Progressive
Degenerative		1. Vascular disorders a. Infarction b. Hemorrhage	Storage diseases
Anomalous		1. Cerebral malformation a. Lissencephaly b. Porencephaly	Hydrocephalus
Metabolic	1. Hypoglycemia 2. Hepatic encephalopathy 3. Uremia	1. Hyperthermia 2. Hypoxia	See *Acute Progressive*
Neoplastic			1. Primary a. Glioma b. Meningioma 2. Reticulosis 3. Metastatic 4. Skull origin a. Osteosarcoma b. Chondrosarcoma
Nutritional	Polioencephalomalacia (ruminants)		
Inflammatory	1. Canine distemper 2. Toxoplasmosis 3. Systemic mycoses 4. Bacterial infections 5. Thromboembolic meningoencephalitis (bovine)		1. Canine distemper 2. Feline infectious peritonitis 3. Systemic mycoses 4. Toxoplasmosis 5. Reticulosis 6. Other—prototothecosis
Toxic	1. Lead 2. Hexachlorophene		1. Lead and other heavy metals 2. Hexachlorophene
Traumatic	1. Cerebral edema 2. Hemorrhage 3. Concussion		Subdural hematoma

Figure 13–11. Etiology of occipital cortex disorders.

| Etiologic Category | Acute | | Chronic |
	Progressive	Nonprogressive	Progressive
Anomalous			Hydrocephalus*
Metabolic		Hyperthermia*	
Neoplastic			Any rostrotentorial tumor*
Inflammatory	Abscess (Retrobulbar most common)		
Toxic	Lead*		
Traumatic		Hemorrhage in midbrain	1. Cerebral edema* (bilateral signs) 2. Hematoma* (unilateral signs)

*Oculomotor signs secondary to tentorial herniation.

Figure 13-12. Etiology of oculomotor neuropathy.

ophthalmology discuss these diseases in detail.[5-8]

Metabolic Diseases

A disease that alters the normal biochemical processes of the eye or the central nervous system (CNS) may produce signs of abnormal vision, although other signs usually are more apparent. Diabetes mellitus may cause vascu-

Table 13-2. PRIMARY RETINAL ANOMALIES AND ABIOTROPHIES

Anomalies	Breeds
Retinal dysplasia	Bedlington terriers, Labrador retrievers, Sealyham terriers, Hereford and Shorthorn cattle
Choroid dysplasia and coloboma	Rough- and smooth-coated collies, Shetland sheepdogs, borzois (also reported in beagles, dachshunds, German shepherds, miniature and toy poodles, Charolais and albinotic Hereford cattle)

Abiotrophies	Breeds
Progressive retinal atrophy	Any breed, especially Irish setters, collies, Norwegian elkhounds, poodles
Rod dysplasia	Norwegian elkhounds
Progressive rod-cone degeneration	Poodles (toy and miniature)
Central retinal atrophy	Mostly working dogs, including Labrador retrievers, golden retrievers, border collies, rough-coated collies, springer spaniels, English setters
Hemeralopia (cone degeneration)	Alaskan malamutes, poodles

lar changes, including retinal hemorrhage. Cataracts are common and make retinal examination difficult.

Diseases that affect cortical function may produce blindness with intact pupillary light reflexes. Examples include hypoglycemia, hepatic encephalopathy, and uremia (see Chapters 15 and 17).

Neoplasms

Visual pathway abnormalities are often very helpful for localizing intracranial tumors. Primary tumors of the globe are apparent on a physical examination.[5,6]

Tumors of the pituitary gland may cause visual field deficits from compression of the optic chiasm; however, most pituitary tumors grow dorsally into the hypothalamus instead of spreading out rostrally and caudally. Visual signs therefore are seen very late in the development of the mass.

A lymphosarcoma may infiltrate all portions of the globe. Involvement of the orbit may cause exophthalmos (especially in cattle). Compression of the optic nerves may cause papilledema or atrophy of the optic disk.

Reticulosis, which is considered either inflammatory or neoplastic by various authors, may infiltrate the optic nerves and cause atrophy or swelling of the optic disk, depending on the degree of involvement.

Neoplasia of the CNS will be discussed in Chapter 17.

Nutritional Deficiencies

Animals that are fed normal commercial rations rarely have nutritional deficiencies severe enough to cause CNS abnormality. Hypovitaminosis A causes abnormal bone growth with stenosis of the optic foramen, which secondarily constricts the optic nerve, producing retinal degeneration. This syndrome is seen more commonly in calves than in companion animals.

Feline central retinal degeneration (FCRD) can be produced by diets that are deficient in the amino acid taurine. Cats that are fed commercial dog food exclusively develop FCRD.[9]

Polioencephalomalacia of ruminants is characterized by cerebral necrosis and edema. Signs of cerebral dysfunction, including blindness, are seen. The pupillary light reflexes are usually normal, unless edema has caused tentorial herniation with compression of the oculomotor nerves. The disease is caused by an excess of thiaminase in the rumen, which produces an acute thiamine deficiency (see Chapter 17).

Inflammations

Systemic infectious diseases with CNS involvement frequently affect the visual system. Retinal lesions are common in canine distemper, feline infectious peritonitis, toxoplasmosis, the systemic mycoses, and thromboembolic meningoencephalitis.[10] A fundic examination may confirm the diagnosis.

Optic neuritis includes degenerative, compressive ischemic, and inflammatory conditions of the optic nerve (Fig. 13–7). All but the inflammatory disorders more appropriately should be called *optic neuropathies*. Sudden blindness may be noticed if both eyes are affected. Papilledema and vascular congestion are seen on a fundic examination if that portion of the nerve is affected. Atrophy of the disk is seen as the process resolves. Many of the diseases causing optic neuropathy are not treatable and may lead to death; however, a number of cases are seen without evidence of systemic disease. Edema and inflammation may lead to loss of function of the nerve, regardless of the outcome of the primary dis-

ease. Early treatment therefore should include antiedema doses of corticosteroids (see Chapter 7). Other supportive or antibiotic therapy is given as indicated by the condition of the animal. The prognosis is guarded to poor. In one report of 12 dogs with optic neuropathy, 7 remained alive, and 5 of them were blind. The other 2 had partial vision.[11]

Toxic Disorders

Heavy metal poisoning, especially lead poisoning, may produce cortical blindness (see Chapter 17).

Trauma

Any portion of the visual system may be affected by trauma. Assessing the function of the oculomotor nerve is of primary importance in evaluating patients with head injury. Brain swelling that leads to tentorial herniation compresses the oculomotor nerve at the tentorium cerebelli. One of the earliest signs of tentorial herniation is a fixed, dilated pupil ipsilateral to the herniation (if it is unilateral). A paralysis of the extraocular muscles that produces a ventrolateral strabismus follows the mydriasis. Hemorrhage in the brain stem also produces abnormal pupils. Hemorrhage above or below the oculomotor nucleus (midbrain) may destroy the UMN to the sympathetic pathway, producing small but responsive pupils. Midbrain hemorrhage may cause fixed, dilated pupils if the oculomotor nucleus is destroyed with the sympathetic pathway intact, but most cases have fixed midposition pupils because both pathways are affected. Serial assessment of pupillary function together with mental status, motor function, and other cranial nerve signs is very important for the evaluation of patients with head trauma. Bilateral, fixed, dilated, or midposition pupils from the time of injury strongly suggests brain stem hemorrhage that is often irreversible, and progressive dilatation of the pupils suggests a developing tentorial herniation that may be treatable (see Chapter 14).

CASE HISTORIES

The case histories in this chapter emphasize localization of the lesion. Only the pertinent neuro-ophthalmologic findings will be given. Make your decision before reading the assessment.

Case History 13A

Neurologic Examination

Vision: Normal.
Pupillary light reflexes (PLR): The right pupil is dilated.

	Reaction	
Shine light	OS	OD
OS *	+	−
OD†	+	−

Eye position and movement: Left eye is normal; fixed ventrolateral strabismus in right eye.

Case History 13B

Neurologic Examination

Vision: Normal in left eye; absent in right eye.
PLR: The right pupil is larger than the left.

	Reaction	
Shine light	OS	OD
OS	+	+
OD	−	−

Eye position and movement: Normal.

Case History 13C

Neurologic Examination

Vision: Absent in both eyes.
PLR: The pupil size is normal; the pupils are symmetric.

	Reaction	
Shine light	OS	OD
OS	+	+
OD	+	+

Eye position and movement: The vestibular eye movements are normal. No strabismus, but the animal does not follow moving objects.

---

*Left eye.
†Right eye.

Case History 13D

Neurologic Examination

Vision: Normal in both eyes.
PLR: The pupil size is normal; the pupils are symmetric.

	Reaction	
Shine light	OS	OD
OS	+	+
OD	+	+

Eye position and movement: Medial strabismus of the left eye. Dorsal and ventral movements can be elicited by moving the head. The right eye is normal.

Case History 13E

Neurologic Examination

Vision: Absent in both eyes.
PLR: The pupils are dilated bilaterally.

	Reaction	
Shine light	OS	OD
OS	−	−
OD	−	−

Eye position and movement: Normal eye position and normal vestibular eye movements, but the animal does not follow moving objects.

Case History 13F

Neurologic Examination

Vision: Normal in both eyes.
PLR: The pupil size is normal.

	Reaction	
Shine light	OS	OD
OS	+	+
OD	+	+

Eye position and movement: The eyes are in the normal midposition, but no vestibular eye movements can be elicited.

ASSESSMENT 13A

Right oculomotor nerve (C.N. III) lesion. The unilateral lesion suggests a lesion after the nerve leaves the brain stem, since the nuclei are only millimeters apart.

ASSESSMENT 13B

Right optic nerve or retinal lesion. A funduscopic examination is likely to differentiate between these two disorders.

ASSESSMENT 13C

Bilateral occipital cortex or optic radiation lesions. This finding suggests a diffuse lesion, such as hydrocephalus, encephalitis, or increased intracranial pressure.

ASSESSMENT 13D

Left abducent nerve (C.N. VI) lesion. Isolated lesions of C.N. VI are rare. In a clinical case, other signs of brain stem disease probably would be present.

ASSESSMENT 13E

Optic chiasm, bilateral optic nerve, or bilateral retinal lesions. This situation is one in which two lesions (actually a diffuse disease) are more common than a single chiasmatic lesion. Retinopathies and optic neuropathies are seen more often than are primary lesions of the optic chiasm.

ASSESSMENT 13F

Medial longitudinal fasciculus (MLF) lesion. This lesion is in the tract connecting the vestibular nuclei to the nuclei of C.N. III, C.N. IV, and C.N. VI. Alternatively, there could be a lesion of C.N. III, C.N. IV, and C.N. VI bilaterally. That would be a big lesion! In either case, other signs probably would predominate. MLF lesions usually are associated with severe brain stem lesions (hemorrhage, tumor), and the animal is comatose when these disorders are present.

REFERENCES

1. Kornegay, J. N.: Small animal neuroophthalmology. Comp. Cont. Ed. Pract. Vet. 2:923–928, 1980.
2. Bistner, S. I.: Neuro-ophthalmology. In Hoerlein, B. F.: Canine Neurology: Diagnosis and Treatment, 3rd ed. Philadelphia, W. B. Saunders Co., 1978.
3. deLahunta, A.: Veterinary Neuroanatomy and Clinical Neurology. Philadelphia, W. B. Saunders Co., 1977.
4. Blake, R., and Crawford, M. L. J.: Development of strabismus in Siamese cats. Brain Res. 77:492–496, 1974.
5. Blogg, J. R.: The Eye in Veterinary Medicine. Victoria, Australia, Medor Company PtY Ltd., 1977.
6. Gelatt, K. N.: Textbook of Veterinary Ophthalmology. Philadelphia, Lea & Febiger, 1981.
7. Magrane, W. G.: Canine Ophthalmology, 3rd ed. Philadelphia, Lea & Febiger, 1977.
8. Rubin, L. F.: Atlas of Veterinary Ophthalmoscopy. Philadelphia, Lea & Febiger, 1974.
9. Aguirre, G.: Retinopathies. In Kirk, R. W.: Current Veterinary Therapy VI. Philadelphia, W. B. Saunders Co., 1977.
10. Martin, C. L.: Retinopathies of food animals. In Howard, J. L.: Current Veterinary Therapy: Food Animal Practice. Philadelphia, W. B. Saunders Co., 1981.
11. Fischer, C. A., and Jones, G. T.: Optic neuritis in dogs. JAVMA 160:68–79, 1972.

14

CHAPTER

STUPOR OR COMA

Altered states of consciousness are always related to abnormal brain function. The nomenclature of these disorders is often confusing, because the terms extend beyond simple medical analysis and encompass psychology, philosophy, and other disciplines. The "mind-brain" problem has been receiving increased attention.[1] Applying the terminology used in human medicine to animals is even more difficult. For the purposes of the clinician, the following definitions are adequate:

Normal: The animal is alert, responsive to external stimuli, aware of its surroundings, and responds to commands as expected.

Depression: The animal is lethargic and less responsive to its environment but still has the capability to respond in a normal manner. Most sick animals are depressed.

Disorientation, confusion: Although the animal can respond to its environment, it may do so in an inappropriate manner.

Stupor: The animal appears to be asleep when undisturbed but can be aroused by strong stimulation, especially pain. There is no clear boundary between lethargy and stupor.

Coma: The animal is unconscious and does not respond to any stimulus except by reflex activity. For example, a strong toe pinch may elicit a flexion reflex or may increase extensor posturing but does not cause a behavioral reaction, such as crying, biting, or turning the head.

Confusion, stupor, and coma invariably are related to abnormal brain function.

ANATOMIC DIAGNOSIS: LOCALIZATION

Consciousness is maintained by sensory stimuli that act through the *ascending reticular activating system* (ARAS) on the cerebral cortex (Fig. 14–1). Decreasing levels of consciousness indicate abnormal function of the cerebral cortex or interference with cortical activation by the ARAS.

All sensory pathways have collateral input into the reticular formation of the pons and the midbrain. The reticular formation projects diffusely to the cerebral cortex, maintaining a background of activity through cholinergic synapses on cortical neurons. A balance is maintained between the ARAS and an adrenergic system that projects from nuclei in the midbrain and the diencephalon and that may be considered the sleep system. Alterations in the balance of these two systems can produce signs ranging from hyperexcitability to coma. Narcolepsy, a syndrome of sleep attacks, will be discussed in Chapter 15.

Stupor and coma are caused by (1) diffuse, bilateral cerebral disease; (2) metabolic or toxic encephalopathies; (3) compression of the rostral brain stem (midbrain, pons); or (4) destructive lesions of the rostral brain stem.

An anatomic diagnosis can be made on the basis of motor function and neuro-ophthal-

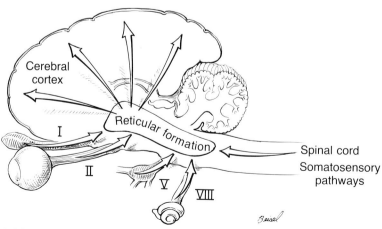

Figure 14–1. Reticular activating system (RAS). The reticular system of the brain stem receives input from most sensory systems. Diffuse projections from the RAS to the cerebral cortex maintain consciousness.

mologic signs (vision, pupils, and eye movements—see Chapter 13 and Table 14–1).

Diffuse cerebral disease usually does not produce localizing signs, although some inflammatory processes may be somewhat asymmetric. Voluntary motor activity and postural reactions are absent or severely depressed. Rhythmic walking movements, reflecting brain stem and spinal cord activity, may be elicited if the animal is suspended in a normal standing posture. Vision is absent, although the pupils are normal. Oculocephalic responses (vestibular eye movements) are normal, but the animal will not follow moving objects. Normal pupils and oculocephalic responses indicate an intact brain stem, whereas loss of vision and voluntary motor activity indicates an abnormal cerebral cortex. Signs of meningeal irritation include pain on palpation of the head and the neck, rigidity of the neck muscles, and resistance to flexion of the neck. Meningeal irritation may be caused by infection or by the presence of blood in the subarachnoid space.

Metabolic or *toxic encephalopathies* usually depress higher (cortical) function early and affect brain stem functions later. They do not produce focal localizing signs. The signs are generally the same as those of diffuse cortical lesions but may have other components, de-pending on the cause. For example, barbiturates may cause depression of the spinal reflexes, organophosphate insecticides may cause muscle fasciculation and autonomic signs, and a number of toxins may cause seizures. Specific entities will be discussed in Chapter 17.

Compression of the brain stem may be caused by a mass (tumor, abscess) adjacent to the brain stem or by herniation of the cerebral cortex under the tentorium cerebelli, which secondarily compresses the brain stem.

The skull forms an inelastic case around the brain. Any developing mass (tumor, abscess, hematoma), increase in the volume of the brain (cerebral edema), or deformation of the skull must displace cerebrospinal fluid (CSF), blood, or nervous tissue. There is approximately 7 ml of CSF in the average dog. Blood volume is maintained nearly constant up to pressures equaling arterial pressure. Increased pressure causes displacement of the cerebral hemispheres caudally under the tentorium cerebelli, resulting in compression of the brain stem (Figs. 14–2 and 14–3). Unilateral masses produce a herniation on the same side, whereas cerebral edema usually causes a bilateral herniation.

If the pressure continues to rise, or if the

Table 14–1. SIGNS OF LESIONS CAUSING STUPOR AND COMA

	Motor Function	Vision	Pupils	Eye Movements
Severe diffuse cerebral cortex lesions	Tetraparesis (may have walking movements, but they are poorly coordinated), postural reaction absent	Absent	Normal	Normal, but no visual following
Metabolic or toxic encephalopathy	Tetraparesis without increased extensor tone, reflexes may be depressed	Absent	Usually normal, but may be altered in intoxication	Normal, but no visual following; absent in deep coma
Bilateral compression of rostral brain stem	Tetraparesis, increased tone in extensor muscles (decerebrate rigidity)	Absent in herniation, present in primary brain stem lesions	Dilated or mid-position, unresponsive	Bilateral ventral lateral strabismus, poor vestibular eye movements
Unilateral compression of rostral brain stem	Hemiparesis or tetraparesis, increased extensor tone on affected side	Present—may be contralateral loss in herniation	Dilated, ipsilateral	Ipsilateral ventrolateral strabismus, poor vestibular eye movements
Destructive lesion, rostral brain stem	Tetraparesis, increased extensor tone (decerebrate rigidity)	Present—animal may not respond if comatose	Midposition unresponsive	No vestibular eye movements, may have bilateral ventrolateral strabismus

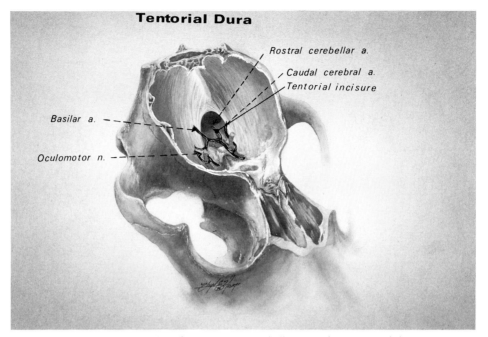

Figure 14–2. Increased pressure rostral to the tentorium cerebelli causes herniation of the cerebral cortex under the tentorium, resulting in compression of the brain stem.

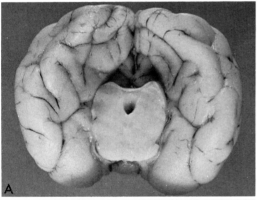

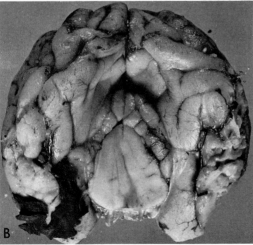

Figure 14–3. Caudal view of the brain, transected at the midbrain. *A.* Normal brain. Note the open mesencephalic aqueduct. *B.* Severe cerebral edema has caused herniation of the cerebrum under the tentorium cerebelli, resulting in compression and distortion of the brain stem. The mesencephalic aqueduct is closed, causing further increases in intracranial pressure. (From Oliver, J. E., Jr.: Neurologic emergencies in small animals. Vet. Clin. N. Amer. 2:341–357, 1972. Used by permission.)

Table 14–2. SIGNS CHARACTERISTIC OF PROGRESSIVE BILATERAL TENTORIAL HERNIATION*

Level	Consciousness	Pupils	Eye Movements	Motor Function	Autonomic Responses
Early diencephalic	Apathy	Small but reactive	Normal	Hemiparesis	Normal to irregular response
Late diencephalic	Stupor	Small but reactive	Normal	Hemiparesis to tetraparesis	Cheyne-Stokes respiration
Midbrain	Coma	Dilated bilaterally	Poor, vestibular eye movements	Decerebrate rigidity	Hyperventilation
Pons	Coma	Midposition unresponsive	Vestibular eye movements absent	Flaccid paralysis	Rapid, shallow response
Medulla	Coma	Midposition, dilated terminally	Absent	Flaccid paralysis	Irregular to apnea, pulse slowing

*Modified from Plum, F., and Posner, J.: The Diagnosis of Stupor and Coma. Philadelphia, F. A. Davis Co., 1966 and Oliver, J. E., Jr.: Neurologic emergencies in small animals. Vet. Clin. N. Amer. 2:341–357, 1972.

Table 14–3. SIGNS CHARACTERISTIC OF PROGRESSIVE UNILATERAL TENTORIAL HERNIATION*

Level	Consciousness	Pupils	Eye Movements	Motor Function	Autonomic Responses
C.N. III	Normal to stupor	Ipsilateral dilatation	Normal to slight lateral strabismus	Normal to hemiparesis	Normal
Early midbrain	Stupor	Ipsilateral to bilateral dilatation	Ipsilateral ventrolateral strabismus	Hemiparesis, ipsi- or contralateral	Normal
Late midbrain	Coma	Dilated bilateral to fixed midposition	Ventrolateral strabismus to fixed midposition	Decerebrate rigidity	Hyperventilation
Pons	Coma	Midposition unresponsive	Vestibular eye movements absent	Flaccid paralysis	Rapid, shallow respirations
Medulla	Coma	Midposition, dilated terminally	Absent	Flaccid paralysis	Irregular to apnea, pulse slowing

*Modified from Plum, F., and Posner, J.: The Diagnosis of Stupor and Coma. Philadelphia, F. A. Davis Co., 1966 and Oliver, J. E., Jr.: Neurologic emergencies in small animals. Vet. Clin. N. Amer. 2:341–357, 1972.

mass starts in the caudotentorial compartment, the cerebellum may herniate through the foramen magnum, compressing the medulla oblongata. The respiratory pathways are blocked, resulting in death.

The signs of brain stem compression from tentorial herniation are outlined in Tables 14–2 and 14–3. Masses that compress the brain stem usually cause similar signs, although the animal's mental status is not altered as severely, because the cerebral cortex is not directly affected. The involvement of C.N. III is particularly important to the clinician, because it is one of the earliest detectable signs of herniation. In some cases, pupillary dilatation may be preceded by a slight pupillary constriction. Either of these signs indicates impending deterioration of the patient, and treatment must be instituted quickly.

Destructive lesions of the brain stem are most frequently parenchymal hemorrhages following head injury. Neoplasia and inflammation also may produce a destructive lesion. Table 14–4 lists the signs of a focal lesion at various levels of the brain stem.

ETIOLOGIC DIAGNOSIS: RULE-OUTS

The causes of stupor and coma are classified in Table 14–5 according to the presence or absence of focal, lateralizing, or meningeal signs and the onset and the progression of the signs.

Table 14–4. SIGNS CHARACTERISTIC OF FOCAL BRAIN STEM HEMORRHAGE AT ONE LEVEL*†

Level	Consciousness	Pupils	Eye Movements	Motor Function	Autonomic Responses
Diencephalon	Apathy to stupor	Small, but reactive	Normal	Hemiparesis to tetraparesis	Normal to Cheyne-Stokes respiration
Midbrain	Stupor to coma	Bilateral dilated or midposition unresponsive	Ventrolateral strabismus, bilateral	Decerebrate rigidity	Hyperventilation (variable)
Pons	Coma	Midposition unresponsive	Vestibular eye movements absent	Decerebrate rigidity to flaccid paralysis	Rapid shallow respiration, loss of micturition reflex
Medulla	Coma	Midposition, dilated terminally	Absent	Flaccid paralysis	Irregular to apnea

*Modified from Oliver, J. E., Jr.: Intracranial Injury. *In* Kirk, R. W.: Current Veterinary Therapy VII. Philadelphia, W. B. Saunders Co., 1980.
†Assuming a large intramedullary hemorrhage confined primarily to one level. The most frequent is in the caudal midbrain and the pons following acute head injury. Asymmetric or smaller lesions will produce less severe signs.

Table 14–5. ETIOLOGY OF STUPOR AND COMA*

	Focal or Lateralizing Signs		
	Acute Progressive	*Acute Nonprogressive*	*Chronic Progressive*
Degenerative		Vascular hemorrhage embolism	
Neoplastic	Metastatic		Primary Gliomas Meningiomas Reticulosis
Traumatic	*Epidural, subdural hematoma* Cerebral edema	*Parenchymal hemorrhgae*	Subdural hematoma (rare)

	No Focal or Lateralizing Signs, But with Evidence of Meningeal Irritation		
	Acute Progressive	*Acute Nonprogressive*	*Chronic Progressive*
Inflammatory	*Meningitis*		
Traumatic		Subarachnoid hemorrhage	

	No Focal, Lateralizing, or Meningeal Signs		
	Acute Progressive	*Acute Nonprogressive*	*Chronic Progressive*
Degenerative			Storage diseases
Anomalous		Malformation of brain Lissencephaly Hydranencephaly Otocephaly	*Hydrocephalus*
Metabolic	*Hypoglycemia* *Hepatic encephalopathy* Uremic encephalopathy Diabetic coma Heat stroke Hypoxia		
Nutritional	*Thiamine deficiency* (polioencephalomalacia)		
Idiopathic	Epilepsy (postictal)		
Inflammatory	Encephalitis		Encephalitis
Toxic	Heavy metals Barbiturates Carbon monoxide		Heavy metals
Traumatic	*Cerebral edema*		

*_Italics_ incidate most common diseases clinically.

Focal or Lateralizing Signs

ACUTE PROGRESSIVE

Trauma

Head injuries in domestic animals are most often the result of motor vehicle accidents. Most of the available information relates to dogs, but other species respond similarly to injuries of the brain.[2]

The terms that are commonly used in describing head injury are defined in Table 14–6. The differentiation of concussion from contusion is far from clear and has no significance for clinical management. Cerebral edema can be assumed to exist in any patient with neurologic signs following head injury. The most common types of intracranial hemorrhage are subarachnoid and intramedullary. Surgical treatment is of no benefit in either case.

The differentiation of the signs of diffuse cerebral and focal brain stem lesions from the signs of tentorial herniation has been discussed earlier (see Tables 14–1 through 14–4 and Figs. 14–2 and 14–3).

The treatment of a head injury cannot be separated from the management of the whole patient. Multiple system injuries are common in animals that have been hit by cars. The owner may be instructed by telephone to establish a patent airway by extending the animal's head and pulling the tongue forward if the animal is unconscious. The animal should be carried on a piece of plywood or some sim-

Table 14-6. TERMINOLOGY OF HEAD INJURY

Concussion: Transient loss of consciousness without structural pathology.

Contusion: Pathologic alterations in the brain, including edema, petechial hemorrhage, disruption of nerve fibers, and so forth.

Coup and Contrecoup: Injuries at the point of impact (coup) and at the opposite pole of the brain (contrecoup).

Cerebral Edema: An increase in intracellular (gray matter) and extracellular (white matter) fluid, present in most head injuries.

Hemorrhage:

Epidural: Bleeding between the dura and the calvarium. It usually is caused by a skull fracture with laceration of a meningeal artery. Relatively rare in animals.

Subdural: Bleeding between the dura and the arachnoid. It usually is caused by disruption of the bridging veins, so it develops slowly. Relatively rare in animals.

Subarachnoid: Bleeding into the subarachnoid space. It usually is caused by disruption of the veins or the arteries of the arachnoid. Relatively common in animals.

Intramedullary (intracerebral): Bleeding into the tissue of the brain. It usually is caused by disruption of the intramedullary vessels. Relatively common in animals.

Skull Fractures:

Linear: Fractures of the calvarium that are not displaced.

Depressed: Fractures of the calvarium that encroach on the brain.

---

ilar rigid support to avoid displacement of the spinal column.[3]

The priorities for management on presentation of the animal to the veterinary clinic are (1) maintenance of adequate ventilation by endotracheal catheter or tracheostomy if necessary and (2) treatment of shock. An intravenous catheter should be established, and lactated Ringer's solution should be administered in order to maintain a route for other medications. Intravenous corticosteroids (dexamethasone, 1 to 2 mg per kg) usually are given for shock and are probably beneficial in the reduction and the prevention of traumatic cerebral edema. The efficacy of corticosteroids in trauma-induced edema has been questioned.[4,5] Other studies, however, have provided objective evidence of reduced intracranial pressure with high doses.[6] Mannitol (0.25 to 1 gm per kg) should be given intravenously if the patient is comatose but not if the patient is hypovolemic.[7]

The extent of the injury must be determined quickly. Cardiopulmonary function, internal hemorrhage, and fractures of the limbs or the spinal column should be evaluated.[3] The nervous system then should be evaluated as has been described previously. Evaluations of the level of consciousness, pupillary function and eye movements, dysfunction of other cranial nerves, and motor function are adequate for the assessment of the level and the extent of the damage to the central nervous system (CNS).

A flow chart relating the neurologic assessment to the treatment is presented in Figure 14-4. Radiography should be performed on the patient with minimal deficits (alert or depressed) in order to detect skull fractures, and

Table 14-7. COMPARISON OF ACUTE BRAIN STEM HEMORRHAGE WITH TENTORIAL HERNIATION FOLLOWING HEAD INJURY*

	Brain Stem Hemorrhage	Tentorial Herniation
Onset	Early	Delayed
Course	Static to progressive	Progressive
Pupils	Constricted early, dilated late	Unilateral dilatation, progression to bilateral dilatation
Consciousness	Stuporous to comatose	Alert or apathetic, progressing to coma
Muscle Tone	Decerebrate rigidity or flaccid paralysis	Normal or weak, progressing to decerebrate rigidity and then to flaccid paralysis
Reflexes	Usually symmetric	Often unilateral asymmetry

*From Oliver, J. E., Jr.: Neurologic emergencies in small animals. Vet. Clin. N. Amer. 2:341–357, 1972. Used by permission.

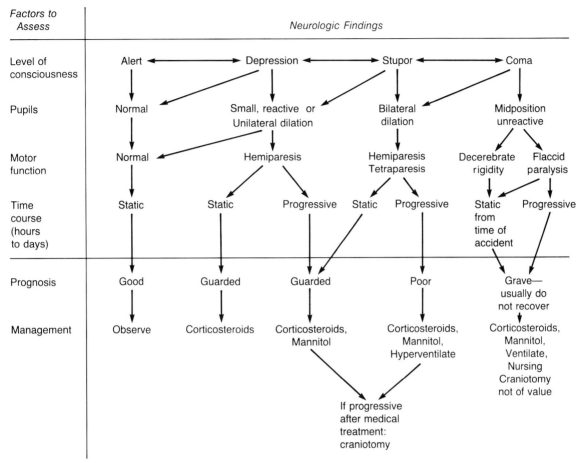

Figure 14–4. Management of intracranial injury. (Modified from Oliver, J. E., Jr.: Intracranial injury. *In* Kirk, R. W. (ed.): Current Veterinary Therapy VII. Philadelphia, W. B. Saunders Co., 1980).

the animal should be observed closely for 24 to 48 hours for progressive signs. Depressed skull fractures in conscious patients are elevated surgically when the animal is stable. Animals with linear fractures do not need surgery unless progressive signs indicate continuing intracranial hemorrhage. Open fractures are debrided and closed as early as possible.

Stuporous or comatose patients require more critical assessment and care and have a poorer prognosis. Brain stem hemorrhage usually can be differentiated from tentorial herniation from the time course of the neurologic signs (Fig. 14–5 and Table 14–7). Intramedullary brain stem hemorrhage, which usually occurs in the midbrain or the pons, produces coma immediately after the trauma, and there is little or no improvement in this case (Fig. 14–6). Tentorial herniation may develop from cerebral edema (usually bilateral) or from rostrotentorial hemorrhage (epidural, subdural). The

progression of signs is usually characteristic (see Tables 14–2 and 14–3). Animals with brain stem hemorrhage rarely recover, and those that do usually have severe neurologic deficits. Tentorial herniation must be managed early in order for the treatment to be successful. Severe tentorial herniation with compression and distortion of the brain stem produces secondary brain hemorrhages that are irreversible. In addition, increased pressure transmitted to the caudotentorial compartment produces cerebellar herniation through the foramen magnum, causing death by interference with the medullary respiratory centers (Fig. 14–7).

Brain stem hemorrhage is treated as was outlined previously: corticosteroids, mannitol, ventilation, and nursing care. The initial management of tentorial herniation involves the same procedures. If the signs do not improve or if progression is observed in the first few hours, craniotomy for evacuation of the

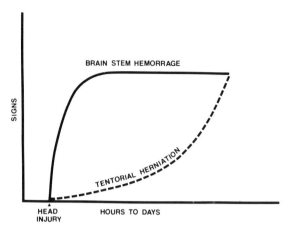

Figure 14–5. Sign-time graph of head injury. Tentorial herniation and brain stem hemorrhage may be differentiated by the clinical course. (From Oliver, J. E., Jr.: Neurologic emergencies in small animals. Vet. Clin. N. Amer. 2:341–357, 1972. Used by permission.)

Table 14–8. ETIOLOGY OF VASCULAR DISEASE IN THE BRAIN

Hemorrhage
   Trauma
   Infectious disease (septicemia, infectious canine hepatitis)
   Toxins (warfarin)
   Neoplasia
   Disseminated intravascular coagulopathy
   Idiopathic thrombocytopenic purpura

Infarction
   Septic emboli (endocarditis, septicemia, thromboembolic meningoencephalitis)
   Neoplasia (metastases)
   Parasites (*Dirofilaria*)
   Idiopathic feline cerebral infarction
   Vasospasm, vascular insufficiency, heart failure
   Emboli secondary to surgery (air, fat, clot)

hematoma and relief of intracranial pressure is indicated. The techniques have been described by Hoerlein.[8]

The management of the comatose patient must include maintaining hydration and nutrition; regulating body temperature; providing adequate ventilation (including hyperventilation in the early stages); preventing decubital ulcers by frequent turning, meticulous cleaning of the skin, and cushioning with sponge rubber or fleece pads; and maintaining urinary and fecal elimination.

The management of the comatose patient can be time-consuming and expensive but is rewarding when successful.

ACUTE NONPROGRESSIVE

Degenerative Diseases

Vascular diseases are classified as degenerative, although primary vascular changes, such as arteriosclerosis, are rare in animals. Atherosclerosis can be produced with atherogenic diets and may be more common in animals with hypothyroidism.[9–11] Most vascular lesions are caused by emboli from sepsis or neoplasia. Fibrocartilaginous emboli from degenerating disks cause infarction in the spinal cord (see Chapter 9). The causes of vascular diseases are listed in Table 14–8.

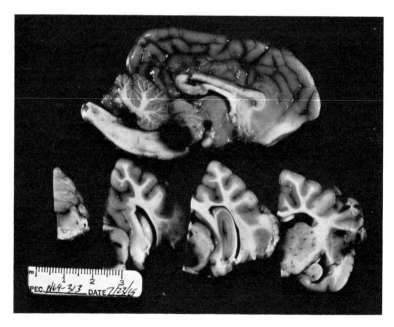

Figure 14–6. Brain stem hemorrhage in a boxer dog that was hit by a car. The hemorrhage extends from the caudal midbrain into the middle of the pons. The sulci and the gyri of the cortex are prominent, indicating minimal brain swelling. There is no evidence of tentorial herniation. (Compare the brain stem section second from the right with that in Fig. 14–3.) (From Oliver, J. E., Jr.: Neurologic examination. VM/SAC 67:654–659, 1972. Used by permission.)

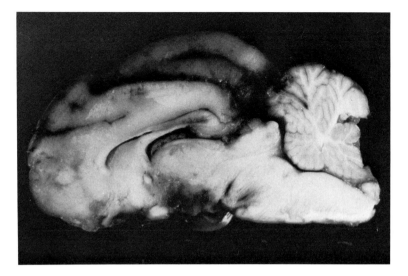

Figure 14–7. Brain of a cat with head trauma. There is tentorial herniation with compression of the rostral cerebellum and foramen magnum herniation with compression of the caudal cerebellum and the brain stem. (Courtesy of Dr. Joe N. Kornegay.)

A *stroke*, or a *cerebrovascular accident* (CVA), is an acute onset of neurologic deficit from spontaneous intracranial hemorrhage or occlusion of an intracranial blood vessel by a thrombus or an embolus. The term *apoplexy* originally was used to mean massive intracranial hemorrhage but is sometimes used synonymously with *stroke*. *Cerebral vasospasm* is a temporary constriction of an intracranial artery, causing transient ischemia. A vasospasm is difficult to document clinically. Transient loss of consciousness (syncope) is usually caused by a cardiac arrhythmia, not by a vasospasm (see Chapter 15).

Hemorrhage in the brain is usually caused by trauma. All other causes of hemorrhage

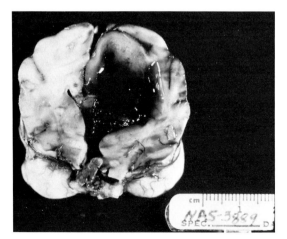

Figure 14–8. Massive hemorrhage in an oligodendroglioma in a Samoyed. There were no clinical signs prior to an acute episode related to the hemorrhage.

combined have a much lower incidence than does trauma. Small hemorrhages (petechiae) are seen on examination of the brain with inflammation as the primary problem, but other pathologies predominate.[12] Hemorrhage producing stroke syndromes probably is seen most often in neoplasms that have compromised an artery (Fig. 14–8). Systemic coagulation disorders, such as disseminated intravascular coagulopathy (DIC) or idiopathic thrombocytopenic purpura (ITP), usually are recognized by systemic signs.[19]

An infarction is usually caused by septic emboli, frequently in association with endocarditis (Fig. 14–9). Cardiomyopathy should be considered in small animals with suspected cerebral infarctions. Thromboembolic meningoencephalitis (TEME) is an acute disease of cattle that is characterized by infarcts produced by septic emboli. The disease is caused by *Hemophilus somnus* and usually is seen in feedlot cattle. Cerebral signs predominate, but brain stem infarctions may produce focal signs (see Chapter 17). Metastatic neoplasia or parasites, including the microfilaria of *Dirofilaria immitis,* are less common causes of vascular occlusion.[13,14] Air, fat, or blood clots may be introduced into the circulation during surgical procedures. Air emboli are of particular concern during vascular surgery of the head and the neck.

Idiopathic feline cerebral infarction has been described as a distinct syndrome. The etiology of the infarction has not been established, although vasculitis and thrombosis have been reported as causes.[15] There is no breed, sex, or age predilection. It has not been correlated

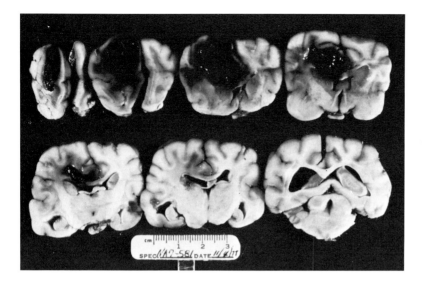

Figure 14–9. Hemorrhagic infarct in a dog with endocarditis. There is a cingulate herniation across the midline.

with feline cardiomyopathy, although an association with this disorder should be considered in the differential diagnosis. The lesions are often confined to the distribution of the middle cerebral artery (Fig. 14–10). The rostral and caudal cerebral arteries are affected less often, possibly because they anastomose with each other, offering a source of collateral circulation, except in their terminal branches (Fig. 14–11).[16]

Clinical signs of hemorrhage and infarction depend on the location and the extent of the involvement. In all cases of vascular occlusion or hemorrhage, a sudden onset with little or no progression is characteristic. Depending on the state of oxygenation and other factors, neuronal death begins in 3 to 10 minutes. Because most vascular lesions are unilateral,

clinical signs are frequently more severe or are confined entirely to one side. Diffuse cerebral or rostral brain stem lesions may cause loss of consciousness that may persist (coma) or may be transient. Hemiparesis is frequent, and behavioral changes may be present.

The management of the unconscious patient is discussed in the section on trauma in this chapter. Less severe lesions are usually not life-threatening; however, the amount of residual damage may be dependent on the adequacy of therapy. Corticosteroids should be given in antiedema doses (1 to 2 mg per kg dexamethasone) in order to control edema.[17,18] Adequate ventilation must be assured if respiration is compromised. Anticoagulants generally are not used unless a clotting problem is known (DIC). If the source of the problem such as bacterial endocarditis, can be identified, specific antibiotic therapy is instituted.[19]

Most animals that are diagnosed clinically as likely to have CVAs recover. Unless the lesion is large or involves the brain stem, neurologic function is adequate for survival. An idiopathic feline cerebral infarction is characterized by massive cortical damage that causes seizures or behavioral disorders, which often are unacceptable in a pet.

CHRONIC PROGRESSIVE

Neoplasia

Neoplasms of the brain may cause stupor and coma, depending on the location, the rate of growth, the development of cerebral edema, and alterations in circulation. A sudden onset

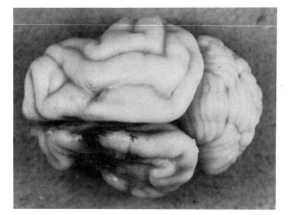

Figure 14–10. Infarction of the left cerebral hemisphere of a cat.

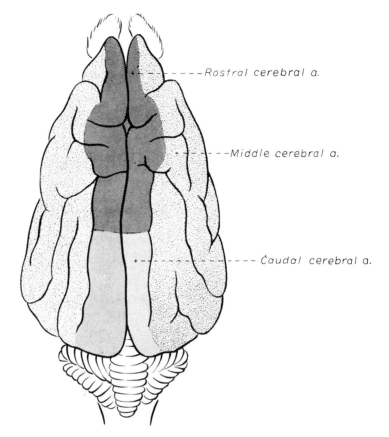

- - - - Rostral cerebral a.

- - - - Middle cerebral a.

- - - - Caudal cerebral a.

Figure 14–11. Areas of the brain supplied by the cerebral arteries. (From Evans, H. E., and Christensen, G. C.: Miller's Anatomy of the Dog, 2nd ed. Philadelphia, W. B. Saunders Co., 1979. Used by permission.)

of stupor or coma has been seen in cases of acute hemorrhage into a cerebral brain tumor. The signs were attributed to an acute increase in intracranial pressure (see Fig. 14–8). Neoplasia will be discussed in Chapter 17.

No Focal or Lateralizing Signs, But Evidence of Meningeal Irritation

ACUTE PROGRESSIVE

Inflammation

Inflammatory diseases of the CNS may affect both the nervous tissue and the meninges,

Table 14–9. CAUSES OF STUPOR AND COMA IN INFLAMMATION

Direct effect on neurons
Cerebral edema
Increased intracranial pressure from increase in CSF volume
Vasculitis or embolism causing hypoxia
Systemic metabolic abnormalities

although one of these entities may be more severely involved than the other. Stupor or coma is the result of one or more of the pathologic changes listed in Table 14–9.

Viral agents tend to have a greater effect on the nervous tissue, with only minimal involvement of the meninges. Vasculitis is common with virus infection. Bacterial and fungal agents produce a greater meningeal reaction. The formulation of a diagnosis usually requires an analysis of CSF (see Chapter 6).

The management of patients with stupor or coma secondary to inflammatory disease includes the treatment of the primary disease, if possible, and the management of the increased intracranial pressure. Cerebral edema should be treated with corticosteroids (dexamethasone, 1 to 2 mg per kg) only if the animal is stuporous or worse. Depression of the immune system is a serious side effect of corticosteroids in a patient with infectious disease; however, the consequence of not treating the increased intracranial pressure is worse, namely, death of the animal. (See Chapter 17 for a complete discussion of inflammatory diseases.)

No Focal or Lateralizing Signs

ACUTE PROGRESSIVE

Inflammation

Many of the viral encephalitides cause depression, stupor, or coma. They will be discussed in Chapter 17.

Metabolic Diseases

Nervous tissue depends upon a continuous supply of glucose and oxygen for normal function. It is protected from toxic substances by the blood-brain barrier (see Chapter 1). Alterations in brain metabolism can cause severe clinical signs, ranging from depression to coma and from tremors to seizures. The most common metabolic problems causing stupor or coma are listed in Table 14–5. Hypoglycemia will be discussed in Chapter 15. Hepatic encephalopathy, uremic encephalopathy, and diabetic coma will be discussed in Chapter 17.

Heat stroke is an acute failure of the heat-regulating mechanisms of the body, which results in a body temperature that exceeds 105 degrees F.[20] High ambient temperature, high humidity, and poor ventilation are the enciting factors. Brachycephalic breeds are especially susceptible. A long-haired coat, obesity, and a high fever also may predispose to heat stroke.[8]

The primary mechanism for dissipation of heat in dogs and cats is panting. The air flow is unidirectional—in through the nose and out through the mouth. The large surface area of the nasal turbinates promotes heat exchange.[21] Prolonged panting causes a respiratory alkalosis that later is modified by a metabolic acidosis, presumably from increased muscular activity. If hyperthermia continues, two major complications are seen, either of which can cause death. Cerebral edema and disseminated intravascular coagulopathy (DIC) occur frequently, although the precise cause is not known. Although all of the CNS is involved, the neurons of the cerebral cortex and the cerebellum seem to be most susceptible to permanent damage.[22,23] The formulation of a diagnosis of heat stroke is based on the clinical signs and the elevation of the body temperature.

The three major objectives of treatment are reduction of body temperature, prevention of cerebral edema, and management of DIC if it develops. A corticosteroid should be given intravenously in an antiedema dose (dexamethasone, 1 to 2 mg per kg). The clinician lowers the body temperature by immersing the animal in cold or iced water. The rectal temperature should be monitored continuously by thermistor or at 10-minute intervals. In order to prevent hypothermia, cooling is stopped when the rectal temperature reaches 103 degrees F. Ice water enemas may be used in refractory cases, but they prevent accurate monitoring of body temperature unless an esophageal thermistor is available. If shivering interferes with the cooling process, a tranquilizer (acetylpromazine, 0.1 mg per kg) may be given.

If the animal shows evidence of cerebral edema, especially if signs of tentorial herniation are present (see Table 14–2), mannitol (0.25 to 1 gm per kg) should be administered intravenously. If serious blood loss or DIC is a complication, mannitol should not be given.[7,20] Corticosteroids should be administered every 8 hours.

Intravenous fluids should be given if hemoconcentration or peripheral circulatory failure is present. Overhydration must be avoided. Ringer's solution is the fluid of choice unless specific replacement therapy can be determined by serum electrolyte determination.

Hemorrhagic diarrhea, petechiae, or excessive bleeding from venipuncture sites signifies the onset of DIC. Intravenous heparin (50 to 150 IU per kg) therapy should be instituted immediately. Coagulation studies can confirm the presence of DIC.[20,24,25]

The patient should be monitored carefully for at least 24 hours after normothermia is achieved so that recurrences can be avoided. The prognosis for patients with heat stroke is relatively good if they are treated early, before signs of cerebral edema or DIC develop.

Hypoxia is an inadequate supply of oxygen for normal brain function. Arterial oxygen tension levels below 50 mm Hg are detrimental to brain function. Increased levels of carbon dioxide have a profound effect on cerebral blood flow. Since there are no oxygen reserves in the brain, merely a few minutes of hypoxia can cause irreversible damage. More than 10 minutes of hypoxia produces neuronal death. The cerebral cortex is most susceptible to hypoxic damage, and the lower brain stem is most resistant.

The most frequent causes of hypoxia in animals are listed in order of importance in Table 14–10.

In spite of the almost universal use of inhalation anesthesia with controlled ventilation, complications of anesthesia are common. Car-

Table 14-10. CAUSES OF HYPOXIA

Anesthesia	Paralysis of respiration
Cardiopulmonary failure	Carbon monoxide
Suffocation	Cyanide

diac arrhythmias, overdose of the anesthetic agent, improper intubation, and faulty apparatus are but a few of the problems encountered. Meticulous attention to detail in the administration and the monitoring of anesthesia is essential.

Heart, lung, and peripheral circulatory failure rival anesthesia as the most common cause of hypoxia. Heart and lung disease may cause a mild to severe hypoxemia. If the condition does not cause unconsciousness, the danger of cerebral damage is low. Shock may cause profound cerebral hypoxia and irreversible damage to the brain. A primary concern in the management of shock is the maintenance of adequate ventilation. The management of the various forms of cardiopulmonary failure is beyond the scope of this text.[19]

Suffocation is a less frequent problem in animals. Examples of causes are aspiration of vomitus (especially in injured or anesthetized animals), aspiration of foreign bodies, and drowning.

Paralysis of respiration may occur with lesions of the CNS between the medullary respiratory centers and the origin of the phrenic nerve at C5–C7 (sometimes C4). The lesion may affect the respiratory center directly, or it may interrupt the descending pathway in the cervical spinal cord and produce the same effect: apnea. Lesions in the lower cervical (C7) or the upper thoracic region may block the pathway to the intercostal innervation, but the intact phrenic pathway will allow diaphragmatic ("abdominal") breathing to occur. The most common cause of this lesion is trauma. If the damage to the CNS is irreversible, life can be maintained only by use of a respirator. Generalized lower motor neuron (LMN) disease also may cause respiratory paralysis through its effect on both the intercostal nerves and the phrenic nerve (see Chapter 10).

Carbon monoxide poisoning is seen occasionally in animals that have been transported in a car trunk. Carbon monoxide combines with hemoglobin, preventing the formation of oxyhemoglobin. The animal typically has bright red mucous membranes and rapid, shallow respiration. Transfusion of fresh (not stored) whole blood and administration of oxygen may be effective if hypoxia has not persisted for too long.

Cyanide poisoning is rare. Cyanide interferes with the cellular utilization of oxygen through blockage of the cytochrome system.[19]

Nutritional Diseases

Thiamine deficiency may cause stupor or coma, especially in ruminants. Polioencephalomalacia, a symmetric laminar necrosis of the cerebral cortex, is seen in cattle, sheep, and goats. Increased intracranial pressure is common. Thiamine deficiency will be discussed in Chapter 17.

CHRONIC PROGRESSIVE

Toxic Disorders

A large number of toxic agents may produce stupor and coma, especially in the terminal stages (see Chapter 17). An overdose of certain drugs, including barbiturates, tranquilizers, or narcotics, may produce stupor or coma as a primary effect. The drugs may have been given deliberately or may have been ingested accidentally. Historical information may be clear ("he ate my bottle of pills") or misleading ("we never have anything like that around"). A comparison of the signs of coma caused by drugs with those of coma caused by structural changes in the brain is provided in Table 14–1. Spinal reflexes and respiration are depressed more severely by sedative drugs than by most structural lesions, whereas pupillary responses are less affected.

Most patients that have overdosed on CNS depressants can be saved with proper management. If the animal is not in coma, attentive nursing is usually all that is necessary. Gastric lavage is performed if the drug was ingested recently. The maintenance of adequate respiration is the most important consideration for patients in coma. Controlled respiration through an endotracheal catheter is essential. Diuresis is promoted by the intravenous administration of glucose or mannitol. (For specific therapy, see Finco and Low.[26]) Urine output must be monitored through an indwelling urethral catheter. The excretion of many agents (e.g., barbiturates) is dependent on the rate of urine formation. Hydration and acid-base balance must be maintained. Periodic evaluation of serum electrolytes and blood gases is of great benefit in the management of persistent coma. The combination of diuresis and controlled ventilation can lead to serious changes in a short time.

Stimulant drugs have been used in the past but appear to be of little benefit, since they do not affect the rate of metabolism or execretion of most drugs.

Degenerative Diseases

Storage diseases, inherited degenerative diseases with accumulation of metabolic products in neurons, may cause depression or stupor. The animal may be in a coma terminally. Other signs, such as ataxia or seizures, are more common in the early stages of the disease (see Chapter 17).

Anomalies

Hydrocephalus is an enlargement of the cerebral ventricular system secondary to an increased amount of CSF. Excessive CSF may be the result of obstruction to flow (noncommunicating or obstructive hydrocephalus), poor absorption, or increased production (communicating hydrocephalus). Hydrocephalus may be seen in any species.

Most of the CSF is produced by the choroid plexus in the lateral, third, and fourth ventricles, but a substantial portion travels through the ependyma lining the ventricles and the subarachnoid space around the brain and the spinal cord. CSF flows from the lateral ventricles through the interventricular foramina to the third ventricle. It continues caudally through the mesencephalic aqueduct to the fourth ventricle and into the subarachnoid space through the lateral apertures of the fourth ventricle. In the subarachnoid space, most of the fluid moves around the brain stem into the rostrotentorial compartment. Most of the absorption occurs through the arachnoid villi in the dorsal sagittal sinus (Fig. 14–12).

Overproduction of CSF by a choroid plexus papilloma is rare. Communicating hydrocephalus from decreased absorption of CSF is usually the result of inflammation of the meninges. Inflammation is usually caused by infectious diseases, such as canine distemper, but may be secondary to subarachnoid hemorrhage or to foreign materials, such as radiographic contrast materials injected in the subarachnoid space.[8] Obstruction of the flow of CSF occurs most commonly at the mesen-

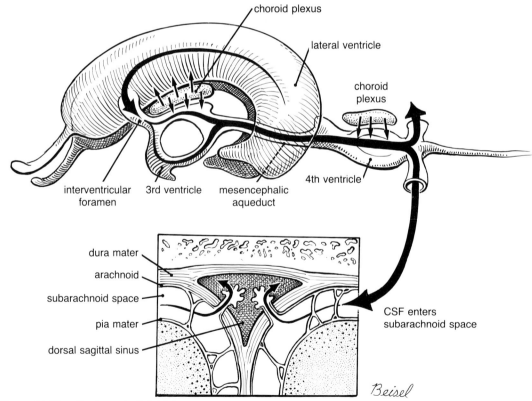

Figure 14–12. Cerebrospinal fluid is produced in all areas of the central nervous system. The bulk of the fluid flows from the lateral ventricles to the third ventricle to the mesencephalic aqueduct and continues from the fourth ventricle to the lateral apertures and then to the subarachnoid space, where it is absorbed.

Table 14–11. BREEDS OF DOGS AT AN INCREASED RISK FOR HYDROCEPHALUS*

Maltese	Toy poodle
Yorkshire terrier	Cairn terrier
English bulldog	Boston terrier
Chihuahua	Pug
Lhasa apso	Pekingese
Pomeranian	

*Modified from Selby, L. A., Hayes, H. M., and Becker, S. V.: Epizootiologic features of canine hydrocephalus. Am. J. Vet. Res. 40:411–413, 1979.

cephalic aqueduct. Malformations of the aqueduct range from complete absence to stenosis. Obstruction of the aqueduct also can be secondary to inflammation or compression by a mass. For example, brain stem tumors that cause obstruction of the aqueduct produce hydrocephalus.

Most cases of hydrocephalus that are seen in veterinary practice are congenital. The disorder may be caused by environmental or genetic factors. Hereditary hydrocephalus has been reported in Hereford cattle.[27] There have not been enough studies of the pathology of congenital hydrocephalus in the dog to determine the primary defect. Some patients have stenosis or atresia of the mesencephalic aqueduct, but others do not. Multiple branching of the aqueduct, called "forking," has been reported in both dogs and human beings.[28,29] A statistically significant correlation between small body size and hydrocephalus has been demonstrated in dogs (Table 14–11).[30]

Ventricular enlargement without clinical signs is a common finding in some toy breeds, especially Chihuahuas. A kennel of Chihuahuas was studied by Redding.[8] Subclinical hydrocephalus was common. Behavioral changes could be correlated with abnormal electroencephalograms (EEGs) in many instances. A selective breeding program using the EEG for screening of breeding animals reduced the incidence of hydrocephalus. Redding concluded that the dogs had a compensated hydrocephalus (a balance between production and absorption of CSF) that could be decompensated by relatively mild changes, such as trauma or infection. These observations correlate with our clinical impression. Redding also observed a high incidence of enlargement of the foramen magnum (occipital dysplasia—see Chapter 11) in these dogs. Whether this abnormality is related to the cause of hydrocephalus or whether it is secondary to increased pressure is still debatable.

The clinical signs are related to (1) the age of onset, (2) the degree of imbalance between production and absorption of CSF, and (3) location of the defect (communicating or noncommunicating).

Congenital hydrocephalus is usually recognized in the very young animal. The increase in intracranial volume occurs before the sutures of the skull have closed, allowing for enlargement of the calvarium. The enlargement of the head, the open sutures and fontanelles, and the poor development of the animal may be recognized shortly after birth. Affected dogs are usually presented to the veterinarian when they are between 2 and 3 months of age (Fig. 14–13). Palpation of the skull may reveal the open sutures and fontanelles. In compensated hydrocephalus the fontanelle may be open, but there is no tension as the brain is palpated. Active hydrocephalus with increased pressure often causes a bulging of the soft tissue through the fontanelle, and palpation reveals the increased tension. The head is enlarged. The prominent frontal areas encroach on the orbits, causing a ventrolateral deviation of the eyes. Oculomotor nerve function (pupils and eye movements—see Chapter 13) is usually normal, indicating that the eye deviation is mechanical, not neurologic, in origin. The widening of the skull is detected by palpation of the parietal area where the space between the skull and the zygomatic arch is narrowed. Head pain may be evident in some animals when the skull is palpated.

Young animals with hydrocephalus usually are smaller and less developed than their littermates. They are often depressed, have episodic behavioral changes (such as aggression or confusion), and frequently have seizures (see Chapter 15). Their mental development is retarded, so they do not learn as readily as their littermates. Visual deficits with normal pupillary responses are common because of damage to the optic radiation and the occipital cortex (see Chapter 13). Motor function may range from almost normal operation to severe tetraparesis. Papilledema may be seen on fundic examination in a small percentage of the cases.

Hydrocephalus in the adult animal is more difficult to recognize. The skull is normal because the sutures have fused prior to the increase in pressure. The clinical signs develop more rapidly and are more severe, but they are dependent on the relative balance of production and absorption of CSF. Seizures are a frequent sign in the early stages. Depression,

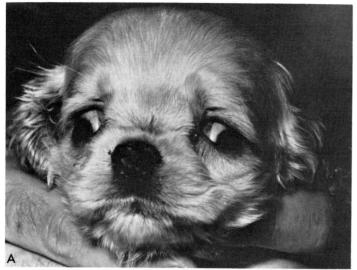

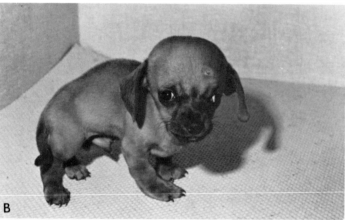

Figure 14–13. Cocker spaniel (*A*) and dachshund (*B*) puppies with hydrocephalus. The large, rounded head and the ventrolateral deviation of the eyes are characteristic.

which may progress to stupor or coma, is common. Since hydrocephalus in the adult is usually secondary to inflammation or a mass, signs of the primary problem may predominate early in the course of the disease. Complete obstruction of the CSF causes a rapidly progressive hydrocephalus, which may cause tentorial herniation, cerebellar herniation, or both (see Figs. 14–2 and 14–3 and Tables 14–2 and 14–3).

The diagnosis of hydrocephalus in the young animal is relatively certain if the characteristic signs are present. Although the clinical signs of severe hydrocephalus are very typical, less severe involvement may present a more subtle picture. Behavioral changes or seizures may be the only complaint. In these cases, ancillary studies are necessary in order to confirm the diagnosis.

An EEG is the first test used in our clinic, because it is noninvasive and the recordings are usually characteristic. High-voltage, slow-wave activity (25 to 200 μv, 1 to 6 Hz) that is hypersynchronous (similar in all leads) may be seen both in dogs that are awake and in those that are anesthetized. A fast component (10 to 12 Hz) often is superimposed on the slow waves. In severe hydrocephalus, in which the large slow waves (1 to 4 Hz) predominate, the EEG is sufficient for diagnosis. Earlier forms, in which faster activity is more prominent, may be confused with inflammatory disease. Since many veterinary practices do not have EEG capabilities, the diagnosis must be confirmed by other procedures.

Radiographs of the skull may demonstrate changes that are compatible with hydrocephalus. If expense is a consideration, radiographs are not essential, and the diagnosis can be confirmed by ventricular tap. Skull radiographs can confirm open suture lines and fontanelles. Increased intracranial pressure for an extended period causes thinning of the skull with loss of the normal digital impressions on the inner surface of the calvarium. The cranial vault has a "ground-glass" appearance (Fig. 14–14 A). Rostral displacement and thinning of the wing of the sphenoid bone also may be seen.

The diagnosis can be confirmed in severe cases by a ventricular tap. A spinal needle is inserted directly into the ventricle (see Chapter 6).[31] The depth that is necessary to obtain fluid provides an estimate of the thickness of the cerebral cortex. Normal animals have a lateral ventricle that is only a few millimeters thick. Careful needle placement is required to obtain fluid. Severe hydrocephalus causes thinning of the cerebral cortex (Fig. 14–15) so that fluid may be obtained within 0.5 to 1.0 cm of the inner surface of the skull. If it is neces-sary to go deeper than 1.0 to 1.5 cm to obtain fluid, a pneumoventriculogram is performed in order to confirm the ventricular enlarge-ment. The distances given are primarily for toy-breed dogs or cats; those for larger ani-mals of any species may vary somewhat. Fluid never should be aspirated with a syringe, be-cause the cerebral cortex may collapse, causing a subdural hematoma (Fig. 14–16). Fluid may be allowed to escape under its own pressure, providing some therapeutic benefit in addi-tion to establishing the diagnosis. Analysis of the CSF may be useful for formulating an eti-ologic diagnosis (see Chapter 6).

If the results of the ventricular tap are not diagnostic, a pneumoventriculogram is per-formed (see Fig. 14–14 B and Chapter 6).[32] Pos-itive contrast ventriculography may be neces-sary to determine whether the hydrocephalus

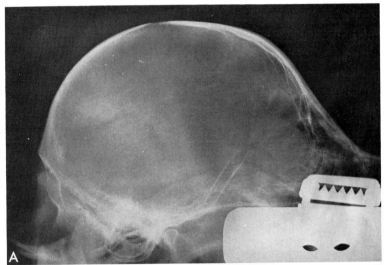
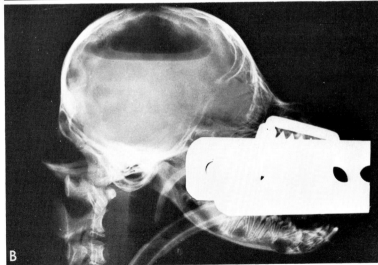

Figure 14–14. *A.* Radiograph of a hydrocephalic dog. Notice the "ground-glass" appearance of the calvarium, caused by loss of the digital impressions from chronic increased pressure. The fontanelle is open on the dorsum of the skull, and the osseous tentorium is ab-sent. *B.* Pneumoventriculogram of a dog with hydrocephalus.

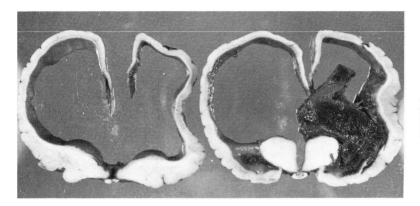

Figure 14–15. Severe hydrocephalus in a Chihuahua. Notice the thinning of the cerebral cortex. There is an intraventricular hematoma.

is communicating or noncommunicating. Since therapy generally will be the same in either case, the increased risks involved in the use of positive contrast material usually are not justified.

The treatment of hydrocephalus depends on the cause of the disorder and the status of the animal. Acquired hydrocephalus in the adult animal requires resolution of the inciting factor. Neoplasia will be discussed in Chapter 17. An inflammatory disease may cause permanent reduction of absorptive capacity, and the hydrocephalus must be managed separately. Presenting hydrocephalic patients usually fit into one of the following categories: (1) acute with rapid progressing signs in a previously normal animal or one that previously has been static, (2) having chronic progressive deterioration, or (3) having static signs that may be mild to severe.

Acute progressive signs indicate a poor prognosis and the need for vigorous treatment. A ventricular tap should be done, and fluid should be allowed to flow under its own pressure with the animal in sternal recumbency and the head elevated slightly above the shoulders. Fluid should not be aspirated. An osmotic diuretic (mannitol, 1 gm per kg) should be given slowly by intraveneous drip to reduce cerebral edema. A corticosteroid (dexamethasone, 1 mg per kg) should be given to reduce CSF production and edema. The dosage of mannitol should be repeated twice at 6-hour intervals. Corticosteroids should be given every 8 to 12 hours with the dosage reduced by half after three doses and on each succeeding dose. Anticonvulsants should be used if needed. If the animal survives and the neurologic status permits, the same long-term treatment should be provided as for chronic progressive cases.

Animals with chronic progressive hydro-

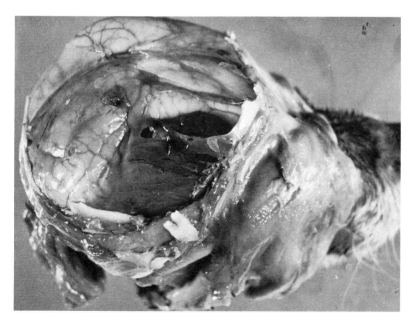

Figure 14–16. A dog with hydrocephalus, with a large subdural hematoma that resulted when too much fluid was aspirated from the lateral ventricle. (From Oliver, J. E., Jr., and Knecht, C. D.: Diseases of the brain. *In* Ettinger, S. J.: Textbook of Veterinary Internal Medicine, 1st ed. Philadelphia, W. B. Saunders Co., 1975. Used by permission.)

cephalus, as indicated by the history and serial neurologic examinations, may be treated medically or surgically. Progression should be stopped, and some clinical improvement should be seen as a result of treatment. The owner must be made aware, however, that the animal will not be totally normal. If the neurologic status is too poor for the animal to function as a pet, then treatment should not be continued. Medical treatment usually is tried first. Low-dose corticosteroid therapy has been effective in approximately 60 per cent of the cases treated by Harrison.[8] Dexamethasone should be given orally at a dosage of 0.25 mg per 5 kg bid. Other corticosteroids may be used in equivalent dosages. Clinical improvement is expected within three days. If improvement is seen, the dosage should be reduced by half after one week. After another week one dose should be given every other day. If signs are stable, medication may be discontinued and repeated only as signs develop. Many animals stabilize in remission and only occasionally require medication. Others may require continuous medication, in which case signs of Cushing's disease may appear. The objective of medical treatment is to provide remission of signs with the least possible amount of medication.

Surgical treatment is reserved for those cases that cannot be stabilized medically. Surgical treatment consists of a drain tube from the lateral ventricle through a one-way valve to the right atrium or the peritoneal cavity. The major disadvantages of surgery are the expense and the postoperative complications. The various shunt systems cost $150 or more, making the total procedure very expensive, especially when one considers that the animal may not be normal. The complications include the necessity to replace the tubing as the animal grows, the occlusion of the tubes by fibrous tissue or clots, and sepsis. The shunts can be very effective and have functioned well in some dogs for up to 8 years.[8] See Hoerlein for a description of the surgical procedure.[8]

Other anomalies of the brain may cause alterations in mental status (see Table 14–5). Some are so grossly abnormal that they are not usually compatible with life, such as hydranencephaly and otocephaly. Others are more typically characterized by seizures and will be discussed in Chapter 15.

CASE HISTORIES

The cases in this chapter have the common sign of alteration in mental status. After you read the history and the results of the examination, make a problem list, localize the lesion, list the rule-outs and formulate a plan for the diagnosis of each, and make a prognosis. Then read our assessment and the results of the diagnostic procedures.

Case History 14A

Signalment

Canine, boxer, female, 6 months old.

History

The dog was hit by a car 6 hours before presentation. She was unconscious after being hit and has not regained consciousness.

Physical Examination

The dog is unconscious in lateral recumbency. The temperature is 100.6 degrees F, the pulse is 75, and the respirations are 25 and shallow. The color of the membranes is good, and the capillary refill time is rapid. There is a small abrasion on the muzzle on the left side. There are no palpable fractures or luxations. Heart and lung sounds are normal.

Neurologic Examination

The dog is unconscious and does not respond to painful stimuli, except for the withdrawal reflexes. All four limbs are in rigid extension. When the dog is forced to flex the limbs, there is considerable resistance to a point, and then they collapse. The postural reactions are absent. When the animal is moved into an erect position, the head and the neck arch dorsally. The myotatic reflexes cannot be evaluated because of the rigid extension of the limbs. Strong stimuli cause an increase in extension followed by a brief partial flexion that reverts to extension almost immediately. Tests for vision are negative. The pupils are small, symmetric and slightly reactive. In a darkened room, they dilate only slightly (about 2 to 3 mm). Vestibular eye movements are absent. The globes are in the center of the palpebral fissure. The palpebral reflex is present but weak. There is no evidence of conscious perception of pain from a pinch of the face or a stimulation of the nasal mucosa. The gag reflex is present. The tongue retracts symmetrically, but there are no licking movements.

Case History 14B

Signalment

Canine, Samoyed, male, 4 years old.

History

The dog has hip dysplasia, but there were no other significant medical problems. At 8:00 a.m. the dog started walking aimlessly, bumping into walls and doors. Within one-half hour the rear limbs began to abduct, and the dog fell. When the owner picked him up, he growled. At 9:00 a.m. the dog was seen by the referring veterinarian, who reported the following:

Mental status: The dog is depressed.

Posture and gait: The dog is unable to walk and falls to the right side.

Postural reactions: All are very poor to absent on the right front and the right rear limbs and normal on the left front and the left rear limbs.

Spinal reflexes: All are normal.

Cranial nerves: The menace reaction is poor bilaterally; otherwise, the reactions are normal.

The dog was brought to our clinic at 6:00 p.m., 10 hours after the onset of the signs.

Neurologic Examination

The dog is in coma. The temperature is 105 degrees F. There is minimal increase in extensor tonus of the limbs. The postural reactions are absent. The spinal reflexes are normal. The menace reaction is absent. The pupils are widely dilated and unresponsive to light. The eyes are deviated ventrolaterally and do not respond to head movements. The palpebral reflex is present, but there is no behavioral response to a pinch of the face or a touch of the nasal mucosa. There is a weak gag reflex and good retraction of the tongue.

Case History 14C

Signalment

Canine, Chihuahua, male, 3 months old.

History

Lack of coordination and intermittent depression began at age 2 months. The dog has had no known illnesses, and his vaccinations have been given on schedule.

Physical Examination

The head is dome-shaped with a large, open fontanelle. The only other abnormalities appear on the neurologic examination.

Neurologic Examination

The dog is depressed and does not seem to have a normal awareness of his environment. Loud noises produce a startle reaction, but the response is not oriented toward the sound. The dog can walk but is reluctant to do so. Once he starts walking, he progresses to a wall and then stands with his head against the wall. Some dysmetria and a mild ataxia are present. The postural reactions are depressed—worse in the pelvic limbs than in the thoracic limbs. The spinal reflexes are normal. There is no menace reaction, and the dog does not appear to be able to see. The visual placing reaction is absent, although the tactile placing reaction is present but slow. The pupillary reflexes are normal. The eyes

appear deviated ventrolaterally, although vestibular eye movements are present in all directions. Other cranial nerves are normal. Sensation is intact, although reactions to painful stimuli are slow and poorly directed.

ASSESSMENT 14A

The dog is in coma and exhibits decerebrate rigidity. Decerebrate rigidity is caused by loss of the voluntary upper motor neuron (UMN) pathways with retention of the reticulospinal and vestibulospinal pathways, which are facilitory to the extensor motor neurons. The loss of postural reactions confirms the absence of voluntary UMN pathways. The arching of the head and the neck is opisthotonos. The spinal reflexes are difficult to assess when the limbs are in extensor rigidity, but it is apparent that the extensor neurons are intact. The visual tests will be negative in an unconscious animal, since we depend on behavioral responses for our assessment. The pupillary reactions indicate that the oculomotor nerve is intact bilaterally. The small size of the pupil suggests loss of sympathetic input or irritation of the oculomotor nerve. The symmetry suggests that it is a loss of sympathetic tone. The absent eye movements indicate paralysis of C.N. III, C.N. IV, and C.N. VI or a lesion of the medial longitudinal fasciculus (MLF) connecting those nuclei with the vestibular nucleus. Since the parasympathetic component of C.N. III is functional, a lesion of the MLF is more likely. Other cranial nerves appear relatively normal, considering the level of consciousness.

Localization: Brain stem, caudal to C.N. III (midbrain), rostral to C.N. VII (rostral medulla), including the midline MLF and a large portion of the reticular activating system (coma). Therefore, it probably is a large intramedullary lesion of the pons.

Rule-outs: Trauma is known, An acute onset of coma without improvement for 6 hours suggests brain stem hemorrhage rather than tentorial herniation. The clinical signs also agree with this hypothesis. Tentorial herniation usually affects C.N. III early. The signs indicate a lesion of the pons rather than the midbrain, which is compressed by tentorial herniation. There are no simple diagnostic tests to confirm intramedullary hemorrhage of the brain stem. The alternatives are to treat and observe for change or to use other tests to rule out epidural or subdural hemorrhage absolutely. Radiographs could detect skull fracture, but this finding probably would not alter the plan.

Skull radiographs were taken, and it was found that a linear fracture extended across the floor of the cranial vault—a basilar fracture. Basilar fractures have been associated with severe brain lesions in the cases we have seen.

Prognosis: Poor.

Plan: Treat medically (corticosteroids, mannitol, intravenous fluids, nursing) and observe for 48 hours.

Results: The dog's neurologic status did not change in 48 hours. The owners requested euthanasia. The brain is shown in Figure 14–6.

ASSESSMENT 14B

Localization: The lesion involves the brain stem. Dilated pupils (C.N. III) and coma (reticular activating system) indicate that there is midbrain involvement. C.N. V and C.N. VII are intact (palpebral reflex), indicating that the pons and the medulla (also C.N. IX, C.N. X, C.N. XII) are intact. The progression of signs from the cerebrum (pacing, blindness, postural reaction deficits) to the midbrain suggests tentorial herniation. The early signs were unilateral, indicating a left cerebral lesion with rapid progression to bilateral tentorial herniation.

Rule-outs: The sudden onset of severe signs usually indicates trauma or vascular lesions. The dog was in the house and had not been out since the night before, making trauma unlikely. Severe cerebral vascular lesions in dogs are unusual, but this hypothesis seems most likely. Vascular lesions may be associated with other pathologies, such as parasites or neoplasia.

Rule out (1) vascular lesion and (2) trauma.

Plan: Spontaneous epidural or subdural hemorrhages have not been reported in dogs. Parenchymal hemorrhages are not likely to be helped by surgery. These factors, plus the severity of the signs, made the prognosis very poor. The animal was given intensive medical treatment (mannitol, corticosteroids, fluids) and was monitored carefully until the next day. The temperature cycled frequently, varying from 101 degrees to 107 degrees F. There was no change in the neurologic status after 18 hours, and the owner requested euthanasia.

Necropsy: The dog had an oligodendroglioma of the left cerebrum with a massive hemorrhage (see Fig. 14–8).

ASSESSMENT 14C

The primary problems are depression, loss of vision, and postural reaction deficits with no paresis. All of these conditions are compatible with lesions above the brain stem. Postural reaction deficits without paresis usually are caused by cerebral or diencephalic lesions. Loss of vision with intact pupillary light reflexes indicates that the pathways from the eye to the midbrain and C.N. III are intact, but there is bilateral damage to the lateral geniculate nucleus, the optic radiations, or the cerebral cortex. Intact vestibular eye movements indicate that the brain stem pathways (MLF) and C.N. III, C.N. IV, and C.N. VI are intact. The deviation of the eyes must have another cause. Depression is not localizing but is compatible with diffuse cerebral or diencephalic disease.

Localization: Cerebrum or diencephalon, diffuse.

Rule-outs: The problems are slowly progressive, with an onset at an early age. Inflammatory disease would have to be considered. The inherited degenerative diseases also may cause a syndrome such as this one, but none of these disorders has been reported in the Chihuahua. Hydrocephalus is commonly seen in this breed. The signs are usually cortical in origin. Blindness is frequent. The dog has a dome-shaped head with an open fontanelle, which is typical of congenital hydrocephalus. Many Chihuahuas have these skull changes without enlarged ventricles, however. The deviation of the eyes is seen in hydrocephalics because of the malformation of the bones of the orbit (Fig. 14–13). Hydrocephalus would have to be our first choice until the presence of another condition is proved.

Rule outs: (1) hydrocephalus, (2) inflammation, and (3) degenerative disease.

Plan: Skull radiographs will not reveal much more than we already can see and feel (shape and open fontanelle). An EEG may be useful but probably will not be absolutely diagnostic because the dog is immature, and we can expect high-voltage slow waves in a normal 3-month-old dog. The most direct diagnostic test for hydrocephalus is a ventricular tap with a pneumoventriculogram if the tap is not diagnostic. The tap can be made through the lateral margin of the open fontanelle. If fluid is obtained with the needle inserted less than 2 cm, then the ventricles are enlarged. If there is doubt, 2 ml of air can be injected and a radiograph made to confirm the size of the ventricles. The CSF that is obtained can be analyzed. A cisternal tap is contraindicated, because it may cause cerebral herniation if hydrocephalus is present. Degenerative diseases cannot be diagnosed except by biopsy or necropsy in most cases.

Prognosis: Guarded.

Plan:
1. Rule out hydrocephalus—ventricular tap, CSF analysis, pneumoventriculogram.
2. Rule out inflammation—CSF analysis.
3. Rule out degenerative diseases—exclusion.

Results: Under general anesthesia, a ventricular tap was performed. Fluid was obtained with the needle only 1 cm below the scalp. The owners refused treatment for the dog, and he was destroyed.

Many dogs with this degree of abnormality will improve with treatment; however, vision may be permanently lost. If vision is present, the prognosis is much better.

Also review Case History E in Chapters 2, 3, 4, and 6.

REFERENCES

1. Popper, K. R., and Eccles, J. C.: The Self and Its Brain. New York, Springer Publishing Co., Inc., 1977.
2. Oliver, J. E., Jr.: Intracranial injury. In Kirk, R. W.: Current Veterinary Therapy VII. Philadelphia, W. B. Saunders Co., 1980.
3. Oliver, J. E., Jr.: Neurologic emergencies in small animals. Vet. Clin. North Am. 2:341–357, 1972.
4. Cooper, P. R., Moody, S., Clark, W. K., Kirkpatrick, J., Maravilla, K., Gould, A. L., and Drane, W.: Dexamethasone and severe head injury. J. Neurosurg. 51:307–316, 1979.
5. Tornheim, P. A., and McLaurin, R. L.: Effect of dexamethasone on cerebral edema from cranial impact in the cat. J. Neurosurg. 48:220–227, 1978.
6. James, H. E., Langfitt, T. W., and Kumar, V. S.: Analysis of the response to therapeutic measures to reduce intracranial pressure in head injured patients. J. Trauma 16:437–441, 1976.
7. Parker, A. J.: Blood pressure changes and lethality of mannitol infusion in dogs. Am J. Vet. Res. 34:1523–1528, 1973.
8. Hoerlein, B. F.: Canine Neurology: Diagnosis and Treatment. Philadelphia, W. B. Saunders Co., 1978.
9. Belza, J., Rubinstein, L. J., Maier, N., and Haimovici, H.: Experimental cerebral atherosclerosis in dogs. Ann. NY Acad. Sci. 149:895–906, 1968.

10. Detweiler, D. K., Ratcliffe, H. L., and Luginbuhl, H.: The significance of naturally occurring coronary and cerebral arterial disease in animals. Ann NY Acad. Sci. 149:868–881, 1968.

11. Fankhauser, R., Luginbuhl, H., and McGrath, J. T.: Cerebrovascular disease in various animal species. Ann NY Acad. Sci. 127:817–860, 1965.

12. Easley, J. R.: Necrotizing vasculitis: An overview. JAAHA 15:207–211, 1979.

13. Patton, C. S., and Garner, F. M.: Cerebral infarction by heartworms (*Dirofilaria immitis*) in a dog. JAVMA 5:600–605, 1970.

14. Segedy, A. K., and Hayden, D. W.: Cerebral vascular accident caused by *Dirofilaria immitis* in a dog. JAAHA 14:752–756, 1978.

15. deLahunta, A.: Feline ischemic encephalopathy: A cerebral infarction syndrome. *In* Kirk, R. W.: Current Veterinary Therapy VI. Philadelphia, W. B. Saunders Co., 1977.

16. Rasmussen, T. B.: Experimental Ligation of the Cerebral Arteries of the Dog. Thesis, University of Minnesota, St. Paul, MN, 1938.

17. Anderson, D. C., and Cranford, R. E.: Corticosteroids in ischemic stroke. Curr. Concepts Cerebrovasc. Dis. Stroke 13:19–24, 1978.

18. Patten, B. M., Mendell, J., Bruun, B., Curtin, W., and Carter, S.: Double-blind study of the effects of dexamethasone on acute stroke. Neurology 22:377–383, 1972.

19. Ettinger, S.: Textbook of Veterinary Internal Medicine. Philadelphia, W. B. Saunders Co., 1975.

20. Schall, W. D.: Heat stroke. *In* Kirk, R. W.: Current Veterinary Therapy VII. Philadelphia, W. B. Saunders Co., 1980.

21. Schmidt-Nielsen, K., Bretz, W. L., and Taylor, C. R.: Panting in dogs: Unidirectional air flow over evaporative surfaces. Science 169:1102–1104, 1970.

22. Hanneman, G. D., Higgins, E. A., Price,, G. T., Funk-houser, G. E., Grape, P. M., and Snyder, L.: Transient and permanent effects of hyperthermia in dogs: A study of simulated air transport environmental stress. Am. J. Vet. Res. 38:955–958, 1977.

23. Mehta, A. C., and Baker, R. N.: Persistent neurological deficits in heat stroke. Neurology 20:336–340, 1970.

24. Perchick, J. S., Winkelstein, A., and Shadduck, R. K.: Disseminated intravascular coagulation in heat stroke. Response to heparin therapy. JAMA 231:480–483, 1975.

25. Krum, S. H., and Osborne, C. A.: Heatstroke in the dog: A polysystemic disorder. JAVMA 170:531–535, 1977.

26. Finco, D. R., and Low, D. G.: Intensive diuresis in polyuric renal failure. *In* Kirk, R. W.: Current Veterinary Therapy VII. Philadelphia, W. B. Saunders Co., 1980.

27. Axthelm, M. K., Seipold, H. W., and Phillips, R. M.: Congenital internal hydrocephalus in polled Hereford cattle. VM/SAC 76:567–570, 1981.

28. Russell, D. S.: Observations on the Pathology of Hydrocephalus. Medical Research Council Special Report No. 265. London, Her Majesty's Stationery Office, 1949.

29. Sahar, A., Hockwald, G. M., Kay, W. J., and Ransohoff, J.: Spontaneous canine hydrocephalus cerebrospinal fluid dynamics. J. Neurol. Neurosurg. Psychiatry 34:308–315, 1971.

30. Selby, L. A., Hayes, H. M., and Becker, S. V.: Epizootiologic features of canine hydrocephalus. Am. J. Vet. Res. 40:411–413, 1979.

31. Savell, C. M.: Cerebral ventricular tap: An aid to diagnosis and treatment of hydrocephalus in the dog. JAAHA 10:500–501, 1974.

32. Oliver, J. E., Jr., and Conrad, C. R.: Cerebral ventriculography. *In* Ticer, J. W.: Radiographic technique in small animal practice. Philadelphia, W. B. Saunders Co., 1975.

Epilepsy is a disorder of the brain that is characterized by recurring seizures. *Seizures, fits,* and *convulsions* are synonymous terms used to describe the manifestations of abnormal brain function that are characterized by paroxysmal stereotyped alterations in behavior. Narcolepsy is a disorder of the brain that is marked by sudden recurring attacks of sleep. Narcolepsy will be discussed at the end of this chapter.

A seizure has several components. The actual seizure is called the *ictus*. Prior to the seizure (preictally), there may be a period of altered behavior, called the *aura*. People with seizures report varying sensation, apprehension, and so forth during the aura. Animals may hide, appear nervous, or seek out their owners at this time. The ictus usually lasts for 1 to 2 minutes, but there is considerable variation. Following the seizure (the postictal phase), the animal may return to normal in seconds to minutes or may be restless, lethargic, confused, disoriented, or blind for minutes to hours.[1] The aura and the postictal phase do not have any relationship to the severity or the cause of the seizures.[1]

Seizures may occur in any animal, but they have been reported more frequently in the dog.

ANATOMIC DIAGNOSIS

Seizures are always a sign of abnormal brain function. The dysfunction may be from a primary lesion in the brain or may be secondary to a metabolic abnormality (e.g., hypoglycemia, toxicity).

Two components are recognized as the basis for seizure disorders: the *seizure focus* and the *spread* of the abnormal activity to other areas of the brain. The paroxysmal alterations in behavior are associated with synchronous excessive discharge in large aggregates of neurons—the seizure focus.[2] If the activity of the seizure focus spreads to other parts of the brain, a generalized cerebral dysrhythmia results, which produces the behavioral change that is recognized as a seizure.

Seizure foci apparently are present in many individuals who do not have seizures. Some populations of neurons in the brain (e.g., the hippocampus) are much more likely to develop seizure activity than others. The seizure focus has been studied extensively in a variety of experimental models and in naturally occurring epilepsy. Neurons in seizure foci are characterized by large-amplitude, prolonged-membrane depolarizations with associated high-frequency bursts of spikes. These changes

cause paroxysmal discharges in the electroencephalogram (EEG).[2] The number of epileptic neurons correlates with the frequency of seizures.

Seizures can be generated in any individual by pharmacologic, metabolic, or electrical changes; however, the threshold of stimulation required varies widely. Normal individuals may require potent convulsant drugs (e.g., pentylenetetrazol) or electric shock to exceed the threshold. A lower seizure threshold may allow production of convulsions by conditions such as fever, photic stimulation, or minor alterations in body chemistry (e.g., hypoglycemia, hypocalcemia, hyperventilation). Finally, there are those individuals who have seizures with no apparent stimulus. The range from normal individuals to those who have spontaneous fits is a continuum without sharply defined boundaries. The threshold for seizures may be an inherited trait.

The behavioral changes of seizures are composed of one or more of the following involuntary phenomena: (1) loss or derangement of consciousness or memory (amnesia), (2) alteration of muscle tone or movement, (3) alteration of sensation, including hallucinations of special senses (e.g., visual, auditory, olfactory), (4) disturbances of the autonomic nervous system (e.g., salivation, urination, defecation), and (5) other psychic manifestations, abnormal thought processes, or moods (recognized as behavioral changes, e.g., fear, rage).[3]

It should be noted that *one or more* of the aforementioned changes is present in a seizure. For example, loss of consciousness is usually associated with a generalized motor seizure but may not be a part of a convulsion

SEIZURES AND NARCOLEPSY

Table 15–1. CLASSIFICATION OF SEIZURES: CLINICAL SIGNS*

Clinical Manifestation	EEG	Etiology	Anatomic Location
Generalized Seizures, Bilateral Symmetric Seizures, or Seizures Without Local Onset			
Tonic-clonic (grand mal, major motor)	Generalized dysrhythmia from onset, symmetric, often normal interictal unless they are activated or have organic or toxic origin.	1. Genetic predisposition 2. Diffuse or multiple organic lesions 3. Toxic or metabolic	1. Unlocalized 2. Diencephalic (centrencephalic)
Absences with or without motor phenomena (petit mal)—rare or rarely recognized in animals	Generalized three per second spike and wave dysrhythmia, symmetric (human)	Usually genetic (human)	1. Unlocalized 2. Diencephalic (centrencephalic)
Partial Seizures or Seizures Beginning Locally			
Partial motor (may generalize to tonic-clonic seizure)—signs depend on site of discharge.	Focal dysrhythmia (spikes, slow waves), may generalize secondarily	Acquired organic lesion, see Tables 15–2 and 15–3	Focal cortical or subcortical
Psychomotor (may generalize or appear as complex behavioral change—running, fear, aggression)	Dysrhythmia related to temporal lobe (unproven in animals)	Acquired organic lesion. See Tables 15–2 and 15–3	Limbic system (hippocampus, temporal or pyriform lobe)

*Modified from Oliver, J. E., Jr.: Seizure disorders in companion animals. Comp. Cont. Ed. Small Anim. Pract. 2:77–86, 1980.

with behavioral manifestations. Behavioral or psychic changes are not necessarily seizure disorders; however, if the changes are paroxysmal, seizures are strongly considered.

The classification of seizures based on clinical signs is useful from a descriptive standpoint and also may be helpful in localization (Table 15–1).[4]

Gastaut has proposed that generalized seizures be called *primary generalized epilepsy* if no etiology can be ascertained and *secondary generalized epilepsy* if any organic cause can be found.[5] Primary generalized epilepsy includes essential epilepsy, true epilepsy, idiopathic epilepsy, genetic epilepsy, and centrencephalic epilepsy. Partial or focal seizures are usually acquired, thus ruling out primary generalized epilepsy.[6]

Generalized Seizures

Tonic-clonic seizures (grand mal, major motor) are the most frequently recognized convulsions in animals. The seizure frequently is preceded by an aura. The animal falls and becomes unconscious, the limbs are extended rigidly, opisthotonos usually is seen, and respiration stops (apnea). The tonic phase is usually brief (10 to 30 seconds) and is rapidly followed by clonic limb movements in the form of running or paddling activity. Chewing movements of the mouth are common. Visceral activity may start in the tonic or clonic phase of the ictus and may include pupillary dilatation, salivation, urination, defecation, and piloerection. The clonic phase may alternate with tonic activity. The ictus usually lasts 1 to 2 minutes. The postictal phase may be a few minutes of rest followed by normal activity or may include confusion, disorientation, restlessness and pacing, and blindness lasting for minutes to hours.

Careful questioning of the owner is required in order to determine if the seizure starts as generalized, symmetric activity or if it has a focal component. The aura should not be confused with focal seizure activity. Any indication of focal motor activity, such as chewing, forced turning of the head, or clonic jerks of muscle groups, indicates a focal component, even if it generalizes secondarily.

Absences, or *petit mal seizures,* either are very uncommon in animals or, more likely, are uncommonly recognized. They are characterized by a brief (a matter of seconds) loss of contact with the environment, but without motor activity. Variations seen in human beings include minor motor components, such as facial twitching, loss of postural tone, and autonomic activity. Redding has reported one dog with absence attacks and characteristic EEG changes (4 Hz spike-wave complexes).[7] Unless these attacks are frequent or the owner is very observant, they are usually unrecognized.

Primary generalized seizures cannot be localized anatomically. Whether the seizure focus is single or multiple, the generalized signs preclude localization.

Partial Seizures

Partial motor seizures (focal motor, Jacksonian) reflect the activity of a local seizure focus in an area producing motor activity. Movements are restricted to one part of the body, such as the face or one limb. Partial seizures frequently spread, resulting in a generalized convulsion. The focal component of the seizure onset is the key differential feature. Since partial seizures are invariably acquired, primary generalized epilepsy is not considered in the differential diagnosis.

The true Jacksonian seizure (which includes a focal onset followed by a slow progression of motor activity to adjacent structures, ultimately terminating in a generalized motor seizure) is rare in animals. The motor area of the cerebral cortex of domestic animals is small, allowing convulsion activity to generalize rapidly. Patients with partial motor seizures are more likely to have focal EEG abnormalities in interictal periods than are those with generalized seizures. Partial sensory and autonomic seizures are not commonly recognized. Psychomotor seizures may have a predominance of autonomic signs.[5,8] Animals that have repetitive episodes of "fly-biting" may be having focal sensory seizures in the visual cortex; however, psychomotor seizures with a sensory component are the generally accepted explanation.

Partial motor seizures are presumed to arise from a seizure focus near a primary motor area, usually the frontal cortex. In animals, partial motor seizures are indicative of a pathology in the contralateral cerebral hemisphere (e.g., a left thoracic limb seizure indicates a right cerebral cortex lesion).

Psychomotor seizures (partial seizures with complex symptomatology, behavioral seizures, emotional disorders) are paroxysmal episodes of abnormal behavior. Examples include hysteria, rage, autonomic reactions (such as salivation), and hallucinations (such as "fly-biting").

Differentiating psychomotor seizures from functional behavioral changes may be difficult. Psychomotor seizures usually will be preceded by an aura and followed by a postictal phase. The ictus is stereotyped and repetitive. Autonomic components of the ictus are common.

Psychomotor seizures indicate an abnormality in the limbic system. The most frequent locations are probably the hippocampus, the amygdala, and the temporal cortex. These areas commonly are involved in inflammatory diseases, such as canine distemper and rabies, and are damaged in tentorial herniation of any cause (see Chapters 14 and 17).

ETIOLOGIC DIAGNOSIS: RULE-OUTS

Seizures may be caused by any process that alters normal neuronal function. As with all neurologic diseases, the differential diagnosis is formulated in broad categories. The most likely diseases within each category then are considered. Tables 15–2 and 15–3 outline the major categories of diseases that are likely to produce seizures.

Genetic

Primary generalized epilepsy (idiopathic, cryptogenic) is inherited and has no demonstrable pathologic cause. Although it may occur in a number of of species,[9] the most comprehensive studies have been those of human beings (see Robb for a review[10]) and dogs.[9,11–15]

In animals, primary generalized epilepsy usually occurs in the form of generalized tonic-clonic seizures. Absence attacks are common in human beings but are apparently rare in dogs.[6] Breeds of dogs that are known to have a genetic basis for epilepsy are listed in Table 15–4. Also listed are those breeds reported to have a high incidence of seizure disorders but for which genetic studies have not been documented. Whether these breeds have genetic epilepsy has not been proved.

An inherited epilepsy also has been reported in Brown Swiss and Swedish Red cattle.[16] A hereditary syndrome characterized by recurrent seizures and the gradual development of cerebellar ataxia occurs in purebred and crossbred Aberdeen Angus cattle. The seizures start in young calves but decline in frequency in those that survive to approximately 15 months of age. Most cattle are clini-

Table 15–2. CAUSES OF SEIZURE DISORDERS OF DOGS AND CATS*

Classification	Most Frequent Causes	Diagnostic Tests†
Genetic	Genetic	Breed, age, history
Degenerative	Storage disease	
	glycoprotein (Lafora's disease)	Breed, biopsy
	lipids	Breed, biopsy
Developmentally anomalous	Hydrocephalus	PE, EEG, ventriculography
	Lissencephaly	Breed, PE, EEG
	Porencephaly	Ventriculography
Infectious	Viral: canine distemper, rabies, feline infectious peritonitis	History, EEG, CSF analysis CSF analysis
	Bacterial: any type	CSF analysis
	Mycotic: cryptococcosis	CSF analysis
	Protozoal: toxoplasmosis	CSF analysis, titer
Metabolic	Electrolyte: hypocalcemia	Serum calcium levels
	Carbohydrate: hypoglycemia, functional insulinoma	Fasting blood glucose levels Fasting blood glucose levels
	Cardiovascular: arrhythmia, vascular disorder	EKG Arteriography
	Renal	PE, BUN levels, UA
	Hepatic: cirrhosis	PE, BSP test, SGPT levels, serum NH_3 levels
	Portocaval shunt	Same + angiography
Neoplastic	Primary: gliomas, meningiomas	NE, EEG, radiography
	Secondary: metastatic	Same
Nutritional	Thiamine	History, response to treatment
	Parasitism (multiple factors)	PE, response to treatment
Toxic	Heavy metal: lead	History, blood lead levels
	Organophosphates	History, NE
	Chlorinated hydrocarbon	History, NE
	Strychnine	History, NE
	Tetanus	History, NE
Traumatic	Acute: immediately after head injury	History, PE
	Chronic: weeks to years after head injury	History, EEG

*Modified from Oliver, J. E., Jr.: Seizure disorders in companion animals. Comp. Cont. Ed. Small Anim. Pract. 2:77–86, 1980.

†PE = physical examination, EEG = electroencephalography, CSF = cerebrospinal fluid, BUN = serum urea nitrogen, EKG = electrocardiography, UA = urinalysis, BSP = Bromsulphalein, SGPT = serum alanine transaminase, NE = neurologic examination.

cally normal by 2 years of age. Pathologic changes have been found in the Purkinje cells of the cerebellum.[17]

The first seizure in a dog with primary generalized epilepsy usually occurs between the ages of 6 months and 5 years.[6,18–20] In a large beagle colony, 29 dogs had their first seizure at a mean age of 30 months (range 11 to 70 months).[12] Many dogs with abnormal EEGs did not have fits by 6 years of age but may have been at risk for future seizures. The incidence of convulsions in each of three different reports was approximately 1 per cent.[1,20,21] The incidence rate was significantly higher in male dogs than in female dogs in a large beagle colony.[12]

The clinician can make a diagnosis of pri-

mary generalized seizures only by excluding other causes. There are no positive diagnostic findings that will substantiate the diagnosis. The breed, the age, and the history may be highly suggestive, especially if there is a familial history of seizures (Tables 15–5 and 15–6). EEG abnormalities are not consistent.[6,14,22,23] Activation techniques may prove useful for detecting latent abnormalities.[14,23]

Degenerative

Deficiencies in specific enzymes cause abnormal cellular metabolism with the accumulation of metabolic products within the neurons. These storage diseases may produce

Table 15–3. CAUSES OF SEIZURE DISORDERS OF LARGE ANIMALS

Classification	Most Frequent Cause	Diagnostic Tests*
Genetic	Genetic (bovine)	Breed, age, history
Degenerative (see Chapter 17)	Storage disease (bovine)	Breed, biopsy
Anomalous (see Chapter 14)	Hydrocephalus	Breed, PE, EEG
	Hydranencephaly	
Inflammatory (see Chapter 17)	Infectious bovine rhinotraceitis	History, PE, CSF analysis
	Pseudorabies (bovine, porcine)	
	Rabies (all)	
	Thromboembolic meningoen-cephalitis (bovine)	
	Hog cholera	
	Viral encephalitis (equine)	
	Bacterial meningoencephalitis (all)	
	Aberrant parasites (all)	
Metabolic (see Chapter 17)	Electrolyte: hypocalcemia, hypomagnesemia	Serum calcium levels, serum magnesium levels
	Carbohydrate: hypoglycemia,	Blood glucose levels
	ketosis (bovine)	Ketones
	Pregnancy toxemia (ovine)	History
	Water intoxication (bovine, porcine)	History
	Salt poisoning (porcine)	History
	Hepatic encephalopathy	PE, BSP test, serum NH_3 levels
Neoplastic	Primary (primarily equine)	NE, CSF analysis
	Secondary: metastatic	
Nutritional (see Chapter 17)	Thiamine (ruminants)	History, response to treatment
Toxic (see Chapter 17)	Heavy metals: lead, arsenic	History, blood lead levels
	Organophosphates	
	Chlorinated hydrocarbons	
Traumatic	Acute (all)	History, PE, NE

*PE = physical examination, EEG = electroencephalography, CSF = cerebrospinal fluid, BSP = Bromsulphalein, NE = neurologic examination.

Table 15–4. GENETIC EPILEPSY: PRIMARY GENERALIZED EPILEPSY*

Genetic Factor Proved or Highly Suspicious
 Alsatian (German shepherd)[9]
 Beagle[12,38]
 Keeshond[39]
 Tervuren (Belgian) shepherd[11]
Breeds Reported to Have a High Incidence of Seizure Disorders[1,6,7,13,19]
 Poodle
 Wire-haired Terrier
 Cocker spaniel
 Saint Bernard
 Irish Setter
 Collie
 Boxer
 Dachshund
 Miniature schnauzer

*Modified from Oliver, J. E., Jr.: Seizure disorders in companion animals. Comp. Cont. Ed. Small Anim. Pract. 2:77–86, 1980.

seizures as one part of the clinical syndrome (see Chapter 17).

Developmental

Disorders in this group may or may not be inherited but are distinguished from primary generalized epilepsy (genetic) by involving demonstrable pathologic changes in the brain. Hydrocephalus is the most common developmental disorder causing seizures (see Chapter 14). Other developmental defects that may produce convulsions are lissencephaly and porencephaly (see Tables 15–5 and 15–6).

Lissencephaly is a congenital absence of the convolutions of the cerebral cortex.[7,24] It has been reported in Lhasa apso dogs and in one cat. Affected animals may have behavioral,

Table 15–5. COMMON CAUSES OF SEIZURES AT DIFFERENT AGES[*]

	Younger Than 1 Year
Degenerative	Storage diseases
Developmental	Hydrocephalus
Toxic	Heavy metals—lead
	Organophosphates
	Chlorinated hydrocarbons
Infectious	Canine distemper, encephalitis
Metabolic	Hypoglycemia—transient, enzyme deficiency
	Portocaval shunt, hepatic encephalopathy
Nutritional	Thiamine, parasitism
Traumatic	Acute
	1 to 3 Years
Genetic	Primary generalized epilepsy (may start at approximately 6 months)
	Others as above
	Older Than 4 Years
Metabolic	Hypoglycemia—secondary to insulinoma
	Cardiovascular—arrhythmia, thromboembolism
	Hypocalcemia—hypoparathyroidism
Neoplastic	Primary or metastatic brain tumor

*Modified from Oliver, J. E., Jr.: Seizure disorders in companion animals. Comp. Cont. Ed. for Small Anim. Pract. 2:77–86, 1980.

visual, and slight proprioceptive deficits in addition to seizures.

Porencephaly is a cystic malformation of the cerebrum that usually communicates with the ventricle or the subarachnoid space. It may be congenital or acquired (degenerative).

Infectious

Any infectious disease has the potential to cause seizures if it invades the central nervous system (CNS). The mose prevalent diseases are listed in Tables 15–2 and 15–3. Canine distemper is probably the most common cause of seizures in dogs. The CNS manifestations may appear without any noticeable clinical illness. The diagnosis may require an EEG.[7,25] Infectious diseases will be discussed in Chapter 17.

Metabolic

Failure of one of the major organs or the endocrine glands may produce alterations in electrolytes or glucose or the accumulation of toxic products, which results in seizures (see Tables 15–2, 15–3, and 15–5).[26] Some animals

Table 15–6. CAUSES OF SEIZURES BY BREED PREDISPOSITION[*]

Breed	Cause
Alsatian (German shepherd)	Genetic
Beagle	Genetic
Belgian (Tervuren) shepherd	Genetic
Boston terrier	Hydrocephalus, neoplasia
Boxer	Neoplasia
Cairn terrier	Globoid cell leukodystrophy
Chihuahua	Hydrocephalus
English setter	Lipodystrophy
German shepherd (Alsatian)	Genetic
German short-haired pointer	Lipodystrophy
Irish setter	Genetic (suspected)
Keeshond	Genetic
Lhaso apso	Lissencephaly
Miniature pinscher	Hydrocephalus
Miniature schnauzer	Hyper-lipoproteinemia, portocaval shunts
Pekingese	Hydrocephalus
Poodle, miniature and standard	Genetic (suspected)
Poodle, toy	Hydrocephalus
Saint Bernard	Genetic (suspected)
West Highland white terrier	Globoid cell leukodystrophy
Yorkshire terrier	Hydrocephalus

*Modified from Oliver, J. E., Jr.: Seizure disorders in companion animals. Comp. Cont. Ed. Small Anim. Pract. 2:77–86, 1980.

have a lower seizure threshold, and relatively minor alterations may cause fits in these instances. The major metabolic disorders will be discussed in Chapter 17.

Neoplastic

Intracranial neoplasia, either primary or metastatic, may cause seizures. The seizure activity is caused by an abnormality in neurons adjacent to the neoplasm that are compressed or distorted or that have an insufficient blood supply. The tumor is not electrically active.

Seizures may be the first sign of brain tumor. A neurologic deficit may not be apparent until weeks to months after the onset of seizures, especially if the mass is in the cerebral cortex. Arteriography, ventriculography, or a brain scan may be required for formulation of a diagnosis. Neoplasia will be discussed in Chapter 17.

Nutritional

Seizures may be the terminal manifestation of a number of nutritional disorders. The B-complex vitamins are most frequently incriminated. Thiamine deficiency causes polioencephalomalacia in ruminants. Similar lesions are seen in dogs and cats with thiamine deficiency, except that the lesions are predominately in the brain stem nuclei.

Animals that are fed most commercial rations do not develop thiamine deficiencies. Dogs that are fed only cooked meat develop paraparesis that progresses to convulsions. Early treatment with thiamine reverses the clinical progression of the disease. Thiamine deficiency in cats has been attributed to cat foods with fish as an ingredient that contain thiaminase. Supplementation with thiamine has eliminated the problem. Cats typically have a seizure syndrome that is characterized by flexion of the head to the sternum, ataxia, behavior changes, dilated pupils and, eventually, coma. Since thiamine toxicity is unlikely, it is best to give thiamine to all cats with seizures. A dose of 50 to 100 mg is given intravenously the first day; thereafter, daily intramuscular injections are given until a response is obtained or another diagnosis is established.[1]

Toxic

Many toxins affect the CNS, and most can cause seizures. The diagnosis usually depends on the history, the identification of the toxic substance from analysis of body tissues or intestinal contents, and the animal's response to treatment.

Lead poisoning is a frequent intoxication in animals. Other clinical signs may include depression, tremor, and ataxia, which sometimes is associated with gastrointestinal signs. Seizures are often psychomotor. Peripheral blood changes may include nucleated erythrocytes (RBCs) and basophilic stippling of RBCs without anemia. The changes in the RBCs are transient and may not be present in chronic lead poisoning. Blood lead determination is diagnostic. Calcium ethylenediamine–tetra-acetic acid (CaEDTA) is used in treatment.[7]

Strychnine causes a tonic seizure that is exacerbated by stimulation. The animal remains conscious unless respiration stops. Strychnine blocks inhibitory interneurons in the spinal cord, causing a release of motor neuron activity.

Organophosphate and chlorinated hydrocarbon insecticides are a common cause of seizures. Toxic disorders will be discussed in Chapter 17.

Traumatic

Seizures may be seen immediately after an acute head injury as a result of a direct effect on neurons. Post-traumatic seizures may occur many weeks to several years after a head injury. Post-traumatic epilepsy may be focal or generalized, depending on the location of the brain lesion. The focus develops secondarily to a scar in the brain at the site of the initial injury. The focal abnormality may be recognized on EEG. The diagnosis is based on the correlation of historical information with the development of seizures and the elimination of other causes. The treatment is directed at controlling the seizures.[4,27]

PLANS FOR DIAGNOSIS AND MANAGEMENT OF SEIZURE DISORDERS

Most animals with seizures present with a similar history—episodic convulsions. Therefore, a protocol for diagnosis and management that includes a defined data base is useful.[4,19]

Data Base

The recommended data base is formulated at three levels (Table 15–7). The minimum data base (MDB) can be obtained at any veterinary clinic with an adequate clinical pathology service. The specific chemistry analyses that are performed can be modified to fit those available in an automated service. The only expense other than the initial examination is the cost of laboratory studies. The risk to the patient is minimal.

The MDB screens for primary neurologic disease (neurologic examination) and metabolic or systemic disorders (physical examination, laboratory examination).

The more complete data base includes cerebrospinal fluid (CSF) analysis, skull radiography, and EEG (see Table 15–7). CSF analysis and radiography can be performed at most

Table 15-7. DATA BASE FOR SEIZURE DISORDERS*

Minimum Data Base
Patient profile
  Breed, age, sex
History
  Immunizations: kind, dates, by whom
  Age of onset
  Frequency, course
  Description of seizure
    General or partial; duration; aura; postictus; time
    of day; relation to exercise, food, sleep, or stimuli
  Previous or present illness or injury
  Behavioral changes
Physical examination
  Complete examination of systems, including specifi-
  cally:
    Musculoskeletal: size, shape of skull, evidence of
      trauma, atrophy of any muscles
    Cardiovascular: color of mucous membranes, evi-
      dence of arrhythmias, murmurs
Funduscopic examination
Neurologic examination
  Complete examination with emphasis on cerebral
  signs, including:
    Vision, pupils
    Tactile and visual placing
    Hopping
    All cranial nerves
    Spinal reflexes
Clinical pathology
  CBC   Urinalysis
  BUN levels   Alkaline phosphatase levels
  Calcium levels SGPT levels
  Fasting blood glucose levels
  Others if indicated
More Complete Data Base
  CSF analysis: cell count, total and differential; protein
  levels; pressure
  Skull radiographs: ventrodorsal, lateral, frontal
  EEG
If Focal Brain Disease Is Suspected
  Contrast radiography
  Brain scans

*Modified from Oliver, J. E., Jr.: Protocol for diagnosis of seizure disorders in companion animals. JAVMA 172:822–824, 1978.

clinics, but EEG usually is not available, except at referral centers. These tests are performed when the MDB indicates the presence of neurologic disease or if the seizures have not been controlled with medication. These procedures are not recommended as a part of the MDB because of the low yield in animals with normal findings on the MDB, the increased risk because anesthesia is required, and the increased cost to the client.

Procedures to evaluate structural alterations in the brain, including contrast radiography and radioisotopic brain imaging, are reserved for animals with a high probability of focal brain disease. The only exception is ventricu-lography, which may be used to make a definitive diagnosis of hydrocephalus. These procedures are more dangerous and more expensive and generally should be performed at the referral center (see Chapter 6).

Plan for Management

An MDB should be completed for every patient having more than one seizure. Patients having only one isolated seizure should be given thorough physical and neurologic examinations. If no abnormalities are found, the owners should be advised to watch for further seizures.

Information from the MDB yields one of three findings: (1) a definitive diagnosis, (2) a possible cause of the seizures that requires further tests to confirm, or (3) no suggestion of the cause (Fig. 15–1).

Seizures occur episodically; therefore, the veterinarian frequently must evaluate an animal without ever seeing a convulsion. The history must be taken carefully and must include a complete description of the fits and their frequency, duration, and severity. The first goal is to determine that the animal is having convulsions. For example, transient vestibular dysfunction and drug reactions may resemble seizures. The most frequent problem to be confused with seizures is syncope (transient loss of consciousness). Syncope is caused by a loss of the blood supply to the brain or hypoglycemia. Cardiac arrhythmia is the most common cause.

The history also provides information related to the onset and the progression of the disease (Fig. 15–2). Seizures, by definition, are acute in onset; however, the owner may be able to recognize a chronic progression of signs with seizures being only one component. The diagnostic tests that are most likely to be useful in each disease are listed in Tables 15–2 and 15–3. The MDB will rule out most metabolic diseases. Other diseases may or may not be suggested by the MDB.

If there are no positive or suggestive findings on the MDB, the animal should be treated with anticonvulsants. If the seizures are not controlled with anticonvulsants, a more complete data base should be obtained. Chronic encephalitis and occult hydrocephalus usually are detected with EEG and are among the most common causes of seizures refractory to medication.

Some breeds have primary generalized epilepsy that is difficult to control. The most com-

Minimum Data Base

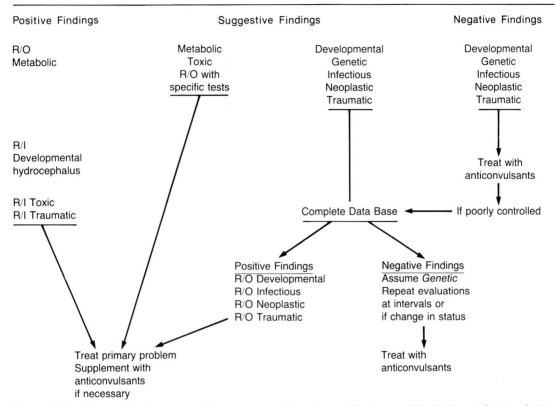

Figure 15–1. Plan for the diagnosis and management of a patient with seizures. R/O = Rule out: Positive findings confirm the diagnosis; negative findings eliminate the diagnosis. R/I = Rule in: Positive findings confirm the diagnosis; negative findings are *not* adequate for diagnosis. (Modified from Oliver, J. E., Jr.: Protocol for diagnosis of seizure disorders in companion animals. JAVMA 172:824, 1978.)

mon examples are German shepherds, Saint Bernards, and Irish setters.[1,6]

Negative findings on the complete data base for an animal that has been poorly controlled with anticonvulsant medication suggest a poor prognosis. The treatment may be altered by changing the dosage or the drugs, combining drugs, or changing the schedule of administration. Periodic re-evaluation may reveal a progressive disease that was missed originally.

Contrast radiography and radioisotope brain scans are indicated if evidence of focal brain disease or hydrocephalus exists. Mass lesions or alterations in the ventricular system are necessary in order for these tests to be positive.

PLANS FOR TREATMENT

The probability of successful treatment depends more on successful client education than any other single factor. Treatment failures are usually the result of (1) a progressive disease,

(2) refractory epilepsy, or (3) inadequate client education. A progressive disease is identified by repeated examinations. Refractory epilepsy is expected in the breeds that have been listed previously. Client education is a variable that the clinician can control.

The client should understand what successful treatment is. We consider a successful treatment to be: (1) one that reduces the frequency of seizures, (2) one that shortens the duration of seizures, or (3) one that reduces the severity of seizures. It should be noted that elimination of seizures is not listed. Complete elimination of seizures is certainly a goal, but it is not an expectation.

The client should be given some basic rules for treating epileptics:
1. Do not judge the efficacy of the medication for at least 2 weeks. Give the medication a chance.
2. Do not change or discontinue the medication suddenly. Status epilepticus may follow.

	Acute *Nonprogressive*	Acute *Progressive*	Chronic* *Progressive*
Developmental	Genetic epilepsy Lissencephaly Porencephaly	Hydrocephalus	
Degenerative			Storage diseases Demyelinating diseases
Infectious		Viral: canine distemper feline infectious peritonitis Bacterial: any Mycotic: any Protozoon: toxoplasmosis	
Metabolic		Hypocalcemia Hypoglycemia Cardiac arrhythmia Hepatic encephalopathy Renal failure	Hepatic encephalopathy
Neoplastic		Metastatic	Primary
Nutritional		Thiamine deficiency	Parasitism (Puppies)
Toxic		Organophosphates Chlorinated hydrocarbons Strychnine Tetanus	Heavy metals
Traumatic		Head injury: immediately after injury	Head injury: weeks to years after injury

*Seizures may have an acute onset, but the syndrome as a whole is chronic.

Figure 15–2. Causes of seizures. (From Oliver, J. E., Jr.: Seizure Disorders in Companion Animals. Comp. Cont. Ed. for Small Animal Pract. 2:77–86, 1980. Used by permission.)

3. Phenothiazine tranquilizers are *contraindicated* in epileptics.
4. Allow for changes in the animal's environment (e.g., give more medication when increased excitement is expected).
5. Medication may be required for life. Do not wean the animal off the drugs too soon.
6. No single drug or combination works in all cases. Adjustments in the dosage, the schedule, or the drugs probably will be required. Finding the right combination is something of a research project.

We usually do not recommend treatment for animals that have had only one seizure. We usually do not treat animals while we are establishing a diagnosis, unless the seizures are frequent and severe (more than one per day).

We do recommend treating seizures if they are recurrent or intense, especially if they tend to cluster (several in one day). Owners should be advised that each time a seizure discharge spreads, it increases the probability that it will spread again.

The final decision on treatment must be made by the client. In essence, *if the client feels that the seizures are more of a problem than is giving the medication, then treatment is in order.* Clients with small dogs in large yards will tolerate more seizures than will those with giant breeds in small apartments.

The ideal anticonvulsant would suppress seizures completely without side effects or toxicity. Unfortunately, such a drug is not known. Three primary drugs are used in the chronic treatment of seizures: phenobarbital, primidone, and phenytoin (diphenylhydantoin). Additionally, diazepam and short-acting barbiturates may be used in the treatment of status epilepticus.

Phenobarbital is generally the first drug used. Phenobarbital raises the threshold for seizure discharge and inhibits the spread of discharge from the epileptic focus.[28] It is safe and inexpensive and has few side effects other than sedation. An initial period of sedation usually is followed by a return to normal activity in a few days. Polyphagia, polydipsia, and polyuria may be seen in some patients. The usual dosage is 1 to 2 mg per kg, given bid.

If phenobarbital is not effective, primidone is used. A portion of the primidone molecule is metabolized to phenobarbital, and the remainder is phenylethylmalonamide (PEMA). The phenobarbital component has been reported to be as little as one fourth and as much as three fourths of the total.[1,28,29] Primidone at a dosage of 50 mg per kg per day produces effective blood levels of phenobarbital (greater than 10 μg per ml). Although primidone and PEMA concentrations are much lower, they may have an additive effect.[30] The major action of primidone probably is suppression of the epileptic focus. The efficacy of primidone in patients with seizures has been demonstrated clinically for years. It is probably the most effective drug available for seizures resulting from encephalitis. Side effects include depression, polydipsia, polyphagia, and hepatic necrosis. The side effects may be dramatic, but they are usually transient. The usual dosage is 50 mg per kg per day, divided into three doses. One half to twice this dosage may be used, depending on the individual animal's response. Larger animals should be started on a lower dose until tolerance is induced. Primidone is not approved for use in food animals or horses, because the dosage and the anticonvulsive effects are unknown.

Phenytoin is probably the most widely used anticonvulsant in human beings. Its use in animals is being questioned because of studies showing marked species differences in the metabolism of the drug. The pharmacokinetics vary, depending on the route of administration, pretreatment, and treatment with other drugs. The action of the drug also varies among individuals, even of the same breed.[31] The approximate plasma half-life of phenytoin is 22 to 28 hours in human beings, 3 to 4 hours in dogs, and 24 to 108 hours in cats. Human beings therefore should be placed on a once- or twice-a-day schedule, and dogs should be medicated three times daily. The drug is not recommended for cats until chronic toxicity studies have been performed. Phenytoin has not been approved by the Food and Drug Administration for use in cats. The combination of phenytoin and phenobarbital may reduce the half-life of phenytoin further.

In addition, blood concentrations of phenytoin in the dog do not reach therapeutic levels (10 μg per ml, based on human clinical and canine research data) at the same dosages prescribed for human beings.[30] Laboratory studies indicate that at least 30 mg per kg tid is needed to reach therapeutic levels in the dog.[31,32] In another study, therapeutic levels were achieved with 3 to 5 mg per lb tid, but the reported concentrations were only 1.5 to 3.0 μg per ml.[33] Clinical studies are needed to resolve the problem. Until these reports are available, we recommend that phenytoin be used only after phenobarbital and primidone have proved unacceptable. Side effects of phenytoin have been rare, but the reason for this finding may be that the dosage has been far too low to be therapeutic. Ataxia, elevated liver enzymes, and gingival hyperplasia have

been reported. The recommended dosage varies from 5 to 50 mg per kg tid. Phenytoin is not approved for food animals or horses. It has been used with beneficial effects in some horses at a dosage of 20 mg per kg bid.

Mephobarbital is longer-acting than phenobarbital and is given once daily. Its efficacy is essentially the same as that of phenobarbital because it is metabolized into two molecules of phenobarbital. It offers a once-a-day medication schedule at a greater expense.

Diazepam is used in the treatment of status epilepticus and may be administered in conjunction with other drugs in the treatment of epilepsy. The duration of action is short, requiring tid or qid administration. Phenobarbital and diazepam are the only anticonvulsants recommended for cats (Table 15–8).

Other drugs that may be of benefit but that have not been cleared for use in animals include paramethadione,[34] carbamazepine,[35] and sodium valproate.[36] Progestational agents have been beneficial in some cases, especially for patients with psychomotor-type seizures.

Table 15–8. PROTOCOL FOR ANTICONVULSANT MEDICATION*

Dogs
Seizures Fewer Than 1 Per Week
Phenobarbital, 1 to 2 mg per kg bid. Reduce dosage after 1 week if sedation is a problem. Increase to point of sedation if seizures are not controlled.

Primidone, 10 to 20 mg per kg tid. Increase or decrease dosage as for phenobarbital.

If seizures are not controlled with primidone, give phenytoin, 30 to 50 mg per kg tid. Increase dosage if seizures are not controlled. Check blood levels if possible, adjusting the dosage to provide 10 μg per ml.

If seizures are not controlled, try combinations of the above or consider the use of drugs that have not been approved (with the owner's consent), i.e., sodium valproate, 15 to 100 mg per kg tid or paramethadione, 30 to 50 mg per kg divided tid.
Seizures More Than 1 Per Week
Phenobarbital, 2 mg per kg bid or primidone, 10 to 20 mg per kg tid. Proceed as above.
Cats
Phenobarbital as above.

Diazepam, 0.5 to 1 mg per kg bid or tid. (May be combined with phenobarbital.)
Horses and Food Animals
Phenobarbital as above.

Phenytoin, 20 mg per kg bid, for horses only (not approved or tested).

*Modified from Oliver, J. E., Jr.: Disorders in companion animals. Comp. Cont. Ed. Small Anim. Pract. 2:77–86, 1980.

Table 15-9. PROTOCOL FOR TREATMENT OF
STATUS EPILEPTICUS*

1. Stop the seizure. Administer diazepam, 10 to 50 mg
   in 10 mg boluses, intravenously. Diazepam usually
   gives at least temporary remission, allowing time for
   succeeding steps. If not, administer phenobarbital
   sodium (10 mg per kg, intravenously). If neither is effective, administer sodium pentobarbital to effect (estimated dosage 10 to 15 mg per kg). Pentobarbital
   must be given cautiously, because diazepam and
   phenobarbital may potentiate its effect. Ultrashort
   barbiturates should not be used, because they may
   potentiate seizure activity.
2. When the seizures have stopped, assure ventilation
   of the patient. An endotracheal tube should be
   placed if the patient is unconscious.
3. Place an intravenous catheter, draw blood for hematology and chemistry analyses, and start a drip with
   lactated Ringer's solution. Measure blood glucose
   levels as soon as possible.
4. Give 50 per cent dextrose intravenously (2 to 3 ml for
   toy breeds, 50 ml for giant breeds). If the seizures are
   not violent or if there are interictal quiet periods,
   you may perform steps 3 and 4 first. Hypoglycemia is
   the one cause of status that can be treated directly.
5. If you suspect hypocalcemia, give an intravenous calcium preparation. Monitor the heart rate.
6. Once the seizures are under control, evaluate the animal to try to determine the cause of the fits. If a
   cause can be found (e.g., toxicity), it should be
   treated specifically.
7. Monitor the body temperature. If it reaches 105 degrees F, cool the animal with ice to a temperature of
   103 degrees F. Maintain the temperature in a normal
   range.
8. Continue to control the seizures. Intravenous or intramuscular phenobarbital should be given until oral
   medication can be used.

*Modified from Oliver, J. E., Jr.: Seizure disorders in
companion animals. Comp. Cont. Ed. Small Anim. Pract.
2:77–86, 1980.

A protocol for the treatment of seizures is
outlined in Table 15–8.

Status epilepticus is the condition of rapidly
recurring convulsions without complete recovery between seizures.[37] This is a serious
emergency that can result in death of the patient. Causes of status epilepticus include (1)
toxicities or metabolic abnormalities, (2) withdrawal of anticonvulsant medication, (3) ineffective anticonvulsant medication, and (4)
progressive brain disease. A protocol for the
treatment of status epilepticus is presented in
Table 15–9.

NARCOLEPSY

Narcolepsy is a disorder of the brain characterized by recurring sudden attacks of
sleep.[40] Cataplexy (loss of muscle tone) commonly accompanies the attacks. Two other
components that have been described in human beings—sleep paralysis and hallucinations—are difficult to verify in animals because of the subjective nature of the
conditions.[41]

Dogs with narcolepsy typically have episodes in which they suddenly fall asleep, often
while excited or during emotional stimulation. Eating is the most common precipitating
factor in reported cases. The dog will start to
eat and suddenly will fall to the ground asleep.
Noise, shaking, or other stimuli will arouse the
animal, and it often will resume eating, only
to fall again. Continual stimulation, such as
petting or shaking, may prevent the attack. The
episodes often are repeated many times a
day.[40,42–45] Narcolepsy also has been reported
in ponies.[45]

Normal sleep is characterized on the EEG by
a change from low-voltage, fast-wave activity
in the animal that is awake to high-voltage,
slow-wave activity in the animal that is asleep.
Rapid eye movement (REM) sleep develops
after approximately 90 minutes of slow-wave
sleep and may recur intermittently thereafter.
REM sleep is associated with dreaming and is
characterized by eye movements, occasional
facial movements, and desynchronized low-
voltage, fast-wave activity of the EEG.[46]

The sleep attacks of narcolepsy are the same
as REM sleep with no intervening slow-wave
sleep. Partial attacks and cataplectic episodes
may occur without EEG changes.[42,45]

The etiology of narcolepsy is not known. The
disorder has been seen in human beings following CNS infection or trauma, but most
cases are idiopathic.[41] A biochemical basis is
presumed. The reticular activating system of
the rostral brain stem presumably is associated with sleep and the more caudal portions
of the reticular formation in the pons with
cataplexy. Alterations in the balance between
adrenergic and cholinergic systems in the brain
may be the basic pathophysiologic mechanism in narcolepsy.

A genetic basis for narcolepsy in some
breeds is suspected. An autosomal recessive
inheritance is hypothesized in Doberman
pinschers.[45]

A diagnosis usually can be made by observation of the characteristic signs if cataplexy is
a prominent part of the syndrome. In the absence of cataplexy, the problem probably will
not be recognized by the owner. The EEG is
the only available diagnostic test. Sleep begin-

ning with REM sleep is characteristic. Polygraphic recording of electromyography (EMG), eye movements, and EEG simultaneously for extended periods is the most definitive test.[42,45]

The treatment is partially effective. Stimulants such as dextroamphetamine (5 to 10 mg tid) and methylphenidate (Ritalin—5 to 10 mg bid or tid) have stopped the sleep attacks but have produced undesirable behavioral changes in some cases.[40,41,45] An antidepressant (imipramine) at a dosage of 0.2 to 0.8 mg per kg bid or tid is more effective in preventing cataplexy.[45] A combination of methylphenidate and imipramine is recommended to control sleep attacks and cataplexy. Combining amphetamines and imipramine is potentially dangerous, because amphetamines cause a release of catacholamines and imipramine blocks their reuptake. Hypertensive episodes can result. Recently, gammahydroxybutyrate taken at bedtime has been reported to be effective in human beings.[47] Reports of its use in dogs are not available.

A balanced regimen of therapy must be developed individually in order for a relatively normal sleep-wakefulness cycle to be attained.

CASE HISTORIES

Seizures are a common neurologic problem in dogs. Most patients with seizures do not have other neurologic deficits. The following case histories demonstrate the approach to management. Localizing signs of brain disease are not present in these cases, because they are discussed in other chapters. After reading the history and the preliminary laboratory data, develop a plan for further diagnosis or treatment of each case. Then read our assessment.

Case History 15A

Signalment

Canine, miniature poodle, male, 18 months old.

History

The dog has received all vaccinations on schedule and has had no major medical problems. The first seizure occurred 2 months ago. The second seizure was observed last night at approximately 6:00 p.m.

The owner describes the seizure as follows: The dog seemed somewhat apprehensive for approximately 30 minutes, seeking attention from the owner. Suddenly, he fell down, extended all four limbs, and arched the head and the neck. After approximately 30 seconds, he started making running movements of the limbs with some chewing movements of the mouth. There was some salivation, and the dog urinated. The owner tried to hold and rub the dog, and the movements stopped after approximately 1 minute. In about 2 or 3 minutes, the dog was able to get up. He seemed a little disoriented for a few minutes, and then he seemed normal.

Other than during the two seizures, the dog has appeared to be healthy. He is fed a variety of commercial dog foods twice daily. Water consumption and urination are thought to be normal.

Physical and Neurologic Examinations

No abnormalities are found.

Laboratory Examination

The complete blood count (CBC) and the chemistry profile (see Table 15—7) are normal.

Case History 15B

Signalment

Canine, Cairn terrier, male, 6 years old.

History

The dog has had no serious illnesses and has had booster vaccinations annually. Ten weeks ago, the dog had a generalized motor seizure that lasted approximately 5 minutes. The dog seemed blind and confused for approximately 4 hours afterward. Two weeks ago, the dog had a second seizure. Since that time, he has not acted "right." His appetite is diminished, he does not play in the way that he did, and he has urinated and defecated in the house several times, which he had not done for years. Last night, he had another seizure that lasted over 5 minutes. Today he is very depressed.

Physical Examination

No abnormalities are found other than depression.

Neurologic Examination

The dog can be coaxed to walk, but he prefers to lie down. The gait is good, with a suggestion of slight symmetric dysmetria. The limbs seem to be lifted a bit high and to be put down with increased force. There is no ataxia, however. The postural reactions also seem slightly dysmetric. The spinal reflexes are normal, as are the cranial nerves, although the menace reaction seems a little sluggish. This response is considered within normal limits when the depression is taken into account.

Case History 15C

Signalment

Canine, German shepherd, female, 4 years old.

History

All vaccinations, including annual boosters, have been given. There have been no major illnesses. Generalized motor seizures started 18 months ago. The first few were 2 to 3 months apart, but recently they have been 2 to 3 weeks apart. Several recent seizures were prolonged (approaching status epilepticus) and were controlled with general anesthesia. Several anticonvulsants, including phenobarbital, phenytoin, and primidone, in dosages that appear to be adequate, have been used in the last year with no apparent control of the fits. The seizures have occurred at various times of day, including at night, when the dog is asleep. Laboratory evaluations performed on several occasions by the referring veterinarian have not revealed any abnormalities. The owner feels that neither he nor the dog can continue to tolerate these seizures.

Physical and Neurologic Examinations

No abnormalities are found.

Laboratory Examination

No abnormalities are found.

Case History 15D

Signalment

Feline, domestic short hair, female, 14 months old.

History

The cat took up residence at the owner's home 6 months ago. She was vaccinated for the usual feline diseases, including rabies, at that time. She has not been ill except for seizures, which started 6 weeks ago. The first seizure, which occurred in the evening, was described as a brief period during which the cat suddenly looked "glassy-eyed," stiffened all four limbs, and arched the neck. The seizure lasted less than a minute. The second and third fits were similar and were approximately 1 week apart. In the last 3 weeks, the cat has had at least two seizures per week. The last two were generalized motor seizures. The most recent fit was described as starting like the first seizure. The cat then twisted to the right, urinated, and began paddling, first with the right limb and then with all four limbs. The seizure lasted approximately 2 minutes, and the cat acted dazed and depressed for approximately 2 hours.

Physical Examination

No abnormalities are found.

Neurologic Examination

The only abnormality is a slight anisocoria, with the left pupil slightly smaller than the right. Both pupils are reactive to light, although the right seems slightly slower to react than the left. The iris and the fundus appear normal.

Case History 15E

Signalment

Canine, dachshund, male, 6 months old.

History

The dog suddenly developed lethargy and a staggering gait. The owners believe that the onset of signs occurred shortly after he was seen eating some unknown substance in the front yard. An observation of the dog for several days results in the following pattern of behavior: The dog suddenly collapses to the ground while walking. He appears to be asleep for a few seconds and then awakens, gets up, and behaves normally. While eating, the dog collapses with food in his mouth, wakes up in less than a minute, and continues eating. This pattern might be repeated every 2 to 3 minutes during a meal. The dog can be aroused from sleep easily by noise or touch. No other abnormalities are observed. The dog had not been ill previously and has had all vaccinations.

Physical and Neurologic Examinations

Other than the behavior just described, no abnormalities are found.

Laboratory Examination

All tests, including an electrocardiogram, are normal.

ASSESSMENT 15A

The seizures are generalized tonic-clonic (grand mal, major motor—see Table 15–1). To the owner's knowledge, they have occurred twice. The seizures are single and are of short duration. There is no history of illnesses or injuries, and the physical, neurologic, and laboratory examinations are normal. Although a genetic basis for epilepsy has not been demonstrated in miniature poodles, it is suspected because of the relatively frequent occurrence of seizures in this breed without specific etiologic diagnosis.

There is nothing in the data base to justify further diagnostic tests at this time. We would recommend prophylactic medication in order to determine if the seizures can be prevented. If the owner feels that giving medication is a serious problem, we would suggest observing the animal closely for further seizures and then starting medication if another fit occurs. The owner should be warned that the dog probably will have more seizures and that medication is the preferred alternative. The choice of medication is not critical, but we would try phenobarbital first.

ASSESSMENT 15B

A 6-year-old dog with a sudden onset of seizures probably has an acquired brain problem. The disorder appears to be progressive. The depression suggests brain abnormalities, which may be primary or secondary to metabolic or toxic abnormalities. Dysmetria, especially when it is subtle and occurs in a terrier, may or may not be significant. It could indicate a diffuse abnormality with cerebellar involvement. A laboratory profile is indicated.

Laboratory examination:

CBC

Packed cell volume	37%
Hemoglobin	14.5 gm/dl
White blood cells (WBCs)	10,950
Neutrophils	7,400
Lymphocytes	2,400
Monocytes	450
Eosinophils	700
Nucleated RBCs	3/high power field
Some polychromasia	
Serum plasma protein	6.5 gm/dl
Albumin	3.3 gm/dl
Serum urea nitrogen	14 mg/dl
Alkaline phosphatase	80 IU/l
SGPT	30 IU/l
Calcium	9.9 mg/dl
Glucose	95 mg/dl
Urinalysis	Normal

There is no evidence of systemic infectious disease (normal WBCs and differential). Severe liver disease is unlikely (normal SGPT and alkaline phosphatase, serum albumin, serum urea nitrogen levels). Calcium and glucose levels are normal. The only unusual findings are nucleated red blood cells and polychromasia with a normal packed cell volume and hematocrit (no anemia). This finding is suggestive of lead poisoning. A sample of whole blood was submitted, and 65 μg of lead per 100 ml was reported. These results are diagnostic of lead poisoning. Chelation therapy with calcium EDTA was successful. The source of the lead was not found for several weeks, until the owners discovered a thoroughly chewed bowling trophy under a bed.

ASSESSMENT 15C

The history is typical of a form of epilepsy, presumably genetic, that is seen in German shepherd dogs and a few other large breeds (Table 15−6). The seizures begin in early adult life and are severe. They often are multiple and are refractory to anticonvulsant therapy. It would be worthwhile to perform EEG and CSF analysis in order to rule out inflammatory disease, but the results of these tests probably will be normal. An EEG may reveal some nonspecific abnormality, such as diffuse spike discharge. Other than trying increasing doses of anticonvulsants or one of the newer drugs, there is little that the clinician can do. Our experience has been almost uniformly negative.

ASSESSMENT 15D

Seizures in cats usually are caused by organic disease. Unfortunately, most of the causes are diseases with a poor prognosis. The progression from a partial motor seizure to generalized seizures also suggests primary brain disease. Anisocoria frequently is seen in cats that have had positive tests for feline leukemia virus (FeLV).[48] The signs also may be associated with feline infectious peritonitis (FIP—usually the "dry" form). Meningiomas also may cause seizures without other signs in the early stages. The age of the cat is more suggestive of the viral diseases than of neoplasia.

Localization: cerebral or diencephalic; rule-outs: (1) FIP, (2) FeLV, and (3) meningioma.

Plan:

Laboratory examination, titers for FeLV and FIP, CSF analysis, EEG. The significant findings are:

WBCs: 16,800

      6,700 segmented neutrophils

      2,500 bands

      6,000 lymphocytes

      800 eosinophils

Serum protein 9.0 gm/dl

(albumin 3.0, globulin 6.0)

CSF: protein—110 mg/dl

      Cells—total—240/cu mm

          neutrophils—130

          lymphocytes—110

EEG: generalized high-voltage slow waves with spikes randomly superimposed

FeLV: positive

FIP titer: positive at 1:1600

All of the findings are characteristic of FIP. If costs are a factor, the laboratory examination (serum protein) and FeLV and FIP tests are adequate for diagnosis. Treatment of the CNS form of FIP has been uniformly unsuccessful. Many of these cats will have either uveitis or retinal lesions, or both, and a strong presumptive diagnosis can be made on the clinical examination alone.

ASSESSMENT 15E

The behavior of this dog is typical of narcolepsy-cataplexy. The EEG is useful for documenting the changes. Clinical management requires long-term therapy, because the disease is not reversible. A brief trial with therapy at home was unsatisfactory for this client, and euthanasia was performed.

REFERENCES

1. Kay, W. J., and Fenner, W. R.: Epilepsy. *In* Kirk, R. W.: Current Veterinary Therapy VI. Philadelphia, W. B. Saunders Co., 1977.
2. Prince, D. A.: Neurophysiology of epilepsy. Annu. Rev. Neurosci. 1:395–415, 1978.
3. Lennox, W. G.: Epilepsy and Related Disorders. Boston, Little, Brown & Co., 1960.
4. Oliver, J. E., Jr.: Seizure disorders in companion animals. Comp. Cont. Ed. Small Anim. Pract. 2:77–86, 1980.
5. Gastaut, H.: Clinical and electroencephalographical classification of epileptic seizures. Suppl. Epilepsia 10:512–513, 1969.
6. Holliday, T. A.: Seizure disorders. Vet. Clin. North Am. 10:3–29, 1980.
7. Hoerlein, B. F.: Canine Neurology, 3rd ed. Philadelphia, W. B. Saunders Co., 1978.

8. Breitschwerdt, E. B., Breazile, J. E., and Broadhurst, J. J.: Clinical and electroencephalographic findings associated with ten cases of suspected limbic epilepsy in the dog. JAAHA 15:37–50, 1979.

9. Falco, M. J., Barker, J., and Wallace, M. E.: The genetics of epilepsy in the British Alsatian. J. Small Anim. Pract. 15:685–692, 1974.

10. Robb, P.: Epilepsy: A review of basic and clinical research. NINDB Monograph No. 1, DHEW Pub. No. (NIH) 73–415. Washington, D.C., Department of Health, Education and Welfare, 1965.

11. Van der Velden, N. A.: Fits in Tervueren shepherd dogs: A presumed hereditary trait. J. Small Anim. Pract. 9:63–70, 1968.

12. Biefelt, S. W., Redman, H. C., and McClellan, R. O.: Sire and sex-related differences in rates of epileptiform seizures in a purebred beagle dog colony. Am. J. Vet. Res. 32:2039–2048, 1971.

13. Croft, P. G.: Fits in dogs: A survey of 260 cases. Vet. Rec. 77:438–445, 1965.

14. Redman, H. C., and Weir, J. E.: Detection of naturally occurring neurologic disorders of beagle dogs by electroencephalography. Am. J. Vet. Res. 30:2075–2082, 1969.

15. Weiderholt, W. C.: Electrophysiologic analysis of epileptic beagles. Neurology 24:149–155, 1974.

16. Chrisman, C. L.: Epilepsy and seizures. *In* Howard, J. L.: Current Veterinary Therapy: Food Animal Practice. Philadelphia, W. B. Saunders Co., 1981.

17. Barlow, R. M.: Morphogenesis of cerebellar lesions in bovine familial convulsions and ataxia. Vet. Pathol. 18:151–162, 1981.

18. Oliver, J. E., Jr., and Hoerlein, B. F.: Convulsive disorders of dogs. JAVMA 146:1126–1133, 1965.

19. Oliver, J. E., Jr.: Protocol for the diagnosis of seizure disorders in companion animals. JAVMA 172:822–824, 1978.

20. Cunningham, J. G.: Canine seizure disorders. JAVMA 158:589–597, 1971.

21. Eberhart, G. W.: Epilepsy in the dog. Gaines Symposium 18–20, 1959.

22. Redding, R. W.: The diagnosis and therapy of seizures. JAAHA 5:79–92, 1969.

23. Holliday, T. A., Cunningham, J. G., and Gutnick, M. J.: Comparative clinical and electroencephalographic studies of canine epilepsy. Epilepsia 11:281–292, 1971.

24. Greene, C. E., Vandevelde, M., and Braund, K.: Lissencephaly in two Lhasa Apso dogs. JAVMA 169:405–410, 1976.

25. Oliver, J. E., Jr., and Knecht, C. D.: Diseases of the brain. *In* Ettinger, S. J.: Textbook of Veterinary Internal Medicine. Philadelphia, W. B. Saunders Co., 1975.

26. Caywood, D. D., and Wilson, J. W.: Functional pancreatic islet cell adenocarcinoma in the dog. *In* Kirk, R. W.: Current Veterinary Therapy VI. Philadelphia, W. B. Saunders Co., 1977.

27. Fenner, W. R.: Seizures and head trauma. Vet. Clin. North Am. 11:31–48, 1981.

28. Berman, P. H.: Management of seizure disorders with anticonvulsant drugs: Current concepts. Pediatr. Clin. North Am. 23:443–459, 1975.

29. Kutt, H.: Interactions of antiepileptic drugs. Epilepsia 16:393–402, 1976.

30. Yeary, R. A.: Serum concentrations of primidone and its metabolites, phenylethyemalonamide and phenobarbital, in the dog. Am. J. Vet. Res. 141:1643–1645, 1980.

31. Sanders, J. E., and Yeary, R. A.: Serum concentrations of orally administered diphenylhydantoin in dogs. JAVMA 172:153–156, 1978.

32. Sanders, J. E., Yeary, R. A., Powers, J. D., and deWet, P.: Relationship between serum and brain concentrations of phenytoin in the dog. Am. J. Vet. Res. 40:473–476, 1979.

33. Pasten, T. J.: Diphenylhydantoin in the canine: Clinical aspects and determinations of therapeutic blood levels. JAAHA 13:247–254, 1977.

34. Parker, A. J.: A preliminary report on a new antiepileptic medication for dogs. JAAHA 11:437–438, 1975.

35. Troupin, A., Ojemann, L. M., Halpern, L., Dodrill, C., Wilkus, R., Friel, P., and Feigl, P.: Carbamazepine: A double-blind comparison with phenytoin. Neurology 27:511–519, 1977.

36. Nafe, L. A., Parker, A., and Kay, W. J.: Sodium valproate: A preliminary clinical trial in epileptic dogs. JAAHA 17:131–133, 1981.

37. Duffy, F. H., and Lombroso, C. T.: Treatment of status epilepticus. *In* Klawans, H. L.: Clinical Neuropharmacology, Vol. 3. New York, Raven Press, 1978.

38. Koestner, A., and Rehfeld, C. E.: Idiopathic epilepsy in a beagle colony. Argonne Natl. Lab., Biol. and Med. Res. Div. Annu. Report 178–179, 1968.

39. Wallace, M. E.: Keeshonds: A genetic study of epilepsy and EEG readings. J. Small Anim. Pract. 16:1–10, 1975.

40. Knecht, C. D., Oliver, J. E., Redding, R., Selcer, R., and Johnson, G.: Narcolepsy in a dog and a cat. JAVMA 162:1052–1053, 1973.

41. Zarcone, V.: Narcolepsy. N. Engl. J. Med. 288:1156–1166, 1973.

42. Mitler, M. M., Soave, O., and Dement, W. C.: Narcolepsy in seven dogs. JAVMA 168:1036–1038, 1976.

43. Blauch, B. S., and Cash, W. C.: A brief review of narcolepsy with presentation of two cases in dogs. JAAHA 11:467–472, 1975.

44. Katherman, A. E.: A comparative review of canine and human narcolepsy. Comp. Cont. Ed. Pact. Vet. 2:818–822, 1980.

45. Foutz, A. S., Mitler, M. M., and Dement, W. C.: Narcolepsy. Vet. Clin. North Amer. 10:65–80, 1980.

46. Wauquier, A., Verheyen, J. L., Van Den Broeck, W. A. E., and Janssen, P. A. J.: Visual and computer-based analysis of 24 h sleep-waking patterns in the dog. Electroencephalogr. Clin. Neurophysiol. 46:33–48, 1979.

47. Broughton, R., and Mamelak, M.: The treatment of narcolepsy-cataplexy with nocturnal gamma-hydroxybutyrate. J. Can. Sci. Neurol. 6:1–6, 1979.

48. Scagliotti, R. H.: Neuro-ophthalmology. *In* Kirk, R. W.: Current Veterinary Therapy VII. Philadelphia, W. B. Saunders Co., 1980.

Abnormal behavior in domestic animals as a clinical problem has received increasing attention in recent years. Several books and numerous journal articles that deal with specific problems and techniques or modifying behavior are available.[1-9] The primary objective of this chapter is to differentiate organic brain disease that causes abnormalities from behavior that is inherited or learned.

NORMAL BEHAVIOR

The term *behavior* encompasses anything that an animal (or a person) does. The more common forms of behavior with their abnormal modifications are listed in Table 16–1.

Behavior that is typical of a species has been produced by genetic selection. Domestic animals have been selected for their traits that are compatible with human beings. Species-typical behavior is modified by early experience (especially during the critical period of socialization) and by learning throughout life.

The time during which early experience has the greatest influence on later activity has been called the critical period of socialization.[10] For the dog and the cat, this stage begins at approximately 3 weeks of age and lasts until 10 to 14 weeks of age. The peak period for socialization of dogs and cats is when they are between 5 and 8 weeks old. If the dog or the cat is deprived of human contact during this interval, it is likely that the animal never will be properly socialized. Similarly, if it has no contact with other animals during this stage, it is unlikely to have normal relationships with them in later life. Therapy may modify the responses to some extent, but the animal always will exhibit avoidance behavior. Therefore, it is important that dogs and cats receive both human and animal contact when they are between 5 and 8 weeks of age.[11]

ABNORMAL BEHAVIOR

Anatomic Diagnosis: Localization

ANATOMY OF BEHAVIOR

If behavior is defined as anything that an animal does, then it is affected by virtually all of the nervous system. The structures of the brain that are considered to be most important in the organization and control of behavior are collectively called the *limbic system*. The limbic system includes most of the structures of the rhinencephalon (olfactory brain) that are not primarily involved in olfaction.[12] These structures form two rings around the diencephalon

16

CHAPTER

ABNORMAL BEHAVIOR

with connections to nuclear groups in the rostral brain stem, the diencephalon, and the cerebral cortex. The key structures involved in organic brain disease that causes behavioral disorders are the hypothalamus, the hippocampus, the amygdaloid body, and the cingulate and septal areas of the cerebral cortex (see Fig. 3–3).

NEUROLOGIC SIGNS AND BEHAVIOR

Very small lesions in some portions of the limbic system can have profound effects on behavior. Localization of a lesion based on alterations in conduct is nearly impossible, however, because the same change may be produced by lesions in more than one location. Other signs of neurologic deficit must be used in order to localize the lesion precisely (Table 16–2).

SEIZURES

Seizures are common in animals with behavioral disorders caused by organic brain

Table 16–1. BEHAVIOR: NORMAL AND ABNORMAL

Normal	Abnormal
Ingestive	Pica, polydipsia, guarding food
Eliminative	Marking, spraying, urinating, or defecating in the house
Sexual	Hypersexuality, failure to breed
Care-giving (maternal)	Maternal aggressions
Care-soliciting	Submissiveness
Agnostic	Aggression, submissiveness
Group-activity	Poor animal socialization, destructive activity
Shelter-seeking	Guarding nest, hyperactivity
Care of body	Chewing tail or paw

Table 16–2. SIGNS ASSOCIATED WITH LESIONS OF LIMBIC SYSTEM STRUCTURES

Hypothalamus: Endocrine and autonomic disorders (diabetes insipidus; disorders of eating, drinking, and temperature control; Cushing's syndrome). Visual and oculomotor deficits.
Thalamus: Sensory or motor deficits (postural reaction deficits with a relatively normal gait).
Hippocampus and amygdaloid body: Seizures (psychomotor type).
Cerebral cortex, septal area: Pacing, circling.

disease. The hippocampus and the amygdaloid area are especially prone to the generation of seizures. The seizure is frequently of the psychomotor type, having a behavioral component with or without generalization to a tonic-clonic convulsion (see Chapter 15). Seizures must be ruled out in all cases of behavior disorders. If a seizure does not generalize, the behavior change may not appear to be a convulsion, although it will have some components of a fit, which should provide a clue. Seizures have one or more of the following characteristics: pre- or postictal alterations are present, the convulsions are episodic, the animal appears relatively normal between fits and has a lack of awareness during a seizure, there is a lack of purposiveness in the behavior, the activity is stereotyped, and the animal is responsive to anticonvulsant drugs.

Examples of psychomotor seizures include running fits (which cannot be stopped with distraction), aggressive behavior that is not related to any particular stimulus (in which the animal does not seem to know what it is doing), "fly-biting" (from which the animal cannot be distracted), and episodic autonomic signs (such as gastrointestinal disturbances with no evidence of digestive tract disease). Some psychomotor seizures may be triggered by a particular stimulus. We (and others) have seen dogs that developed a stereotyped reaction to feeding that consisted of stalking and attacking the food pan. Some dogs attack themselves, chasing their tails or biting at a spot on one of their legs. Narcolepsy-cataplexy also may be triggered by feeding (see Chapter 15). The episodic and stereotyped nature of the behavior is the key to the recognition of psychomotor seizures.

Etiologic Diagnosis: Rule-outs

DIAGNOSTIC PLAN

The approach for solving a behavioral problem is essentially the same as that for any neu-rologic disorder. The first objective is to rule out systemic disease and organic brain disease (Fig. 16–1). The history, the physical examination, and the laboratory analyses that are recommended for inclusion in the minimum data base for neurologic problems (see Chapter 4) help to rule out systemic disease. These data, plus the results of the neurologic examination, are used in the identification of animals with primary brain disease, although the alterations in behavior may be the only sign in some animals with pathophysiologic changes. As is true for many neurologic disorders, the history may be the most important part of the data base. The history is usually the primary source for recognition of seizure disorders. It also must be used in the differentiation among species-typical activity, inadequate socialization, and learned behaviors. The development of a complete history may require considerable time (more than one session). Unless the client and the veterinarian are willing to spend this time, success may be impossible.

CAUSES OF BEHAVIORAL DISORDERS
Systemic Diseases

Organic diseases other than those of the nervous system may cause abnormal behavior. Some of the more common problems are listed in Table 16–3 and are discussed in Chapters 14, 15, and 17.

Organic Diseases of the Nervous System

Any disease affecting the brain can cause a change in behavior. The recognition of primary brain disease is dependent upon the presence of some neurologic deficit other than the behavioral problem or an episodic disorder indicative of seizures (see Table 16–3). Ancillary studies, such as electroencephalography (EEG) and cerebrospinal fluid (CSF) analysis may be useful for ruling out central nervous system (CNS) disease. See the appro-

Table 16–3. SYSTEMIC DISEASES CAUSING BEHAVIORAL PROBLEMS

Renal disease: polyuria, polydipsia, vomiting
Lower urinary tract disease: incontinence, dysuria
Gastrointestinal disease: anorexia, polyphagia, diarrhea, tenesmus, coprophagy
Liver disease: lethargy, stupor, coma, seizures
Endocrine disease: polyuria, polydipsia, sexual disorders
Dermatologic disease: self-mutilation
Cardiovascular disease: syncope

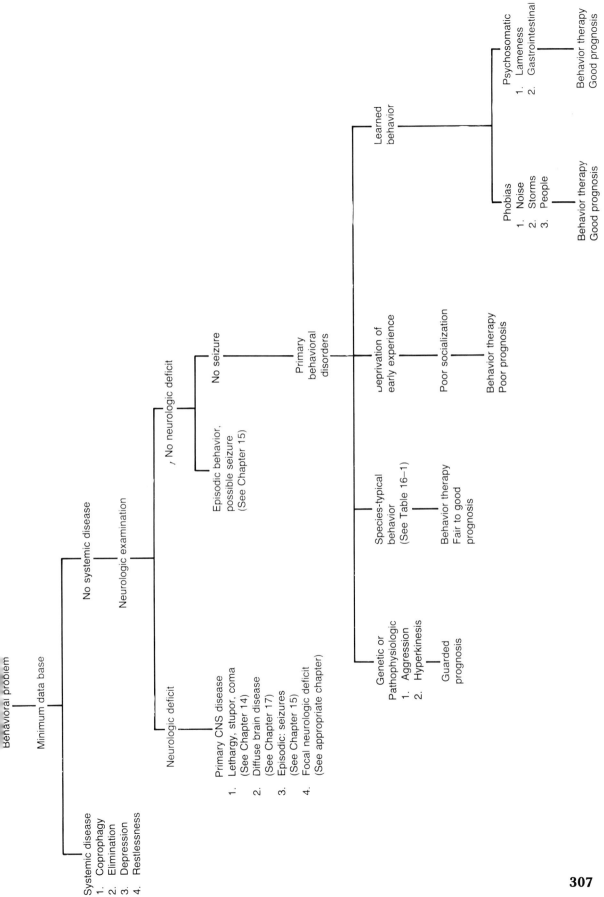

Figure 16-1. Etiologic diagnosis of behavioral disorders.

priate chapter in this text (Chapters 11 through 15 and Chapter 17) for details on the formulation of an etiologic diagnosis if signs of brain disease are present. Many of the diseases causing behavioral problems will be discussed in Chapter 17.

Primary Behavioral Disorders

Behavioral disorders without organic disease may be separated into four major categories (see Fig. 16–1). Overlapping of these classifications is common. For example, aggression and territorial marking are species-typical behavior and are usually abnormal as a result of learned experiences. Some genetic behavioral disorders may have a pathophysiologic basis, but the pathophysiology is not usually manifested other than in the abnormality of the animal's actions.

Genetic transmission of the tendency for unprovoked aggression has been reported in the Bernese mountain dog and in the Saint Bernard. Other breeds may be predisposed to aggressive behavior, especially those that have been bred selectively for guarding and attack purposes. Terriers are more likely to bite than are other breeds.

Neurochemical abnormalities are associated with hyperkinesis and narcolepsy-cataplexy. Research has centered on adrenergic transmitters, although cholinergic mechanisms are important in cataplexy. Additional findings of peptides and opiate-like substances in the nervous system may lead to dramatic changes in the pharmacologic management of behavior disorders.

Species-typical behavior includes all of the normal traits associated with a species. Domestication has modified many of these behaviors in companion and farm animals. An excess or deficit of any normal activity is deemed abnormal. If organic disorders are excluded, most of the inappropriate species-typical traits are learned (see Table 16–1 and Fig. 16–1).

Early experience is important in the development of normal behavior. The most common problem related to early experience is a lack of socialization during the critical period. Animals that are orphaned and deprived of contact with their own species usually do not develop normal interactions in later life. Some breeding problems are rooted in a lack of socialization. More commonly, animals reared without adequate human contact are timid, exhibit submissive urination, and may become fear-biters.

Learned abnormal behavior is common. Learning also reinforces abnormalities that orginate from any of the factors discussed previously. Specific learned behaviors include phobias and psychosomatic disorders. Dogs that are afraid of thunderstorms or other loud noises are encountered frequently. Psychosomatic disorders are less common. Most veterinarians have seen dogs that continue to limp after an orthopedic problem has been resolved. Usually, the patient is a small house pet that has received considerable attention because of the injury. When the dog is hospitalized, the "lameness" disappears. The dog has learned to gain attention from the owner by limping.

Psychosomatic disorders in people encompass a broad range of clinical syndromes, including asthma, vomiting and diarrhea, heart disease, and skin conditions. Psychosomatic disorders can be real medical problems (for example, gastric ulcers and hypertension). We can expect to recognize more of these disorders in animals as our awareness increases.

Treatment of Behavioral Disorders

The treatment of organic diseases that may cause behavioral problems has been discussed in Chapters 11 through 15 and will be considered in Chapter 17. Primary behavior disorders may be treated with psychological techniques, drugs, or surgery. Frequently, a combination of behavioral techniques and drugs is used.

PSYCHOLOGICAL TECHNIQUES

A specific plan for the treatment of abnormal behavior in animals on a clinical basis is in its infancy. Treatment protocols must be carefully developed in order to match the specific problem. It cannot be overemphasized that a specific behavior (for example, aggression) can be caused by a wide variety of abnormalities. Behavioral disorders frequently have more than one component (e.g., in the case of the hyperactive dog that is also destructive and occasionally aggressive).

Behavioral therapy must focus on the cause (stimulus) of the abnormal behavior (response). This approach requires a very careful diagnosis, which should be made primarily on the basis of the history. When dealing with a behavior problem involving a companion animal, the clinician must realize that the animal is part of a social unit. The pet's unnatural behavior is usually a reflection of some abnormal interactions in the family unit. The therapy must involve the family not only in the diagnosis but also in the treatment. Behavioral therapy can be slow and tedious, and the results are not obvious at first. According to Borchelt and Tortora, two rules predict failure.[8] First, the greater the immediate change that is required of the client, the more likely that the treatment will fail. Second, the more complex the procedure, the more likely that it will be misunderstood and that it consequently will fail.[11] Procedures must be simple and must require only small, stepwise changes both in the family and in the animal. Flow charts should be maintained by the client and reviewed periodically by the clinician. These diagrams are valuable for maintaining enthusiasm.[7]

The description of specific behavior techniques is beyond the scope of this book. The serious reader should study several of the references that are listed.[1,3,8]

PHARMACOLOGIC AND SURGICAL THERAPY

Drugs are useful adjuncts to therapy in behavioral disorders but are rarely effective alone. Tranquilizers are the most frequently used complements of treatment. They may be administered to reduce or obliterate the undesired behavior, whereas behavioral techniques are applied to eliminate it permanently. For example, a phobia may be suppressed by tranquilization. The clinician may accomplish desensitization by gradually exposing the animal to increasing stimuli while it is tranquilized. Specific applications are discussed in the references.[1,3,8]

Hyperkinetic dogs may respond to amphetamine therapy. These animals apparently have a genetic disorder in the catecholamine systems of the brain. Learned behavior, lead intoxication, and other environmental causes should be ruled out. The response to therapy is usually dramatic but drug-dependent, and treatment therefore must be continued. A dosage of 0.2 to 1.3 mg per kg of dextroamphetamine administered orally has been recommended.[7]

Hormones also are useful adjuncts to behavior therapy. Alterations in the balance may be achieved by giving a hormone to the animal or by eliminating hormones through neutering. Masculine behavior patterns such as the tendency to roam, aggression against other male animals, urination patterns, and hypersexuality are most readily altered by castration

or the use of progestins. Castration is effective in stopping roaming behavior in over 90 per cent of adult male cats and dogs. The other activities are modified in over half of the animals. Progestins are effective in approximately 50 per cent of the cases.[13] Castration or progestin therapy has less of an effect on other behavioral abnormalities, such as aggression toward human beings.

Redding has described the use of electroconvulsive therapy in the treatment of aggression and other behavioral disorders.[14,15] Controlled studies demonstrating its effectiveness in animals have not been reported. The limited number of cases that have been documented so far indicate that electroconvulsive therapy may be useful.

Prefrontal lobotomy has had varying effects in the treatment of aggression. The resulting alterations in other behaviors may be unacceptable, even if aggression is reduced. Prefrontal lobotomy should be considered a last resort.[16–18]

Olfactory tractotomy was effective in eliminating urine spraying in 6 of 11 male cats and in one female cat. Urine marking was eliminated in one male cat and three female cats (four cases reported). These cats had not responded to neutering or progestin therapy.[19]

CASE HISTORIES

Most of the books listed in the references include numerous case histories. We will limit the cases presented here to those that involve making a decision—is this behavior the result of abnormal brain disease or is it a primary behavioral problem?

Case History 16A

Signalment

Canine, German shepherd, male, 10 months old.

History

For the past 2 months, the owners have observed the following sequence of behavior: The dog sits quietly, looks straight ahead, and then suddenly pricks up his ears, looks quickly to one side, and snaps. The owners best describe this behavior as "fly-catching." The dog seems to bite in the air in all directions. A touch or a command stops the behavior. The periods of abnormal activity have increased from 2 to 3 times daily to 30 to 40 times daily in the 2-month period. The dog has had all vaccinations, has no illnesses, and seems healthy and normal between episodes. He has been obedience-school trained and has shown no aggressive tendencies.

Physical and Neurologic Examinations

No abnormalities are found. The results of funduscopic and otoscopic examinations are normal. During one episode in the examination room, menacing gestures do not elicit a response, although the menace reaction is normal at other times.

Case History 16B

Signalment

Canine, mixed breed hound, female, 10 months old.

History

The dog was obtained from the pound 2 months ago and was given all vaccinations. Until 1 week ago, the dog was normal. At that time, the owners noticed that the dog was less playful and seemed to want to be left alone. The following day, the dog snapped at the owner when he picked up the food dish. Two days later, the dog bit the 6-year-old son when he reached down to pet her. For the past several days, the dog has been very withdrawn and growls when approached.

Physical and Neurologic Examinations

The dog is brought in on a lead and is muzzled prior to the examination. No abnormalities are found. The dog resents all manipulation and growls continuously during the examination.

ASSESSMENT 16A

This syndrome has been observed in a number of dogs by various clinicians. It is presumed to be a form of psychomotor epilepsy. The eyes and the ears have always been normal in the cases that have been observed. Anticonvulsant drugs have been effective in some cases.

ASSESSMENT 16B

Although this dog could have a primary behavioral problem, the history strongly suggests primary brain disease. Since a human being was bitten 4 days ago, rabies must be considered. The owners were advised to consult their physician. The alternatives of confinement with observation or immediate euthanasia with examination of the brain were presented. They elected to leave the dog in the hospital until they talked to their physician. That afternoon, the dog had a generalized seizure. When the owners were informed of the fit, they requested euthanasia. The brain analysis was negative for rabies, but numerous inclusions characteristic of distemper virus were found. The rapid progression of the syndrome is the clue that organic brain disease probably was present. Rabies must be considered as a possible diagnosis until the presence of another disease is proved, especially in a dog with a questionable history of vaccinations.

REFERENCES

1. Voith, V. L., and Hart, B. L.: Behavioral disorders. *In* Hoerlin, B. F.: Canine Neurology: Diagnosis and Treatment, 3rd ed. Philadelphia, W. B. Saunders Co., 1978.
2. Fox, M. W.: Abnormal Behavior in Animals. Philadelphia, W. B. Saunders Co., 1968.
3. Tortora, D. F.: Help! This Animal Is Driving Me Crazy. Chicago, Playboy Press, 1977.
4. Campbell, W. E.: Behavior Problems in Dogs. Santa Barbara, CA, American Veterinary Publications, 1975.
5. Hart, B. F.: Feline Behavior. Santa Barbara, CA, Veterinary Practice Pub. Co., 1978.
6. Beaver, B.: Veterinary Aspects of Feline Behavior. St. Louis, C. V. Mosby Co., 1980.
7. Voith, V. L.: Applied Animal Behavior for the Veterinary Practitioner. Proceedings of Scientific Presentations. Amer. Anim. Hosp. Assoc. 15–38, 1980.
8. Borchelt, P. L., and Tortora, D. F.: Animal Behavior Therapy: The Diagnosis and Treatment of Pet Behavior Problems. Proceedings of Scientific Presentations. Amer. Anim. Hosp. Assoc. 3–11, 1979.
9. Houpt, K. A.: Animal behavior as a subject for veterinary students. Cornell Vet. 66:73–81, 1976.
10. Fox, M. W.: Neuro-behavioral Ontogeny. A synthesis of ethological and neurophysiological concepts. Brain Res. 2:3–20, 1966.
11. Fox, M. W.: Psychosocial and clinical applications of the critical period hypothesis in the dog. JAVMA 146:1117–1119, 1965.
12. deLahunta, A.: Veterinary Neuroanatomy and Clinical Neurology. Philadelphia, W. B. Saunders Co., 1977.
13. Hart, B. L.: Problems with objectionable sociosexual behavior of dogs and cats: Therapeutic use of castration and progestins. J. Comp. Cont. Ed. 1:461–465, 1979.
14. Redding, R. W.: Electroconvulsive therapy. *In* Hoerlein, B. F.: Canine Neurology: Diagnosis and Treatment, 3rd ed. Philadelphia, W. B. Saunders Co., 1978.
15. Redding, R. W.: Electroconvulsive therapy to control aggression in dogs. Mod. Vet. Pract. 57:595–597, 1976.
16. Hoerlein, B. F., and Oliver, J. E., Jr.: Brain surgery. *In* Hoerlein, B. F.: Canine Neurology, Diagnosis and Treatment, 3rd ed. Philadelphia, W. B. Saunders Co., 1978.
17. Allen, B. D., Cummings, J. F., and deLahunta, A.: The effects of prefrontal lobotomy on aggressive behavior in dogs. Cornell Vet. 64:201–216, 1974.
18. Houpt, K. A.: Aggression in dogs. J. Comp. Cont. Ed. 1:1–123–128, 1979.
19. Hart, B. L.: Olfactory tractotomy for control of objectionable urine spraying and urine marking in cats. JAVMA 179:231–234, 1981.

The first step in the management of a neurologic problem is localization of the disease process to a single anatomic site. Localization has been emphasized throughout this book; however, a group of diseases that produce more than one lesion or that affect most of the central nervous system (CNS) simultaneously has not yet been discussed. These disorders are categorized as multifocal, systemic, or diffuse diseases. Some of them initially may appear as focal diseases but progress to affect other structures.

ANATOMIC DIAGNOSIS: LOCALIZATION

The key to the recognition of these diseases is a neurologic examination that indicates the involvement of two or more parts of the nervous system that are not anatomically closely related. The most obvious example is an abnormality in both the brain and the spinal cord. All of the possible combinations of signs of diffuse or multifocal diseases are too extensive to list, but Table 17–1 outlines some of the more common ones. Any time that the neurologic examination does not strongly indicate a single lesion, this group of diseases becomes more likely.

ETIOLOGIC DIAGNOSIS: RULE-OUTS

The major disease categories producing systemic or multifocal signs are degenerative, metabolic, neoplastic, nutritional, inflammatory, and toxic disorders. Some of these diseases may be chiefly focal in the individual animal, such as primary CNS neoplasms, but

17

CHAPTER

SYSTEMIC OR MULTIFOCAL SIGNS

they are capable of affecting any part of the nervous system and therefore are included in this section. Diseases that are primarily skeletal in origin will be mentioned but not discussed. All of these diseases are progressive. The acute or chronic onset and the rate of progression may be of some help in establishing the diagnosis (Table 17–2).

Degenerative Diseases

Primary degenerative diseases of the CNS have been reported with increasing frequency in the past 5 to 10 years, because interest in clinical neurology has increased and pathologic evaluation has improved.

Table 17–1. EXAMPLES OF SYSTEMIC OR MULTIFOCAL SIGNS

LMN signs: more than one location, may include cranial nerves, e.g., diffuse LMN diseases, polyneuropathy (see Chapter 10)
Brain and spinal cord signs: e.g., pelvic limb paresis and seizures
Systemic disease and CNS signs: e.g., fever, anorexia, and ataxia or seizures
Generalized pain: e.g., meningitis
Cerebral cortex and brain stem: e.g., seizures and cranial nerve deficits, blindness, severe gait deficits
Bilateral cerebral cortex: e.g., blindness with normal pupils (may be seen with brain swelling, hydrocephalus, and so forth—see Chapter 14)
Cerebellum and paresis: e.g., head tremor, ataxia, and severe gait deficits and paresis
Ascending paralysis: e.g., pelvic limb paresis progressing to tetraparesis (focal cervical spinal cord must be ruled out)

Table 17–2. ETIOLOGY OF SYSTEMIC DISEASES*

	Acute Progressive	Chronic Progressive
Degenerative		*Storage disease* *Abiotrophy*
Metabolic	*Hepatic encephalopathy* Hypoglycemia Endocrine disease Renal disease	*Hepatic encephalopathy* Endocrine disease
Neoplastic	Metastatic	*Primary* Metastatic
Nutritional		Hypovitaminosis Hypervitaminosis
Inflammatory	*Infectious*	Infection—usually viral
Toxic	Most toxins	*Heavy metals* Hexachlorophene

*Italics indicate most common diseases clinically.

Three groups of diseases will be discussed: (1) storage diseases, (2) abiotrophies, and (3) degenerations of unknown cause. Primary vascular disease has been discussed in Chapter 9 (spinal cord) and Chapter 14 (brain).

STORAGE DISEASES

A large group of diseases are characterized pathologically by the accumulation of metabolic products in cells (Table 17–3). A geneti-cally based deficiency of an enzyme causes an accumulation of the product in neurons, glia, or other cells. The effect of the disease may be caused by the accumulation of the product or may be a direct result of the metabolic distur-bance.[1] The clinical signs and the progression of the disease are dependent on the pathologic process, so many of the conditions are similar. All of the disorders are slowly progressive and lead to the death of the animal. There is no

Table 17–3. STORAGE DISEASES[1,4,28–30]

Storage Product	Disease (Human Eponym)*	Breed/Species
Lipids	**Lipidoses**	
Gangliosides	Gangliosidoses	
GM$_1$	Generalized gangliosidosis Type 1 (Norman-Landing disease)	Beagle dogs,† domestic cats,† Friesian cattle†
	Juvenile GM$_1$ gangliosidosis Type 2 (Derry's disease)	Siamese,† Korat, domestic cats†
GM$_2$	GM$_2$ gangliosidosis Type 1 (Tay-Sachs disease)	German short-haired pointer dogs†
	GM$_2$ gangliosidosis Type 2 (Sandhoff's disease)	Domestic cats†
	Juvenile GM$_2$ gangliosidosis Type 3 (Bernheimer-Seitelberger disease)	Yorkshire swine†
Glucocerebroside	Glucocerebrosidosis (Gaucher's disease)	Sidney Silky terrier dogs†
Sphingomyelin	Sphingomyelinosis (Niemann-Pick disease)	Siamese† and domestic cats, poodle dogs
Galactocerebrosides	Globoid cell leukodystrophy (Krabbe's disease)	Cairn terrier,† West Highland white terrier,† beagle, blue tick hound, and mixed-breed dogs, domestic cats, polled Dorset sheep
Sulfatides	Metachromatic leukodystrophy	Domestic cats
Mucopolysaccharides	**Mucopolysaccharidoses**	
Mucopolysaccharide	Mucopolysaccharidosis VI (Maroteaux-Lamy disease)	Siamese and domestic cats
Carbohydrates		
Glycoprotein	Neuronal Glycoproteinosis (Lafora's disease)	Beagle,† basset hound, poodle dogs
Mannoside	Mannosidosis	Angus cattle,† domestic cats
Glycogen	Glycogenosis Type II (Pompe's disease)	Domestic cats, Lapland dogs, sheep
Ceroid Lipofuscins	**Ceroid Lipofuscinoses**	
Ceroid lipofuscin	Neuronal ceroid lipofuscinosis (juvenile amaurotic idiocy)	English setter,† dachshund, Chihuahua†, spaniel dogs, Siamese cats, cattle, South Hampshire sheep†

*The relation of the animal disease to the human disease has not been firmly established for all of the conditons listed.
†Autosomal recessive inheritance.

treatment known for any of them; however, they are important diseases because (1) they are genetic disorders and can be eliminated by selective breeding; (2) they may be confused with conditions of nongenetic origin, such as viral diseases based on clinical examination alone; and (3) they are important models for diseases of human beings. Colonies of animals with many of these diseases have been established at research institutions.

Gangliosidoses

The most thoroughly studied group of storage diseases in animals is the gangliosidoses. Various forms of this condition are related to defects in particular enzymes in the metabolic cycle of lipids with accumulation of the ganglioside in neurons and other cells. Gangliosidoses have been reported in Siamese, Korat, and mixed-breed cats; German short-haired pointers; beagles; mixed-breed dogs; Friesian cattle; and Yorkshire swine (see Table 17–3).

Cerebellar signs of tremors and ataxia predominate in the early stages of the disease in most animals.[2,3] Progression leads to cerebral and brain stem signs, including dementia, blindness, seizures and, eventually, death. The GM_2 gangliosidosis of German short-haired pointers usually starts with cerebral signs, including nervousness, the inability to learn, dementia, and convulsions.

The feline diseases are usually recognized by the time the cat has reached 4 months of age, whereas the German short-haired pointer disease is apparent when the dog is approximately 6 months of age. The animals are generally severely incapacitated or are dead by the time they are 1 year old.

An autosomal recessive inheritance has been demonstrated in all species that have been studied (see Table 17–3).

The diagnosis is suspected in any young animal that presents with a progressive neurologic syndrome as described. Cerebellar hypoplasia caused by a prenatal viral infection is nonprogressive (see Chapter 11). The diagnosis can be confirmed by biochemical assay of the brain, the liver, the skin, cultured fibroblasts, or purified leukocytes. The assays can be performed at institutions involved in research concerning these diseases.[4]

Ceroid Lipofuscinosis

An autosomal recessive disease of English setter dogs is characterized by accumulations of ceroid and lipofuscin in neurons. The enzyme defect is not known, and there is some controversy regarding the identification of the accumulated product. Signs are first recognized when the animal is 9 to 12 months of age. The dogs are dull and have impaired vision. As the disease progresses, the animal may appear demented and ataxic. Seizures are seen in the later stages. The dogs usually die before they have reached 2 years of age.[5] Similar inclusions have been found in other breeds of dogs and in other species (see Table 17–3). In dachshunds, the disease appears when the animals are older.

Neuronal Glycoproteinosis

Neuronal inclusions that appear to be the same as Lafora bodies in human myoclonic epilepsy have been found in beagles with epilepsy.[6] The disease is inherited as an autosomal recessive condition. The causative relationship of the inclusions to the seizures has not been clearly established. Similar inclusions have been found in older dogs of various breeds with no evidence of clinical disease.

Leukodystrophies

Globoid cell leukodystrophy has been widely reported, primarily in Cairn terriers and West Highland white terriers.[7] It is an autosomal recessive disease in these breeds. It also has been reported in beagles, one blue tick hound, mixed-breed cats, and polled Dorset sheep (see Table 17–3). The disease is characterized by destruction of the white matter with accumulations of macrophages filled with lipid (globoid cells).

Two clinical syndromes are recognized in the early stages of the disease. The combination of pelvic limb paresis and ataxia is probably the most common sign, whereas a cerebellar syndrome is seen in some dogs. Progression to tetraparesis and cerebral signs occurs in either form. Peripheral nerves are affected in many dogs. The diagnosis can be established by enzyme assay in leukocytes or by biopsy of a peripheral nerve.[8]

Other Storage Diseases

Most of the other diseases listed in Table 17–3 have been seen in only a few animals.

ABIOTROPHIES AND OTHER DEGENERATIVE DISEASES

The normal neuron is not capable of dividing and reproducing itself but has the capacity to survive for the life of the animal. An abnormality of the metabolic pathways leads to early death of the neuron. This process is termed *abiotrophy*.[9] Most of the abiotrophies and undefined degenerative diseases have a dominance of cerebellar or spinal cord signs and pathology. The spinal cord diseases have been discussed in Chapters 9 and 10. The cerebellar conditions have been presented in Chapter 11.

All of these diseases are seen in young animals, with the exception of degenerative myelopathy of German shepherd dogs (Table 17–

4). The progression is generally slow (months) but unrelenting.

DIFFERENTIAL DIAGNOSIS OF DEGENERATIVE DISEASES

Many of these diseases have a similar clinical history and course. The findings on a neurologic examination may indicate a predominance of cerebral, cerebellar, or spinal cord signs. These results and the age and the breed of the animal should suggest a small number

Table 17–4. ABIOTROPHIES AND DEGENERATIVE DISEASES OF UNKNOWN CAUSE

Anatomic Location	Disease (Human Disease)*	Breed/Species	Age of Onset
Cerebellum and extra-pyramidal system	Cerebellar abiotrophy	Kerry blue terrier dogs†	8 to 16 weeks
Cerebellum, brain stem, spinal cord	Cerebellar degeneration	Collie dogs†	4 to 12 weeks
Cerebellum	Cerebellar cortical abiotrophy	Gordon setter dogs	6 to 30 months
Cerebellum	Cerebellar degeneration	Airedale, Finnish harrier, beagles, Samoyeds, and Bern running dogs, cattle	Variable
Cerebellum, Purkinje cells	Bovine familial convulsions and ataxia	Aberdeen Angus, Holstein, and Charolais cattle	Newborn
Spinocerebellar tracts	Hereditary ataxia	Smooth-haired fox terrier dogs†	2½ to 4 months
Spinal cord, peripheral nerves, auditory pathways	Hereditary ataxia	Jack Russell terrier dogs†	2 to 6 months
Cerebellum, brain stem, coat color	Hereditary neuronal dystrophy	Domestic cats†	5 to 6 weeks
Cerebellum, white matter	Hereditary quadriplegia and amblyopia	Irish setter dogs†	5 to 6 weeks
LMN	Hereditary neuronal abiotrophy	Swedish Lapland dogs†	4 to 6 weeks
LMN	Hereditary canine spinal muscular atrophy (juvenile spinal muscular atrophy)	Brittany spaniel dogs‡	2 to 8 months
LMN	Stockard's paralysis	Great Dane-bloodhound crossbreeds, Great Dane-Saint Bernard crossbreeds	11 to 14 weeks
Neurons: brain and spinal cord	Neurofibrillar accumulations	Collie dogs, domestic cats	6 to 12 weeks
Myelin of CNS	Dysmyelination	Chow chow, Dalmatian dogs	6 weeks
Myelin of CNS	Demyelination	Miniature poodle dogs	9 weeks to 5 months
Spinal cord	Necrotizing myelopathy	Afghan hound dogs	3 to 13 months
Spinal cord	Degenerative myelopathy	German shepherd dogs, other dogs rarely	Older than 5 years
CNS	Hereditary neuroaxial edema	Polled Hereford cattle	Calves

*The relation of the animal disease to the human disease has not been firmly established for all of the conditions listed.

†Autosomal recessive inheritance.

‡Autosomal dominant inheritance.

of possibilities (see Tables 17–3 and 17–4). In the early stages, neuronal diseases often can be differentiated from demyelinating diseases. Neuronal diseases (storage disease, abiotrophy) are more likely to have cerebral or lower motor neuron (LMN) signs. Demyelinating diseases are more likely to have ascending ataxia and paresis of an upper motor neuron (UMN) type, often with tremors of the limbs. Proprioceptive positioning is commonly affected in demyelinating diseases but is rarely involved in the early stages of neuronal disease.

The degenerative diseases also must be differentiated from inflammatory, neoplastic, and toxic disorders. Specific diagnostic tests are available for most of these conditions and will be discussed later in this chapter.

Metabolic Disorders

Normal nervous system function depends on a closely regulated environment. Conversely, the homeostasis of the body is coordinated by the nervous system through the neuroendocrine, autonomic, and somatic systems. Disorders altering homeostasis often have profound effects on the nervous system.

LIVER DISEASES

Hepatic encephalopathy (HE) is a complex metabolic disorder resulting from abnormal liver function.

Pathogenesis

HE has been reported in three types of liver disease: (1) severe parenchymal liver damage (cirrhosis, neoplasia, toxicosis) (2) anomalous portal venous circulation, and (3) congenital urea cycle enzyme deficiencies (Table 17–5). Parenchymal liver diseases other than cirrhosis (fatty infiltration, chronic active hepatitis, and so forth) usually do not cause hepatic encephalopathy, except in the terminal stages of

Table 17–5. CAUSES OF HEPATIC ENCEPHALOPATHY

Disease	Age of Onset
Parenchymal liver disease	
Cirrhosis	Usually old
Acquired portosystemic shunts	Usually old
Toxicity	Any age
Neoplasia	Usually old
Congenital portosystemic venous shunts	Young
Congenital urea cycle enzyme deficiency	Young

the disease.[31] Pyrrolizidine alkaloids in certain plants, such as the *Senecio* species and the *Crotalaria* species, cause parenchymal liver damage and HE in herbivores.

Parenchymal disease severely reduces the capacity of the liver to perform its normal metabolic functions. Portosystemic venous shunts divert a significant portion of the portal blood past the liver into the vena cava. Potentially toxic substances that normally are absorbed from the gastrointestinal tract and detoxified in the liver enter the systemic circulation. Urea cycle enzyme deficiencies prevent the metabolism of ammonia to urea.

The metabolic changes that cause the clinical syndrome of HE include increased circulating ammonia; short-chain fatty acids; and degradation products of amino acids, including mercaptans, skatoles, and indoles. Altered amino acid and neurotransmitter concentrations in the brain also are found.[10] Ammonia is probably the most important toxic substance, although the level of ammonia in the blood does not necessarily correlate with the severity of the CNS disturbance.

Clinical Signs

Most animals with a liver abnormality that is sufficient to produce HE also have other evidence of poor health. Gastrointestinal disturbances, anorexia, weight loss, stunted growth, ascites, and polyuria-polydipsia are seen in varying combinations.

The neurologic signs are frequently worse after feeding, especially if high-protein food is given. The release of nitrogenous materials into the portal circulation exacerbates the signs. Depression that may progress to stupor and coma is the most common neurologic sign. Other signs of cerebral involvement, such as behavior change, continuous pacing and head pressing, blindness, and seizures, also are common. Frequently, the clinical picture is that of a waxing and waning diffuse cerebral abnormality. The postural reactions and reflexes are only minimally involved, except when the animal is nearly comatose. The cranial nerves are not markedly affected, except that vision may be impaired.

A variety of factors may precipitate the neurologic signs of HE in an animal with marginal liver function (Table 17–6). Any source of protein in the digestive tract is a common cause. Hemorrhage in the gastrointestinal tract, constipation, or increased fatty acids also may precipitate a crisis. Alterations in fluids, electrolytes, or pH may increase the blood and tis-

Table 17–6. MANAGEMENT OF HEPATIC ENCEPHALOPATHY (HE)

Factors That Exacerbate HE	Management of HE
Increased dietary protein and fatty acids	Low-protein, low-fat diet
Bacterial production of ammonia in large bowel	Diet, antibiotics
Constipation leading to bacterial production of ammonia in large bowel	Diet, laxatives, enemas in acute problems, lactulose
Gastrointestinal hemorrhage	Monitoring and treatment of ulcers, bleeding disorders, hookworms, whipworms
Hypokalemia, hypovolemia, alkalosis—aggravated by diuretics	Monitoring and correction of fluid and electrolyte imbalance, use of diuretics with caution or not at all
Stored blood transfusion	Use of fresh blood (only if essential)
Sedatives, narcotics, anesthetics	Use of depressant drugs with extreme caution (in lowest possible dosages), monitoring carefully
Infections, fevers	Monitoring and vigorous treatment

sue ammonia levels. Decreased renal function reduces elimination of ammonia and other metabolites. Fever and infection cause increased tissue catabolism and increased nitrogen release. Stored blood for transfusions may have an excess of ammonia. Depressant drugs directly affect the brain and frequently are metabolized in the liver. The first evidence of hepatic dysfunction often has been poor recovery from anesthesia. Diuretics that often are used to treat ascites may cause HE through their effect on potassium, renal output of ammonia, and alkalosis.

Management

The successful medical management of HE depends on the cause of the liver disorder and the degree of liver malfunction. Animals with marginal liver function may be managed by reducing the sources of nitrogenous products in the gastrointestinal tract (see Table 17–6). A high-carbohydrate, low-fat, low-protein diet with a high biologic value is indicated. If dietary management alone is inadequate, then oral, nonabsorbable antibiotics (such as neomycin) may be used to reduce the bacterial flora that split urea. Mild laxatives or lactulose (a nonabsorbable disaccharide) may be helpful.

Acute crises of HE require more vigorous treatment. Protein sources must be removed completely. Enemas and laxatives are used to remove all nitrogenous material from the gastrointestinal tract. Sedative drugs, methionine, and diuretics are discontinued. Sources of gastrointestinal hemorrhage are corrected if they are present. Dehydration, hypokalemia, and alkalosis are managed with intravenous fluid therapy. Renal output must be maintained in order to eliminate nitrogenous products. Oxygen therapy may be necessary, especially in cases of coma. The treatment of herbivores with HE from pyrrolizidine toxicity is usually hopeless.

Specific treatment of the cause is instituted if possible. Unfortunately, most chronic liver diseases and the urea cycle enzyme deficiency cannot be treated specifically. Portosystemic shunts may be corrected surgically if there is adequate portal circulation to the liver. Partial occlusion of the shunt may be effective. For details of the management of HE, the reader should consult the references.[10,11]

RENAL DISEASES

The terminal stages of renal failure may cause tetany or seizures. Chronic renal disease may be associated with muscle wasting and weakness. Polyneuropathy and polymyopathy have been seen in human beings with chronic renal disease, especially those on hemodialysis, but have not been documented in animals. Alterations in electrolyte metabolism, especially that of calcium, may cause signs that are related to the nervous system (see later in this chapter).

ENDOCRINE DISORDERS

Endocrine disorders that affect electrolyte, calcium, magnesium, phosphorus, and glucose homeostasis may produce neurologic signs in affected animals. In addition, hormonal excess or deficiency may affect the function of nerves or muscle directly. Also, pituitary lesions may cause signs of hormonal and brain dysfunction if the disease extends into the hypothalamus. In this section, specific endocrine and metabolic diseases that produce prominent neurologic signs will be discussed. Readers should seek other textbooks for in-depth descriptions of each disorder.

Tetany

Tetany is the continuous tonic spasm of muscles, muscle twitchings, cramps and, occasionally, convulsions. It may be induced by toxins, hypocalcemia, hypomagnesemia, and acid-base disturbances. When the extracellular fluid concentration of calcium ions (Ca^{++}) falls below normal, the nervous system becomes more and more excitable because of increased neuronal membrane permeability. Nerve fibers become so excitable that they discharge spontaneously, initiating the contraction of skeletal muscle and, eventually, tetany. In all animals except the bovine, hypocalcemia produces few other significant effects, because tetany kills the animal before other signs develop. In cattle, hypocalcemia (paturient paresis) produces an initial period of hyperexcitability and muscle twitches followed quickly by severe paresis.

In ruminant animals, decreased serum concentrations of magnesium also may produce tetany. A low magnesium concentration causes greatly increased irritability of the nervous system, peripheral vasodilatation, and cardiac arrhythmias. In this section, conditions producing hypocalcemia and hypomagnesemia are discussed.

Hypocalcemic Tetanies. Hypocalcemia results in tetany when serum calcium concentrations drop below 6 mg/dl. Calcium ion concentrations control neuronal membrane permeability; however, both protein-bound and ionized calcium are measured when serum calcium levels are quantitated. Thus, in hypoproteinemic conditions, low total serum calcium levels may be encountered without concomitant tetany. In dogs, cats, and horses, hypocalcemic tetany may result from hypoparathyroidism, postparturient eclampsia (rare in cats), terminal renal failure, protein-losing enteropathy, and severe alkalosis.

Postparturient eclampsia (puerperal tetany) in the bitch usually occurs within 3 weeks after whelping. Small-breed dogs with nervous temperaments are more prone to this disorder. The exact mechanism of postparturient hypocalcemia in the bitch is not known; however, calcium losses from fetal ossification and lactation combined with deficient osteoclastic activity or calcium absorption are probably responsible for the altered calcium homeostasis. Although some bitches may become hypoglycemic during puerperal tetany, lowered blood glucose values probably are not important in the production of tetany. Some authors believe that nervous dogs are predisposed to puerperal tetany because they hyperventilate during parturition, inducing a respiratory alkalosis. Alkalosis favors the protein binding of calcium, thus lowering the concentrations of ionized calcium. Since ionized calcium is biologically active, alkalosis would enhance the development of tetany.

The early clinical signs include nervousness, pacing, whining, and panting. Muscle spasm and ataxia are subsequent signs. These early manifestations usually progress to tonic-clonic tetanic spasms. The dogs are often febrile and, in severe cases, major motor seizures may be encountered.

The diagnosis of puerperal tetany is based upon the clinical signs and low blood calcium concentrations. Upon presentation, a blood sample should be collected for calcium analysis. Five to 10 ml of 10 per cent calcium gluconate should be given slowly intravenously while the heart rate and rhythm are monitored simultaneously. Two to 5 ml of 10 per cent calcium gluconate diluted with equal volumes of normal saline can be given intramuscularly to prolong the calcium effect. Severely hyperthermic patients (body temperature greater than 106 degrees F) should be cooled with ice packs or alcohol soaks. Animals that continue to have seizures or that remain excessively irritable or restless can be mildly sedated with diazepam or phenobarbital. For maintenance therapy, puppies should be separated from the bitch for 24 hours and supplemented with bitch's replacement milk. Full nursing should be restricted for an additional 48 hours. Calcium lactate is given in oral dosages of 0.5 to 2.0 gm per day.

Eclampsia of mares is rarely encountered except in draft horses. Most cases reportedly occur in lactating mares near the tenth day post parturition or 1 to 2 days after weaning. Factors that may tend to lead to eclampsia in mares include grazing on a lush pasture, strenuous work, and prolonged transport. Affected mares tend to sweat profusely, develop muscle spasticity of the limbs, and become ataxic. Rapid respirations, muscular fibrillations, and trismus are evident, but there is no protrusion of the membrana nictitans. The rectal temperature is normal or mildly elevated, and the pulse may be rapid and irregular. Swallowing may be impeded, and urination and defecation may cease. Within 24 hours, tetanic convulsions develop, followed by death within an additional 24 hours. The diagnosis is based upon clinical signs and the presence of reduced serum calcium concentrations (4 to 6 mg/dl). Treatment with intravenous calcium solutions produces rapid, complete recovery.

Hypoparathyroidism results in decreased secretion of parathormone (PTH) with subsequent hypocalcemia and hyperphosphatemia. This condition has been recognized and studied most frequently in dogs. Although the exact cause is unknown, the majority of dogs have histologic parathyroid changes indicative of a primary autoimmune disease (lymphocytic-plasmocytic cellular infiltration). A parathyroid deficiency also may occur following thyroid gland surgery. An acute form of the disease is characterized by a sudden onset of tetany or convulsions, or both. A chronic form of the disease is associated with recurrent depression, lethargy, anorexia, vomiting, intermittent facial and forelimb spasm, and latent tetany. Primary hypoparathyroidism is suspected in a dog with persistent hypocalcemia and hyperphosphatemia in the presence of normal renal function. Decreased concentrations of PTH in the presence of hypocalcemia substantiate the diagnosis; however, this test is not widely available for use in the dog.

Primary hypoparathyroidism is treated with drugs to overcome the PTH deficiency. Dihydrotachysterol, ergocalciferol (vitamin D_2) and calcitriol (1,25 dihydroxycholecalciferol) are the products frequently recommended. The clinician must individualize the dosage by following the serum calcium levels of each patient twice a week. Approximate initial dosages of these drugs are: dihydrotachysterol, 0.01 mg per kg per day; ergocalciferol, 1000 to 2000 μ per kg per day; and calcitriol, 0.25 μg once a day. The clinician should monitor the serum calcium concentrations carefully in order to prevent hypercalcemia. The effect of vitamin D therapy may be delayed for 2 to 3 weeks. Calcium supplementation must be administered with caution, since its use with vitamin D increases the probability of hypercalcemic toxicity.

Hypomagnesemic Tetanies. These syndromes occur primarily in ruminants. Several hypomagnesemic conditions have been de-

scribed, including grass tetany, wheat pasture poisoning, milk tetany of calves, and transport tetany. The basic pathophysiology of each is similar and probably is related to decreased dietary intake, reduced mobilization, or increased excretion of magnesium.

Grass tetany occurs in the lactating bovine that grazes in a lush pasture. It also occurs in the pregnant and lactating ewes and occasionally is seen in feeder cattle. Lush pastures are low in magnesium, and when magnesium requirements are increased, (as in the case of the lactating bovine) clinical signs are likely to occur. Early signs include restlessness, extreme alertness, and muscular twitching. Animals may become excitable, belligerent, and even aggressive. Stimulation may induce severe signs of tetany, ataxia, and bellowing. Animals may become recumbent with opisthotonos and paddling movements. The diagnosis of grass tetany is supported by laboratory findings of hypomagnesmia (less than 1 mg/dl), hypocalcemia (less than 7 mg/dl), and high normal levels of potassium. Therapy should correct the immediate ionic imbalance and should supplement the dietary intake of magnesium. Magnesium lactate in a 3.3 per cent solution (2.2 ml per kg), magnesium gluconate in a 15 per cent solution (0.44 ml per kg), and magnesium sulfate in a 20 per cent solution (0.44 ml per kg) can be given slowly intravenously or subcutaneously. Commercial combination solutions also may be used effectively. Magnesium oxide, 1 gm per 45 kg per day, should be force-fed or supplied in blocks containing protein supplements and molasses. Animals on high-risk pastures should be given magnesium oxide or chloride supplements.

Wheat pasture poisoning is very similar to grass tetany, except that it occurs in cattle and sheep that graze in a cereal grain pasture during its early growth. The diagnosis and the treatment are the same as those for grass tetany.

Milk tetany occurs in 2- to 4-month-old calves that are fed only milk. The signs may occur after episodes of diarrhea. The digestive disorders may decrease magnesium absorption, thus complicating the magnesium deficiency. The clinical signs include hyperesthesia, nervousness, recumbency, and seizures. Repeated attacks may occur. The diagnosis is based on the history, the clinical signs, and a serum magnesium concentration of less than 0.7 mg/dl. Calves respond to parenteral magnesium ionic therapy. Susceptible calves should be given supplements of 1 gm per day of magnesium oxide.

Transport tetany occurs following stressful events, such as transportation, vaccination, deworming, adverse weather, and marked dietary changes. It occurs in both cattle and sheep. A dietary reduction in calcium, magnesium, and potassium coupled with stress produces ionic imbalances that result in a wide range of clinical signs, from spastic to flaccid paralysis. The signs usually begin within 24 hours of the stress but may be delayed for 72 hours. Early manifestations include restlessness, anorexia, and excitement. These signs progress to muscular trembling, tooth grinding, ataxia, and recumbency. Opisthotonos, paddling, and coma may develop. The treatment consists of the parenteral administration of polyionic glucose solutions and attentive nursing care.

Generalized Weakness

Many endocrine and metabolic diseases result in generalized weakness because they affect neuromuscular functions. In certain conditions, clinical signs improve with rest and are exacerbated by exercise. The term *episodic weakness* has been applied to this condition (see Chapter 10). In this section, endocrine and metabolic diseases that produce episodic or generalized weakness are discussed.

Parturient Paresis. Parturient paresis, or milk fever, is a hypocalcemic metabolic disorder that occurs in mature dairy cows and sheep, usually within 48 hours of parturition. The affected cows are usually more than 5 years of age, and the incidence is increased in heavy milk producers and in the Jersey breed. Many dairy cows are marginally hypocalcemic at parturition, and any factor that decreases the metabolic adjustment to this hypocalcemia may cause paresis. Such factors include milk yield versus calcium mobilization from bone and gut, calcium to phosphorus ratios in the diet, anorexia and decreased intestinal motility, and dietary pH.

Parturient paresis is characterized by early hypersensitivity and a stiff gait followed by progressive muscular weakness, recumbency, depression, and coma. Stage 1 is often missed and is characterized by apprehension, anorexia, ataxia, and limb stiffness. Stage 2 is marked by recumbency and depression. The head is usually turned to the flank, and there may be an S-shaped curvature of the neck. Other signs include dilated pupils, decreased

pupillary light reflexes, reduced anal reflex, decreased defecation and urination, no ruminal motility, protrusion of the tongue, and frequent straining. Stage 3 occurs in approximately 20 per cent of the cases and is characterized by lateral recumbency; severe depression or coma; subnormal temperature; a weak, irregular heart rate; and slow, irregular, shallow respirations. The pupils are dilated and unresponsive to light. Bloating may occur. Changes in serum ions include hypocalcemia, hypophosphatemia, and hypermagnesemia. With prolonged anorexia, serum sodium and potassium levels may decrease. Intravenous calcium salts, 1 gm Ca^{++} per 45 kg body weight, are usually effective. Calcium borogluconate is commonly used, and a 25 per cent solution contains 10.4 gm of calcium per 500 ml. Milk fever can be prevented in susceptible cows or herds by the administration of vitamin D or its analogues or by manipulation of the prepartum dietary calcium and phosphorus levels.

Ketonemic Syndromes. These diseases occur primarily in ruminants and are characterized by hypoglycemia and the accumulation of ketones in body fluids. Conditions that have been recognized include bovine ketosis (acetonemia) and pregnancy toxemia of cattle, sheep, and goats. Unlike most monogastric animals, ruminants produce most of their glucose supplies from the gluconeogenesis of volatile fatty acids (acetic, propionic, and butyric acids). Nearly 50 per cent of the glucose in the cow is normally derived from dietary propionic acid that is converted to glucose in the gluconeogenic pathway. Reduction of propionic acid production in the rumen can result in hypoglycemia and the subsequent mobilization of free fatty acids and glycerol from fat stores. The liver has a limited ability to utilize these fatty acids because the levels of oxaloacetate are low. Acetylcoenzyme A therefore is not incorporated into the tricarboxylic acid cycle and is converted into the ketone bodies acetoacetate and betahydroxybutarate. When the production of ketones by the liver exceeds peripheral utilization, pathologic ketosis results.

Both ketosis and the primary hypoglycemia are involved in the development of the clinical signs. The most common signs include depression, partial to complete anorexia, weight loss, and decreased milk production. The neurologic signs that are present in some cows include ataxia, apparent blindness, salivation, tooth grinding, muscle twitching, and hyperesthesia. Cows may charge blindly if they are disturbed. The diagnosis of bovine ketosis is based on the presence of elevated ketone levels in blood and milk with concomitant hypoglycemia. The immediate therapy is an intravenous injection of glucose followed by an oral administration of 125 to 250 gm of propylene glycol twice a day. Glucocorticoids are also beneficial in cows that are not septic. Cows with severe nervous signs can be treated with 2 to 8 gm of chloral hydrate orally twice a day for 3 to 5 days.

Pregnancy toxemia is a condition that is closely related pathophysiologically to bovine ketosis. It occurs in ewes during the last 6 weeks of pregnancy, when there is a large demand for glucose by developing fetuses. Pregnancy toxemia occurs in pastured or housed beef cows during the last 2 months of pregnancy. Overweight cows or those bearing twin calves are especially susceptible. In ewes and cows, the basic etiology is nutrition insufficient to maintain normal blood glucose concentrations when fetal glucose demands are high. Hypoglycemia precipitates the ketosis, as has been described earlier in this section. In sheep, clinical signs may develop in a flock and may extend for several weeks. Ewes become depressed and develop weakness, ataxia, and loss of muscle tone. Terminally, recumbency and coma develop. Neuromuscular disturbances include fine muscle tremors of the ears and the lips. In some cases, seizures may develop. "Star-gazing" postures and grinding of the teeth are common. The neurologic signs in cattle include depression, excitability, and ataxia. The diagnosis of pregnancy toxemia is based upon the history, the clinical signs, and the presence of ketosis and hypoglycemia. In sheep, flock treatment consists of increasing the availability of glucose precursors in the diet or by drenching affected ewes twice daily with 200 ml of a warm 50 per cent glycerol solution. The anabolic steroid trienbolone acetate also is beneficial in 30 mg doses intramuscularly. Induction of parturition or fetal removal by cesarean section also may be needed in order to reduce the metabolic drain on the ewe. Cattle are treated by the method described for bovine ketosis. Pregnancy toxemia can be prevented by assuring adequate nutrition during pregnancy.

Diabetes Mellitus. Diabetes mellitus may result in neurologic signs from at least four mechanisms. Insulin deficiency results in a failure of glucose transport into muscle and adipose tissue. An early sign of diabetes may be exercise intolerance and weakness. If severe insulin deficiency occurs, ketonemia develops from a marked increase in lipolysis and serum fatty acids. The ensuing metabolic acidosis results in depressed cerebral function that culminates in coma and death. In the nontreated ketoacidotic dog or cat, hyperkalemia may be a serious complication that depresses neuromuscular and cardiovascular function. With therapy and correction of the acidosis, potassium ions re-enter cells, and hypokalemia may be a complication that fosters muscle weakness and depression. In some animals, the hyperglycemia may be severe, even though acidosis is absent. This syndrome is called *hyperosmolar nonketotic coma.* Clinical signs result from the hyperosmolar effects on the cerebral cortex. On rare occasions, diabetic patients may develop neuropathies with associated LMN signs in affected muscles.

The comatose diabetic animal is a difficult therapeutic challenge. The clinician must exercise great care in performing insulin, acid-base, electrolyte, and fluid therapy. Interested readers should consult other texts for an in-depth discussion of the diagnosis and management of the diabetic patient.

Hypothyroidism. Deficiencies of thyroxine result in a marked decrease in cerebration and basal metabolic rate. Severely hypothyroid dogs may become very depressed or may appear dull and unresponsive. A very low-voltage electroencephalogram (EEG) usually is seen. Myopathies and peripheral neuropathies also rarely occur secondarily to chronic hypothyroidism. The cerebral signs improve dramatically following replacement thyroid medication.

Hyperadrenocorticism. Hyperactivity of the adrenal cortex may result in generalized muscle weakness from the catabolic effects of glucocorticoids, which are secreted excessively in this disease. In addition, some dogs with this condition develop muscle degeneration that is known as *steroid-induced myopathy.* This syndrome has been described in Chapter 10.

Bilateral adrenal cortical hyperplasia is a common cause of canine hyperadrenocorticism. This condition may develop as a consequence of adrenocorticotropic hormone (ACTH)–producing pituitary tumors. Occasionally, these pituitary tumors may grow large enough to produce neurologic signs, including depression, confusion, seizures, and a variety of autonomic nervous system abnormalities. Neurologic signs rarely occur unless the tumor invades the hypothalamus.

Episodic Weakness

In Chapter 10, the problem of episodic weakness was introduced and the primary neuromuscular causes of this problem were discussed. In this section, the endocrinologic and metabolic causes of episodic weakness are described briefly.

Hypercalcemia. An increased concentration of serum calcium may result in neuromuscular, cardiovascular, and renal dysfunction. When the level of calcium in body fluids rises above normal, excitable cell membranes are depressed. Reflex activities of the CNS become sluggish, and muscles also become sluggish and weak. Hypercalcemia also will decrease the QT interval of the heart and will decrease mycardial function. Hypercalcemia impairs the renal concentrating ability. In prolonged hypercalcemia, mineralization of soft tissue may occur. The syndrome of hypercalcemic nephropathy is well documented in animals and culminates in chronic renal failure. In the dog, calcium levels above 12.5 mg/dl result in hypercalcemic signs. In some cases, muscle weakness is markedly worse during exercise and improves with rest.

Several causes of hypercalcemia exist, including primary hyperparathyroidism, pseudohyperparathyroidism, vitamin D intoxication, and iatrogenic calcium therapy. Primary hyperparathyroidism results from autonomously functioning parathyroid adenomas. These tumors secrete PTH in the face of increasing serum calcium concentrations. Certain nonendocrine tumors, such as lymphosarcomas, secrete substances with PTH-like activity that results in hypercalcemia. This syndrome is called pseudohyperparathyroidism. An excessive intake of vitamin D promotes increased absorption of calcium and may produce hypercalcemia.

The symptomatic therapy of hypercalcemia includes diuresis with fluids and furosemide. Cortiosteroids also are beneficial, because they promote the renal excretion of calcium.

Hyperkalemia. Increased serum concentrations of potassium decrease the activity of excitable membranes, especially cardiac muscle. An excessive extracellular concentration of potassium causes cardiac flaccidity and decreases the conduction of cardiac impulses through the atrioventricular (AV) node. Thus, heart rate and cardiac output may be severely depressed. In addition, the contraction of skeletal muscle also may be somewhat depressed. Hyperkalemia therefore manifests itself as generalized weakness that becomes worse with exercise.

Hyperkalemia may occur secondarily to severe acidosis; however, the usual cause is adrenal insufficiency. Adrenal insufficiency may result in aldosterone deficiency, which produces hyperkalemia and hyponatremia. Typical signs include depression, anorexia, vomiting, diarrhea, weakness, bradycardia, and decreased cardiac output. The disease responds well to fluid and replacement adrenocortical hormone therapy.

Hypokalemia. Decreased serum concentrations of potassium decrease the activity of skeletal muscle, because the membranes are hyperpolarized. Muscle weakness, and even paralysis, may occur. The primary causes of hypokalemia include diuretic therapy, vomiting, diarrhea, alkalosis, and excessive mineralocorticoid therapy for adrenal insufficiency. Most patients respond well to potassium supplementation.

Hypoglycemia. Hypoglycemia causes altered CNS function similar to that which occurs with hypoxia. The blood glucose concentration is of prime importance for normal neuronal metabolism, because glucose oxidation is the primary energy source. There are no glycogen stores in the CNS. Glucose enters nervous tissue by diffusion rather than by insulin facilitation. The severity of the CNS signs is related more to the rate of decrease than to the actual concentration of glucose. Sudden drops in glucose levels are more likely to cause seizures, whereas slowly developing hypoglycemia may cause weakness, paraparesis, behavioral changes, or severe depression.

Hypoglycemia in young animals may be secondary to malnutrition, parasitism, stress, or a gastrointestinal abnormality. Puppies frequently present as extremely depressed or comatose. The blood glucose level is usually very low (below 30 mg per 100 ml). A blood sample should be obtained for glucose determination, and intravenous glucose should be administered immediately (2 to 4 ml of 20 per cent glucose per kg). If seizures are present, diazepam should be administered if there is no immediate response to the glucose (see the section on the treatment of status epilepticus in Chapter 15). Continued signs of stupor or coma indicate brain swelling and are treated with corticosteroids and mannitol (see Chapter 14). Dietary regulation, including tube feeding if necessary, must be established in order for normoglycemia to be maintained.

Glycogen storage diseases also have been reported in puppies. Persistent recurrent hypoglycemia, hepatomegaly, acidosis, and ketosis suggest a glycogen storage disease. It is necessary to perform a biopsy in order to make a definitive diagnosis. The management of these cases is frequently unsuccessful.

Adult-onset hypoglycemia usually is caused by a functional tumor of the pancreatic beta cells (insulinoma). The excessive insulin produces an increased transfer of blood glucose into the non-neuronal cellular compartments, resulting in hypoglycemia and abnormal CNS metabolism. Although insulinomas are relatively rare, increasing awareness has resulted in more frequent diagnosis in recent years. Most of the tumors in dogs are carcinomas and have metastasized to the liver and other sites by the time a definitive diagnosis is made.

Seizures are more frequently related to exercise, fasting (or, conversely, eating), and excitement. Other signs, such as weakness, muscle tremor, disorientation, and behavioral changes, are more common. The signs are episodic until irreversible neuronal damage occurs.

Hypoglycemia may mimic the other causes of seizures. Blood glucose concentrations after a 12-hour fast are usually below normal (less than 60 mg per 100 ml). Longer fasts (24 to 48 hours) may be necessary in some cases, but animals should be monitored closely during this time. Plasma insulin levels are more specific for making a diagnosis. Values above 54 μ per ml in a fasting dog are considered abnormal (immunoreactive insulin test—IRI). Serum IRI concentrations are near zero when plasma glucose concentrations are less than or equal to 30 mg/dl. The amended insulin–glucose ratio (AIGR) has been found to be the simplest and most sensitive indication of functional beta-cell carcinoma. The AIGR is obtained by the application of the following ratio:

$$\frac{\text{Serum insulin } (\mu\text{U/ml} \times 100)}{\text{Plasma glucose (mg/dl)} - 30}$$

Normal values are less than 30 μU/mg glucose. The glucagon tolerance test may be used as an alternative procedure but carries a greater risk of profound hypoglycemia during the test.[12]

The management of patients in status epilepticus has been discussed in Chapter 15.

Coma has been discussed in Chapter 14. Surgical removal of the tumor is indicated when the patient's condition has stabilized. The reported incidence of malignancy ranges from 56 per cent to 82 per cent; therefore, the prognosis is poor even with successful removal of the pancreatic focus. Chemotherapy following surgical removal may provide for a longer life.

Neoplasms

Neoplasia affecting the nervous system may be classified conveniently in three groups (Table 17–7). Primary tumors arise from cells that normally are found in the cranial vault, in the spinal canal, or in the peripheral nerves. Secondary tumors metastasize from a primary tumor to the nervous system. Bone tumors of the skull or the vertebrae may be considered a form of secondary tumors. The peripheral nerves may be invaded or compressed by tumors of other structures.

Table 17–7. CLASSIFICATION OF NEOPLASIA OF THE NERVOUS SYSTEM*

Primary Tumors	
Neural tube	
Glial cells	Astrocytomas, oligodendrogliomas, glioblastomas
Ependymal cells	Ependymomas, choroid plexus papillomas
Neurons	Medulloblastomas† ganglioneuromas, gangliomas
Neural crest	
Schwann cells	Schwannomas, neurofibromas
Arachnoid cells	Meningiomas
Other cells	
Connective tissue	Sarcomas
Reticuloendothelial cells	Reticulum cell sarcomas (reticulosis, microglioma)
Adenohypophyseal cells	Pituitary adenomas
Secondary Tumors	
Metastasis	
Bone Tumors	
Primary or secondary tumors of skull or vertebrae	

*Modified from Escourolle, R., and Poirer, J.: Manual of Basic Neuropathology, 2nd ed. Philadelphia, W. B. Saunders Co., 1978.

†Often classified as gliomas.

PATHOGENESIS

Tumors affect the function of the nervous system by (1) destruction of nervous tissue, (2) compression of surrounding structures, (3) interference with circulation and the development of cerebral edema, and (4) disturbance of cerebrospinal fluid (CSF) circulation. Secondary effects may include herniations of the cerebrum under the tentorium cerebelli or the cerebellum into the foramen magnum (see Chapter 14).

Primary tumors usually grow slowly, producing a clinical syndrome of chronic progression. If the mass obstructs or erodes a vessel, the resulting infarction or hemorrhage may produce an acute onset of a severe neurologic deficit (see Fig. 14–4). Secondary tumors, especially those that are highly malignant, also may have a more acute progression. Edema of surrounding tissues is frequent with neoplasia of the CNS. Brain tumors frequently pro-

duce signs of increased intracranial pressure. The progression may be more rapid if there is obstruction of CSF flow with secondary hydrocephalus.

INCIDENCE

The frequency of occurrence of tumors affecting the nervous system of animals is not known. Brain tumors were found in less than 1 per cent of necropsied dogs in several series.[2] A complete evaluation of the nervous system usually is not performed except at referral institutions, which precludes an accurate estimate of the incidence of CNS neoplasia in the general population of any species. Primary tumors of the CNS are infrequently reported in food animals and horses. The relative frequencies of the types of tumors and the relative risk of some breeds of dogs have been established (Tables 17–8 and 17–9).

Brain tumors, primarily gliomas, are found

Table 17–8. ESTIMATED RELATIVE RISK (R) OF CANINE NERVOUS-TISSUE TUMORS FOR ALL BREEDS WITH ≧4 TUMORS OBSERVED, BY BREED AND BY SEX WITHIN TUMOR CATEGORY*

Tumor Category	Risk Category	Cases Observed	R†
Glial (96)	Breed		
	Boxer	33	23.3‡
	Boston terrier	6	5.2‡
	All breeds combined	96	1
	Poodle, miniature or toy	6	0.7
	All other purebred	38	0.7‡
	Mixed breed	13	0.5§
	Sex		
	Female	42	0.8
	Male	54	1
Meningeal (50)	Breed		
	German shepherd	6	1.4
	Poodle, miniature or toy	5	1.1
	All breeds combined	50	1
	All other purebred	32	0.9
	Mixed breed	7	0.6
	Sex		
	Female	26	1.0
	Male	24	1
Peripheral nerve (53)	Breed		
	Beagle hound	4	2.4
	German shepherd	5	1.1
	Mixed breed	14	1.0
	All breeds combined	53	1
	All other purebred	30	0.9
	Sex		
	Female	31	1.3
	Male	22	1

*From Hayes, H. M., Jr., Priester, W. A., and Pendergras, T. W.: Occurrence of nervous tissue tumors in cattle, horses, cats and dogs. Int. J. Cancer 15:39–47, 1975. Used by permission.

†Adjustment made for age and sex in determining breed R and for age and breed in determining sex R.

‡Significantly different (p<0.05) from R = 1.

§Significantly different (p<0.01) from R = 1.

Table 17–9. GLIAL TUMORS IN ALL DOGS BY CELL TYPE AND SITE*

Cell Type	Site	
	Brain	*Spinal Cord*
Astrocytoma	49	9
Ependymoma	14	8
Plexus-papilloma	8	
Oligodendroglioma	2	1
Medulloblastoma	3	
Glioma, undifferentiated	2	

*From Hayes, H. M., Jr., Priester, W. A., and Pendergras, T. W.: Occurrence of nervous tissue tumors in cattle, horses, cats and dogs. Int. J. Cancer 15:39–47, 1975. Used by permission.

Table 17–10. COMMON SITES AND SIGNS OF BRAIN TUMORS

Frontal lobe—cortex	Seizures, abnormal behavior, contralateral postural reactions
Occipital lobe—cortex	Seizures, contralateral visual field deficit
Temporal lobe—cortex	Seizures, abnormal behavior
Basal nuclei and internal capsule	Circling, postural reaction deficits, contralateral visual deficits
Pituitary fossa	Hypothalamic signs: polyuria, polydipsia, changes in eating, sleeping, and behavior patterns, and so forth; later visual deficits
Brain stem	Gait and postural reaction deficits, cranial nerve signs
Cerebellopontine angle	C.N. V, C.N. VII, and C.N. VIII signs, hemiparesis

more frequently in boxers, Boston terriers, and English bulldogs than in other breeds. The incidence of meningiomas is slightly higher in German shepherds, collies, poodles, and cats.[13,14] Plexus papillomas are found most frequently in nonbrachycephalic breeds.[14] Neoplastic reticulosis is seen in all breeds. Spinal cord tumors have not been reported as often as brain tumors, but secondary tumors either from vertebral involvement or by metastasis are seen most frequently.[15] Beagles are slightly more at risk for peripheral nerve tumors.[13]

In general, the risk of neoplasia increases with age. In one study, the risk for glial tumors peaked at 10 to 14 years of age, meningeal tumors at 7 to 9 years, and peripheral nerve tumors at 2 to 3 and 7 to 9 years.

CLINICAL SIGNS

The signs of CNS tumors are dependent on the location of the mass (Table 17–10). In contrast with the other diseases discussed in this chapter, signs of focal abnormality are expected with CNS neoplasia. Metastatic disease and the diffuse neoplastic disorders (reticulosis, lymphosarcoma) are the exceptions. Although there is some evidence that the different types of tumors have sites of predilection, the number of reported cases is too low for predictions to be made with confidence.

Cerebral tumors can become relatively large (greater than 1 cm diameter) before clinical signs are recognized. Seizures may be the first sign of a cerebral tumor. An examination performed at the time of the first seizure may not reveal any neurologic deficits. Medical control of the seizures may be effective at first, but as the tumor expands, seizures usually become more frequent in spite of anticonvulsant medication. A progression usually is recognized over a period of a few months.

In addition to the signs that are related to the location of the lesion (see Table 17–10), signs that are related to the generalized increase in intracranial pressure frequently are present. Depression, and dullness are common, and the animal often appears to have a headache. Papilledema may be seen in some animals.[16]

Many gliomas arise in the deeper structures of the cerebrum, possibly from the cells of the subependymal plate.[17] Involvement of the basal nuclei and the diencephalon is common (Fig. 17–1).

Pituitary tumors in animals tend to expand

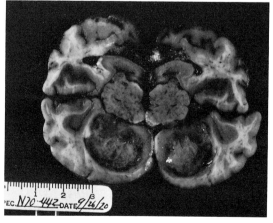

Figure 17–1. A Grade IV astrocytoma in a boxer dog. Note the compression of the brain stem.

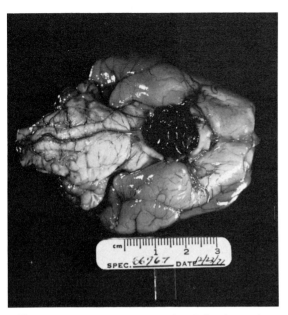

Figure 17–2. A pituitary tumor in a Labrador retriever with visual and postural reaction deficits and Horner's syndrome.

dorsally into the hypothalamus, producing seizures and changes in metabolic and endocrine function in the early stages. These tumors can be quite large before cranial nerve signs or motor signs are observed (Fig. 17–2).

Brain stem tumors are characterized by gait deficits and cranial nerve signs (Fig. 17–3). Behavioral changes and seizures are usually absent in tumors of the brain stem and the cerebellum until the mass affects the reticular activating system or alters intracranial pressure by obstructing CSF circulation.

Spinal cord tumors usually produce signs of a segmental myelopathy. Extramedullary tumors often cause unilateral signs until late in their growth. The unilateral signs are in direct contrast with the usual bilateral signs that are seen with most other spinal cord compressive lesions (e.g., disk luxation). Intramedullary lesions are more likely to produce bilateral signs. Intramedullary tumors rarely cause pain, whereas extramedullary tumors, especially extradural masses, usually do (Table 17–11).[15]

Peripheral nerve tumors other than neurofibromas of the nerve roots have been reported infrequently. Neoplasia must be considered in any mononeuropathy without evidence of trauma (see Chapter 8). Secondary tumors, especially lymphosarcomas, may invade or compress peripheral nerves.

DIAGNOSIS

Brain Tumors

Until localizing signs develop, the diagnosis of a brain tumor may be extremely difficult. The primary groups of diseases that must be

Table 17–11. CHARACTERISTICS OF SPINAL CORD TUMORS*

	Extradural	Intradural-Extramedullary	Intramedullary
Frequency	50%	35%	15%
Tumor types	Bone tumors	Neurofibromas	Gliomas
	Metastatic tumors	Meningiomas	Ependymomas
Rate of growth	Rapid	Slow	Usually slow
Clinical signs			
Pain	Early, severe	Early, variable	Unusual, late
Paresis	Early, rapidly progressive, usually bilateral	Late, slowly progressive, often unilateral	Late, rapidly progressive, usually bilateral
Sensation	Usually intact until late	Usually intact until late	Usually intact until late
Course	Acute onset, rapid progression	Very slow progression	Insidious onset, rapid progression
Diagnosis			
CSF	↑ protein, normal cells	↑ protein, normal cells	↑ protein, normal cells, may be xanthochromia
Radiography	Skeletal lesions	Possibly large intervertebral foramen (neurofibroma)	Possibly widened spinal canal
Myelography	Extradural compression	Variable, may be cupping of dye column	Widened spinal cord, attenuated dye column

*Modified from Prata, R. G.: Diagnosis of spinal cord tumors in the dog. Vet. Clin. North Am. 7:165–185, 1977.

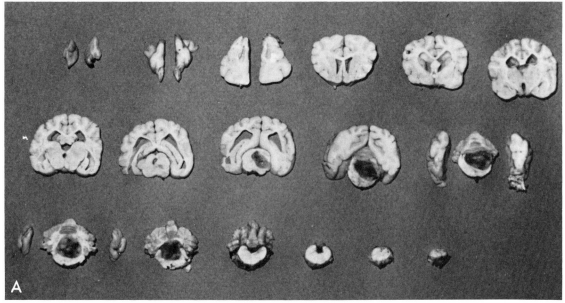

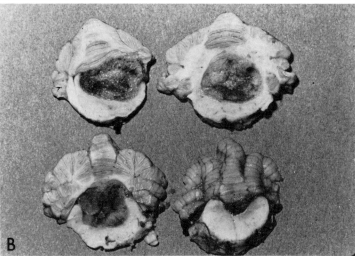

Figure 17–3. *A* and *B*. This oligodendroglioma is in the brain stem, extending from the midbrain to the rostral medulla. The dog had a left facial paralysis, a right hemiparesis, and a forced gaze deviation to the right. This case is an exception to the usual rule of ipsilateral paresis with brain stem lesions, possibly related to the central location of the mass.

ruled out are outlined in Table 17–12. The more common degenerative diseases can be excluded on the basis of age of onset; however, tumors occasionally are seen in young animals. The other diseases, except for inflammation and vascular lesions, may be excluded when focal signs develop. Most inflammatory diseases, with the exception of brain abscesses, are multifocal or diffuse in distribution; however, they may produce focal signs early in the course of the disease. Hemor-

rhages and infarcts are usually acute in onset and nonprogressive.

The most useful diagnostic test available in clinical practice is CSF analysis. Tumors generally cause an increase in pressure and protein with no increase in cells. Inflammatory diseases almost always cause an increase in protein *and* cells with a variable effect on pressure. The risks of a CSF tap must be carefully weighed against the benefits. If there is increased intracranial pressure, the chances of

Table 17–12. DIFFERENTIAL DIAGNOSIS OF BRAIN TUMORS

	Brain Tumor	Degenerative Disease	Metabolic Disease	Inflammatory Disease	Toxic Disease	Vascular Disease
Age	Adult to old	Young	Any	Any	Any	Any
Progression	Slow	Slow	Variable, often waxing and waning	Usually fast	Slow (heavy metals)	Acute onset, not progressive
Focal signs	Yes	No	No	Maybe, especially abscess	No	Yes
CNS	↑Protein, N cells*	↑Protein (variable), N cells	N	↑Protein, ↑Cells	↑Protein, N cells	↑Protein, N cells, may be xanthochromic
EEG	Maybe focal (cortical tumor) or diffuse HVSW†	Diffuse abnormality	Diffuse abnormality	Diffuse abnormality, except abscess	Diffuse abnormality	May be focal abnormality
Contrast radiography	Positive	Negative	Negative	Negative, except abscess	Negative	May be positive

*N = normal.
†HVSW = high-voltage slow waves.

causing a herniation of the brain are very high (see Chapter 6). We have seen cerebellar herniations following CSF taps in animals with no clinical evidence of increased pressure. We also have seen cases in which the patients were strongly suspected of having a tumor but proved to have bacterial infections (abscess and meningitis) and subsequently were cured with medical therapy. Ultimately, the decision must be made with the owner fully informed of the risks. The alternatives to a CSF tap are contrast and isotope radiographic procedures in an attempt to demonstrate a mass. In the case of a serious progressive disease, such as a brain tumor, we recommend doing the tap.

An EEG may aid in the diagnosis of cortical tumors by showing focal abnormality. Increased intracranial pressure often causes generalized high-voltage slow waves. Therefore, we prefer to do an EEG study prior to the CSF tap. EEGs are available only at institutions and in specialty practices.

Radiographic procedures that are useful for the detection of brain tumors include arteri-

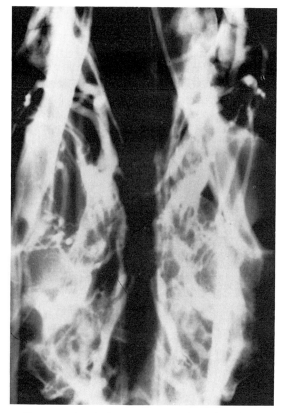

Figure 17–4. A sinus venogram of a dog with a pituitary tumor. Note the bilateral widening of the space between the cavernous sinuses. Compare this figure with Figure 6–5.

ography and radioisotope brain scans for cerebral lesions and sinus venography for lesions on the floor of the skull (Figs. 17–4 and 17–5). Computerized axial tomography may be useful for localizing any mass in the brain but is available at very few institutions.

Spinal Cord Tumors

The localization of spinal cord tumors can be accurate if LMN signs or pain is present. The differential diagnosis of spinal cord tumors is outlined in Table 17–13. Degenerative myelopathy, which occurs primarily in German shepherd dogs, is the only condition that is never painful. Myelitis initially may appear to be a focal disease, but progression to other parts of the spinal cord is the rule. These diseases cannot be differentiated on the basis of clinical evaluation alone.

Radiography is the most useful diagnostic procedure for confirmation of a diagnosis. Vertebral changes may be seen in primary bone tumors, metastatic tumors, and some primary tumors of nervous tissue (see Fig. 9–16). Tumors of the nerve root may cause an enlarged intervertebral foramen (see Fig. 9–18). Slowly expanding tumors in the spinal canal may erode the lamina and the body of the vertebra, giving the appearance of a slightly enlarged spinal canal (see Fig. 9–19). Myelography is necessary in order to confirm these findings, to demonstrate those that do not cause vertebral change, and to define the extent of the mass (Fig. 17–6).

CSF analysis is of limited benefit. Inflammation can be ruled out if there is no increase in cells. The other diseases usually cause an increase in protein with normal cells.

Peripheral Nerve Tumors

Peripheral nerve tumors that do not affect the spinal cord are difficult to diagnose. Any mononeuropathy without evidence of trauma is likely to be caused by a tumor. Peripheral nerve tumors are usually painful.

Electrophysiologic testing is useful for establishing which nerve (or nerves) is involved. A final diagnosis must be made by surgical removal and histopathologic examination.

MANAGEMENT

Brain Tumors

Surgical resection, possibly combined with chemotherapy and radiation, is the only treatment for brain tumors.[2] Successful manage-

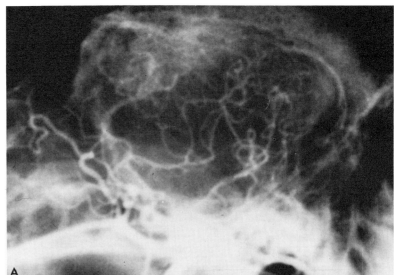

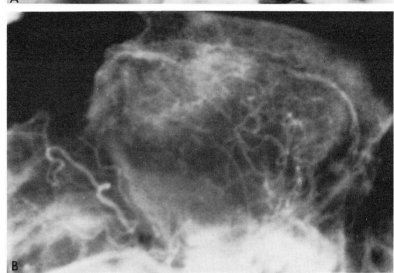

Figure 17–5. Cerebral arteriogram of a dog with a meningioma of the frontal area. *A.* Arterial phase of the arteriogram. There is a diffuse increase in contrast material in the frontal area. *B.* Venous phase of the arteriogram. Although contrast material is now in the veins, the diffuse density (tumor blush) is still present.

Table 17–13. DIFFERENTIAL DIAGNOSIS OF SPINAL CORD TUMORS

| | Spinal Cord Tumor | Degenerative Myelopathy | Inflammation | | Type II Disk |
			Myelitis	Diskospondylitis	
Age	Adult to old	>5 years	Any	Any	>6 years
Progression	Usually slow	Slow	Variable	Variable	Slow
Focal signs	Yes, unless metastatic; may be painful	T3–L3, not painful	Sometimes early, later progresses to other areas; may be painful	Yes, may be multifocal; usually painful	Yes, may be painful
Radiography survey	Sometimes vertebral changes	Normal, frequently have spondylosis	Normal	Characteristic, osteomyelitis	May be normal
Myelography	Defines extent: extradural, intradural, intramedullary	Normal	Normal	May demonstrate extradural compression	Extradural compression at disk space
CSF	↑ Protein, normal cells	↑ Protein (variable), normal cells	↑ Protein, ↑ Cells	Variable	↑ Protein (variable), normal cells

329

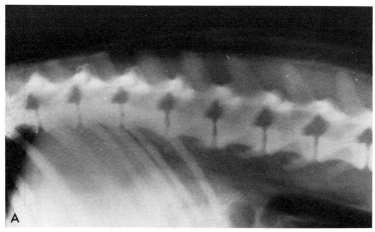

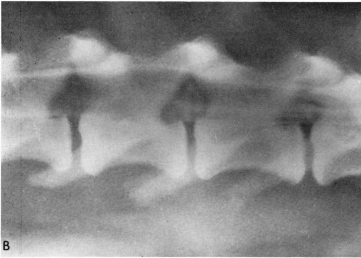

Figure 17–6. *A.* Enlarged spinal canal at L4. The canal is normally larger in this area because of the lumbosacral intumescence. *B.* Myelogram demonstrating an intramedullary mass. Note the thinning of the dye column. There was an astrocytoma in the spinal cord.

ment is unusual, and there have been no reports of any significant numbers of treated patients. The criteria for possible success include (1) a solitary noninvasive tumor, (2) a tumor that is on or near the surface of the cerebral hemisphere, (3) a neurologic status that is compatible with life, (4) accurate localization, (5) careful and complete surgical resection, and (6) intensive postoperative care. Meningiomas are most likely to meet the first two requirements.

Few data are available regarding the medical treatment of brain tumors in animals. Corticosteroids may provide some improvement in clinical signs for a limited time, primarily through the reduction of cerebral edema.

Spinal Cord Tumors

Surgical removal of spinal cord tumors is the treatment of choice. Extradural tumors would seem to be the most favorable for surgical removal. Unfortunately, extradural tumors are usually metastatic, with metastases also present elsewhere, or they are primary bone tumors. The resection of a vertebral tumor is likely to produce an unstable spine. Intradural-extramedullary tumors, which are usually meningiomas or neurofibromas, are more likely to be resectable. An early diagnosis is critical. Intramedullary tumors, usually gliomas, ependymomas, or metastases, are frequently invasive and are not amenable to resection without destruction of the spinal cord. Microsurgical techniques should improve the prognosis for spinal cord tumors significantly.

Peripheral Nerve Tumors

Complete resection of primary peripheral nerve tumors can be readily accomplished with good results. The primary limiting factor is the functional significance of the affected nerve (see Chapter 8). Resection with anastomosis of the nerve is possible if the tumor is not too large.[2] Amputation of the limb with resection of the tumor is the alternative.

Nutritional Disorders

Nervous system disorders caused by nutritional deficiencies or excesses are uncommon in companion animals but more common in food animals. Severe malnutrition can cause a variety of abnormalities that are related to multiple deficiencies. Vitamin deficiencies and excesses are the most common nutritional abnormalities seen in practice.

HYPOVITAMINOSIS

Vitamin A

Deficiencies in vitamin A may produce night blindness. Hypovitaminosis A in young animals may cause excessive thickening of the skull and the vertebrae with secondary compression of nervous tissue (especially of the cranial nerves as they pass through the foramina). Poor absorption of CSF may result in communicating hydrocephalus. Hypovitaminosis A is rare or rarely recognized in companion animals but has been reported in food animals.[2,18]

Vitamin E

A noninflammatory myopathy may be produced by vitamin E deficiency. Although myopathies are seen fairly often, vitamin E deficiencies are rare in companion animals. Calves and sheep have a myopathy associated with a deficiency in vitamin E and selenium. Swine may die suddenly because of the degeneration of cardiac muscle.

Vitamin B Complex

Deficiencies in all of the B vitamins can cause pathologic changes in both the central and the peripheral nervous systems.

Thiamine deficiency has been reported in dogs, cats, and ruminants. The syndrome in dogs progresses from anorexia to pelvic limb paresis, tetraparesis, seizures, and coma in approximately 1 week.[19,20] Malacia and hemorrhage were found in multiple sites in the brain and the spinal cord, with the most severe lesions in the brain stem. Animals that were treated with thiamine recovered. A peripheral neuropathy with LMN paralysis also has been seen.[2] Cats with a thiamine deficiency often have a characteristic ventral flex-

ion of the head and the neck, sometimes causing the chin to touch the sternum. Ataxia and seizures also may be present. The lesions are similar to those that occur in dogs.[21] The deficiency that was observed in dogs was produced by a diet consisting entirely of cooked meat[19] or a specific thiamine-deficient diet.[20] Cat foods with fish as the primary ingredient contain thiaminase, which has been reported to cause the thiamine deficiency in cats.

Treatment should be instituted immediately for any animal that is suspected of having thiamine deficiency. A dosage of 50 to 100 mg should be given intravenously and should be repeated intramuscularly daily until a response is obtained or another diagnosis is established.

Polioencephalomalacia (symmetric necrosis of the cerebral cortex) is caused by a thiamine deficiency in ruminants. The deficiency is the result of an increased breakdown of thiamine in the rumen. Usually, the animals have been moved from a marginal pasture to a lush pasture or have had some similar change in feeding patterns. Animals less than two years of age are most commonly affected.

Clinical signs are primarily cerebral in origin, including depression, pacing, head pressing, blindness, ataxia, odontoprisis, opisthotonos, and seizures. A dorsomedial strabismus that has been attributed to trochlear nerve (C.N. IV) paralysis has been described. Increased intracranial pressure is common and may lead to tentorial herniation.

A symmetric laminar cortical necrosis is the most prominent pathologic finding. Edema of the brain with flattening of the gyri and herniations may be present.

Measurement of transketolase, the thiamine-dependent coenzyme, is helpful for making a diagnosis. The condition should be treated with thiamine, 5 to 10 mg per kg intravenously bid for at least 3 days. Steroids should be given if CNS signs are severe. Severely affected animals may have permanent cortical damage.[22]

Niacin and riboflavin deficiencies are less common, but since animals with thiamine deficiency also may have deficiencies in these vitamins, multiple B-complex preparations are indicated. The diet should be corrected in order to prevent recurrences.

HYPERVITAMINOSIS

Vitamin A

Increased levels of vitamin A have been reported in cats with diets predominantly of

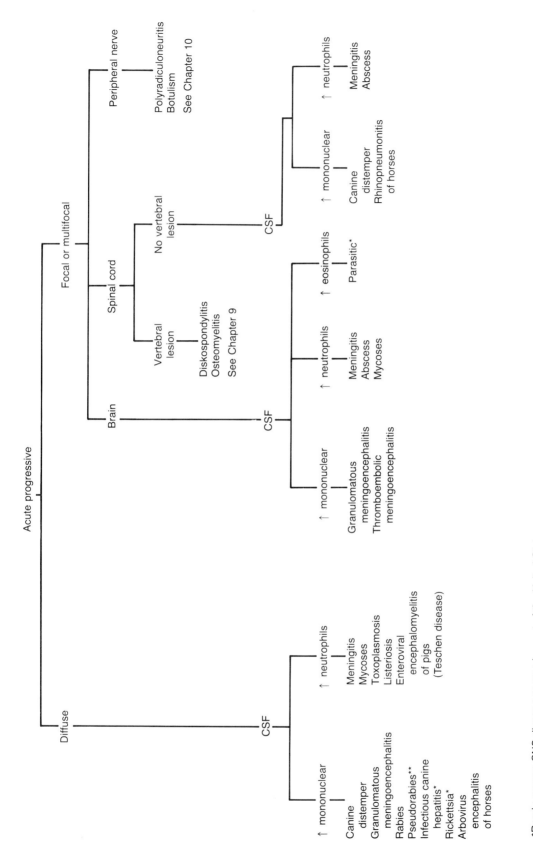

Figure 17–7. Differential diagnosis of inflammatory diseases.
Illustration continued on opposite page

*Rarely causes CNS disease *or* rare in most of the United States

**Rarely causes CNS disease in small animals but not infrequent in food animals

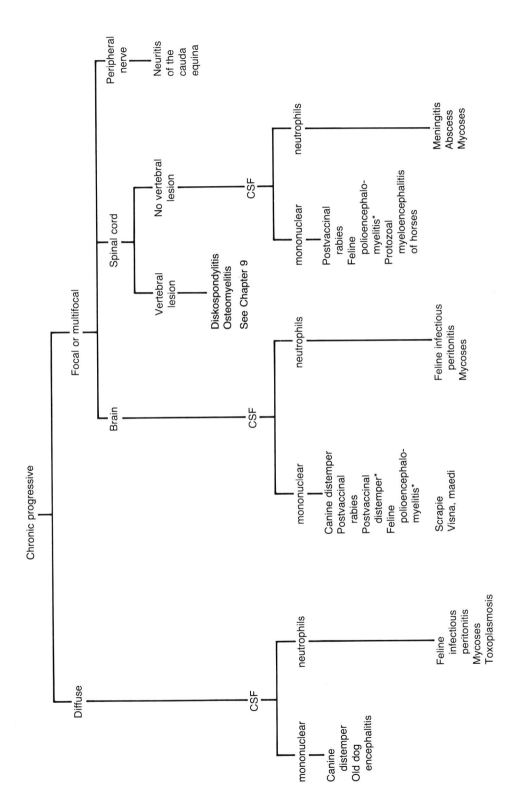

Figure 17-7. *Continued*

*Rarely causes CNS disease or rare in most of the United States

liver. A hypertrophic bone formation on the vertebrae causes an ankylosing spondylosis primarily of the cervical vertebrae but in some cases extending to the lumbar region. The clinical signs primarily are related to the rigidity of the spinal column. Nerve compression occurs in severely affected cats. Alterations in the diet stop the progression of the spondylosis but do not significantly reduce the spondylosis that is present. Anti-inflammatory and analgesic drugs have been recommended, but they must be used with caution, especially in the cat.[2,23]

Inflammatory Diseases

The inflammatory diseases of the nervous system are caused by infectious or parasitic organisms or immune reactions. Canine distemper, feline infectious peritonitis, and bacterial infections, including thromboembolic meningoencephalitis and listeriosis, are common causes of disease. Some of the fungal diseases are common in endemic areas. Most of the other diseases are relatively uncommon, although inflammatory reticulosis and granulomatous meningoencephalomyelitis in dogs are being recognized with increased frequency. Inflammatory diseases are discussed in many textbooks.[2,21–24] The differential diagnosis is outlined in Figure 17–7 and will be discussed in the next section. The more common inflammatory diseases are outlined in Tables 17–14 to 17–21.

DIAGNOSIS

Most of the inflammatory diseases are characterized by an acute onset. All of the inflammatory diseases are progressive. A diffuse or multifocal distribution is characteristic of most of the diseases in this group (Table 17–22). The minimum data base (see Chapter 3) may provide evidence of systemic infection (such as alterations in white blood count), although many primary CNS diseases do not produce a systemic response. Therefore, positive findings in laboratory data are useful, but negative findings do not rule out infectious disease. Focal deficits should be investigated according to the location of the lesion (see Chapters 8 through 16).

CSF analysis is the single most useful test for establishing the diagnosis of inflammatory disease (see Chapter 6). Increases in CSF protein vary from low (50 to 100 mg/dl) in chronic viral diseases to very high (300+ mg/dl) in

bacterial and fungal infections. Characteristic cell changes are: increased mononuclear cells (in viral diseases); increased neutrophils (in bacterial diseases); increased numbers of both mononuclear cells and neutrophils (in mycotic and protozoal diseases and feline infectious peritonitis); and increased numbers of mononuclear cells, neutrophils, and some eosinophils (in parasitic and immune-mediated diseases) (see Fig. 6–1). The presence of neutrophils in the CSF is an indication for bacterial and fungal cultures and bacterial sensitivity tests. Fluorescent antibody techniques on the mononuclear cells in the CSF may be diagnostic of canine distemper.

Toxic Disorders

Toxicities are common in both small and large animals. Many toxic materials produce signs of CNS disorder (many of which are biochemical changes and potentially reversible), whereas others produce structural damage. The more common toxicants are listed in Table 17–23. Toxicologic disorders, including those caused by poisonous plants, are discussed in detail in several books.[2,22,24–27]

DIAGNOSIS

A history of exposure to a toxic agent is the most important factor in the establishment of a diagnosis in cases of poisoning. CNS signs of intoxication include (1) seizures; (2) depression or coma; (3) tremors, ataxia, and paresis; and (4) LMN signs.[27] Animals that present with any of these four signs must be considered as possible poisoning victims until proved otherwise. The primary groups of diseases that are likely to be confused with toxicoses are metabolic disorders and inflammatory diseases.

When an animal presents with signs suggestive of poisoning, the owner must be questioned carefully in an attempt to find a possible source. Animals that present in status epilepticus must be treated immediately, and the history must be obtained later (see Chapter 15). Direct questions regarding agents that are capable of producing the signs must be asked. Owners usually are aware of common agents, such as insecticides and rodenticides, but may have difficulty identifying a source of lead poisoning and may be reluctant to admit a source of drug intoxication.

The clinical signs may be sufficient for the clinician to establish a presumptive diagnosis

Text continued on page 346

Table 17–14. VIRAL DISEASES OF THE CNS[2,12,21–23]

Disease	Cause	Incidence	Clinical Signs and Pathology	Course and Prognosis	Diagnostic Tests	Treatment	Prevention
Canine distemper	Paramyxovirus	Common, dogs	Young dogs: Systemic illness; respiratory, gastrointestinal, and CNS signs. Cerebellum, cerebellar peduncles, optic nerves and tracts, and spinal cord commonly affected. CNS signs may occur early or weeks to months after systemic illness.	Acute to subacute, progressive, poor prognosis if CNS signs	History, EEG, CSF (↑ lymphocytes, ↑ protein), fluorescent antibody (F.A.) (CSF, conjunctiva, peripheral blood), ophthalmoscopy	Supportive antibacterial agents, anticonvulsants	Vaccine
		Common, dogs	Mature dogs: Similar to above or may have CNS disease without systemic illness. May start with focal signs (spinal cord, cerebellum) and progress to involve other areas.	Subacute to chronic, progressive, poor prognosis if CNS signs	History, EEG, CSF (↑ lymphocytes, ↑ protein), ophthalmoscopy	Same	Vaccine
Old dog encephalitis	Distemper virus(?)	Uncommon but not rare, dogs	Mature to older dogs: Cerebral signs at onset (blindness, dementia, head pressing).	Chronic, poor prognosis	History, EEG, ophthalmoscopy, CSF often normal	Supportive	Vaccine
Rabies	Rhabdovirus	Variable, all mammals	Initially behavioral changes. Rapid progression to either furious or dumb form. Furious: restlessness, wandering, biting anything encountered, convulsions. Dumb: progressive paralysis, pharyngeal and hypoglossal paralysis, respiratory paralysis.	Acute, progresses to death in 3 to 8 days from onset	Necropsy: F.A. of brain, mouse inoculation	None	Vaccine

Table continued on following page

Table 17–14. VIRAL DISEASES OF THE CNS [2,12,21-23] *Continued*

Disease	Cause	Incidence	Clinical Signs and Pathology	Course and Prognosis	Diagnostic Tests	Treatment	Prevention
Pseudorabies (Aujeszky's disease)	Herpesvirus	Rare, except in swine	Early excitement, progressing rapidly to coma and death. Intense pruritus and self-mutilation, especially at portal of entry. Dogs and cats usually are infected by eating contaminated pork.	Peracute, progression to death in 1 to 2 days usually.	History, signs, necropsy (F.A.)	None	None available for dogs or cats, vaccine for swine
Infectious canine hepatitis	Canine adenovirus, Type I	Rare CNS, dogs	Affects vascular endothelium, potentially causing signs of CNS disease. Primarily liver, kidney and respiratory signs.	Acute to chronic	Signs, clinical laboratory profile (liver)	Supportive	Vaccine
Feline infectious peritonitis	Coronavirus	Relatively common, cats	Two forms: wet (diffuse, fibrinous peritonitis) and dry (disseminated pyogranulomatous lesions in viscera, CNS, and eye). Dry form may have only CNS signs, which may be focal in onset. Meningeal involvement is common.	Slowly progressive, invariably fatal	Signs, clinical laboratory profile (WBC, neutrophils, plasma protein >8 gm/dl), ↑ globulin, ocular lesions, CSF (↑ protein, ↑ cells, neutrophils or mixed), antibody titer	Supportive	None
Postvaccinal rabies	Inadequately attenuated virus in vaccine	Rare, more common in cats	Progressive ascending paralysis to diffuse meningoencephalomyelitis.	Acute onset, rapid progression, poor prognosis	History, necropsy	None	Use proper vaccine

Disease	Cause	Occurrence	Signs	Course	Diagnosis	Treatment	Prevention
Postvaccinal canine distemper	Inadequately attenuated virus in vaccine(?)	Rare, usually young dogs	Usually occurs 1 to 2 weeks after vaccination. Behavioral changes common. Ataxia, depression, seizures have been reported. Brain stem lesions predominate.	Acute, poor prognosis	History, necropsy	None	None
Encephalitis	Arbovirus	Variable, horses, dogs	Depression, fever, anorexia, lack of coordination, pacing, circling. Primarily cerebral signs.	Acute progressive, recovery variable, may be permanent brain damage	History, CSF, serology, virus isolation	Supportive	Vaccine
Enteroviral encephalomyelitis	Enterovirus	Variable, swine	Pelvic limb ataxia and paresis, paralysis, seizures.	Acute progressive, recovery or progression to death in 1 to 3 weeks	History, virus isolation, serology	Supportive	Vaccine
Rhinopneumonitis	Herpesvirus	Rare, horses	Upper respiratory infection in other horses. Ataxia, cauda equina signs, tetraplegia or paraplegia.	Acute progressive, may progress to recovery or severe signs in 24 hours	History, CSF (xanthochromia, mononuclear pleocytosis, increased protein)	Supportive, corticosteroids	Vaccine
Scrapie	"Slow" virus	Sporadic, sheep >2 years old	Pruritus, ataxia, death. Neuronal and spongiform degeneration of brain.	Chronic progressive, always fatal	History and signs, histopathology	None	None
Visna, maedi	Virus	Variable, sheep >2 years old	Pelvic limb paresis, tremors of lip, progressive paralysis.	Chronic progressive, usually fatal	History, signs, CSF (↑ cells, lymphocytes), histopathology, virus isolation	None	None
Malignant catarrhal fever	Herpesvirus	Sporadic, adult cattle	Depression, blindness, pacing, seizures, death. Nasal and ocular discharge.	Acute progressive, usually fatal	History and signs, histopathology	None	None

Table 17–15. BACTERIAL DISEASES OF THE CNS

Disease	Cause	Incidence	Clinical Signs and Pathology	Course and Prognosis	Diagnostic Tests	Treatment
Meningitis	*Staphylococcus* species, *Pasteurella* species, and others	Uncommon	Generalized or localized (especially cervical) hyperesthesia. Degree of illness variable. Temperature and white blood count may be normal.	Usually acute onset, but may be chronic, prognosis is good with early treatment	CSF (protein often over 200 mg/dl, ↑ cells, primarily neutrophils), culture and sensitivity testing	Antibiotics according to sensitivity, ampicillin, chloramphenicol, trimethoprim
Meningoencephalomyelitis	As in meningitis	Uncommon	As in meningitis, but in addition, signs of brain or spinal cord disease. Often includes blindness, seizures, ataxia, cranial nerve deficits.	Usually acute; prognosis is good with early treatment, but neurologic deficits are common	Same as meningitis, EEG may indicate encephalitis	Same as for meningitis—seizures: diazepam, phenobarbital; acute cerebral edema: mannitol
Abscess	As in meningitis	Rare	May have focal signs or focal signs plus signs of meningitis or meningoencephalitis.	May be chronic, progression may be rapid once signs are obvious	Same as meningoencephalitis	Same as for meningoencephalitis
Vertebral osteomyelitis, diskospondylitis	*Staphylococcus* species, *Brucella canis*, others	Moderately frequent	Pain, usually focal. May or may not have spinal cord compression. Usually clinically ill, often over weeks to months.	Chronic, may become acute when spinal cord is compressed	Radiography, myelography, *Brucella* test	Antibiotics, preferably bactericidal, curretage, decompression if spinal cord is compressed

Disease	Organism	Occurrence	Signs	Course	Diagnosis	Treatment
Tetanus	*Clostridium tetani*	Rare, except in horses	Extensor rigidity of all limbs, often with opisthotonos. Contraction of facial muscles, prolapsed membrana nictitans. Usually an infected wound.	Acute onset, often lasts 1 to 2 weeks, animal may die, prognosis fair if treated	Signs, isolation of *Clostridium* from infected wound	Penicillin, tetanus antitoxin, tranquilizers or muscle relaxants, quiet environment, treat wound, nursing
Botulism	*Clostridium botulinum*	Moderately frequent	LMN-type paralysis, often beginning in pelvic limbs, progressing to tetraparesis in less than 24 hours. Caused by a toxin blocking the neuromuscular junction.	Acute onset, lasts about 2 weeks, good prognosis unless respiratory paralysis is present	Serum, fecal analysis, history, EMG and nerve conduction velocity (NCV)	Enemas and laxatives early, supportive care, antitoxin usually not effective
Thromboembolic meningoencephalitis	*Hemophilus somnus*	Young calves, cold weather, feedlots	Fever, depression, ataxia, lack of coordination, cranial nerve signs.	Acute progressive, animal may recover with treatment	History, CSF (↑ protein, ↑ neutrophils), culture, serology	Antibiotics, vaccine available
Listeriosis	*Listeria monocytogenes*	Sporadic in ruminants, winter and spring	Depression, asymmetric ataxia and paresis, cranial nerve signs, central vestibular signs.	Acute progressive in sheep and goats, more chronic in cattle, poor prognosis if CNS signs are present	History, CSF (↑ protein, ↑ mononuclear cells), histopathology, fluorescent antibody, isolation	Antibiotics, supportive care

Table 17–16. MYCOTIC DISEASES OF THE CNS

Disease	Cause	Incidence	Clinical Signs and Pathology	Course and Prognosis	Diagnostic Tests	Treatment
Cryptococcosis	*Cryptococcus neoformans*	Low, primarily in eastern and midwestern states, but reported throughout United States	Nose and sinuses usually are infected with extension to brain. Ocular lesions and blindness common. CNS involvement common.	Chronic, poor prognosis	Smears and culture of exudate, serum titers, CSF (↑ protein ↑ cells, neutrophils, and mononuclear cells)	Amphotericin B and 5-fluorocytosine
Blastomycosis	*Blastomyces dermatitidis*	Low, primarily in eastern and midwestern states	Rarely involves CNS. Pyogranulomatous encephalitis or single or multifocal granulomas are seen. Frequently involves lungs, skin, and eyes.	Chronic, poor prognosis	See *Cryptococcosis*	Amphotericin B
Histoplasmosis	*Histoplasma capsulatum*	Low, primarily in central United States	CNS involvement uncommon. Involves reticuloendothelial cells of most viscera.	Chronic, poor prognosis	See *Cryptococcosis*	Amphotericin B
Coccidioidomycosis	*Coccidioides immitis*	Low, primarily in southwestern United States	CNS involvement rare. Pulmonary infection common.	Chronic, poor prognosis	See *Cryptococcosis*	Amphotericin B, ketoconizole
Nocardiosis	*Nocardia* species	Low, throughout United States	Systemic disease similar to canine distemper, respiratory or cutaneous forms. CNS abscesses and vertebral osteomyelitis reported.	Chronic, poor prognosis	Smears, cultures. CSF (↑ protein, ↑ cells, neutrophils)	Penicillin, sulfonamides, trimethoprim
Actinomycosis	*Actinomyces* species	Low, throughout United States	Similar to nocardiosis.	Chronic, poor prognosis	Similar to nocardiosis	Penicillin, clindamycin, erythromycin, lincomycin
Paecilomycosis	*Paecilomyces* species	Rare	Disseminated form or diskospondylitis.	Chronic, poor prognosis	Culture, biopsy	?

Table 17–17. PROTOZOAL DISEASES OF THE CNS

Disease	Cause	Incidence	Clinical Signs and Pathology	Course and Prognosis	Diagnostic Tests	Treatment
Toxoplasmosis	*Toxoplasma gondii*	Common infection but infrequent clinical problem	Clinical manifestation usually associated with another disease, such as distemper. CNS, eyes, lungs, gastrointestinal tract and skeletal muscle often affected.	Chronic, fair to poor prognosis	Serum titer, oocysts in stool, biopsy, CSF (↑ protein, ↑ cells: mononuclear cells and neutrophils)	Sulfadiazine and pyrimethamine
Babesiosis	*Babesia canis*	Rare in United States	Parasite of RBC. Rarely causes CNS disease, primarily infarction and hemorrhage. More severe with other infections, such as *Ehrlichia*.	Acute to chronic, poor prognosis	Peripheral blood smears	Berenil and phenmidine
Encephalitozoonosis	*Encephalitozoon cuniculi*	Rare, primarily affects dogs <2 months old	Causes acute encephalitis, ataxia, tumors, behavior changes.	Acute, poor prognosis	None available clinically— serum titers, culture, necropsy	None
Trypanosomiasis	*Trypanosoma cruzi*	Rare in United States	Parasite of RBC disease. Rarely causes CNS disease.	Chronic, fair prognosis	Peripheral blood smears	Diamines, dimedium, quinapyramines
Equine protozoal myeloencephalitis	Probably *Sarcocystis*	Uncommon, horses	Ataxia, paresis, may involve LMN of brachial or lumbosacral plexus and cranial nerves. Multifocal.	Chronic progressive, usually poor prognosis, treatment may arrest progression	History, CSF (↑ mononuclear cells), histopathology	Sulfas and pyrimethamine

Table 17–18. RICKETTSIAL DISEASES OF THE CNS

Disease	Cause	Incidence	Clinical Signs and Pathology	Course and Prognosis	Diagnostic Tests	Treatment
Canine ehrlichiosis	*Ehrlichia canis*	Uncommon in United States, German shepherd more susceptible	CNS signs are unusual. A few animals have CNS and meningeal hemorrhage and nonsuppurative encephalitis or meningitis.	Acute to chronic, fair to good prognosis if treated early	Pancytopenia (WBC), serum titer	Tetracycline
Salmon poisoning	*Neorickettsia helminthoeca*	Rare, Pacific Northwest region	Depression and convulsions terminally. Paresis of pelvic limbs less common. Nonsuppurative meningoencephalitis.	Acute, fair to good prognosis if treated early	History of eating salmon, fluke eggs in feces	Tetracycline
Rocky Mountain spotted fever	*Rickettsia rickettsii*	Rare, regions with *Dermacentor* species ticks	CNS signs unusual. Ataxia, nystagmus, depression.	Acute, good prognosis with treatment	Serum titer	Tetracycline
Sporadic bovine encephalomyelitis (Buss disease)	*Chlamydia psittaci*	Sporadic, young cattle	Respiratory disease, polyarthritis, diffuse cerebral signs.	Acute progressive, mortality approximately 50%	History, CSF ($\uparrow$ protein, $\uparrow$ mononuclear cells), serology	Tetracycline

Table 17–19. PARASITIC DISEASES OF THE CNS IN THE DOG AND THE CAT

Disease	Cause	Incidence	Clinical Signs and Pathology	Course and Prognosis	Diagnostic Tests	Treatment
Dirofilariasis	*Dirofilaria immitis*, microfilaria or abberant adult	Rare, areas with heartworm disease	CNS signs are rare. Microfilaria or migrating adult heartworm may cause infarction. Seizures and other cerebral signs.	Acute onset, prognosis poor	Knott test to confirm heartworm disease, CSF (↑ protein, ↑ cells: some eosinophils would be suggestive), impossible to prove antemortem	None proved
Larva migrans	*Toxocara canis*, larvae	Rare	Granulomas in brain from migrating larvae. Signs related to location of lesions.	Acute or chronic, prognosis dependent on severity of signs	None, necropsy CSF (↑ eosinophils suggestive)	None
Cuterebra	*Cuterebra* species, larvae	Rare	CNS signs depend on location of lesion.	Acute to chronic, prognosis poor	None, necropsy CSF (↑ eosinophils suggestive)	None
Coenurosis	*Coenurus* species cyst	Rare	CNS signs depend on location of lesion.	Acute to chronic, prognosis poor	None, necropsy CSF (↑ eosinophils suggestive)	None

Table 17–20. IMMUNE-MEDIATED DISEASES OF THE CNS IN DOGS AND CATS

Disease	Cause	Incidence	Clinical Signs and Pathology	Course and Prognosis	Diagnostic Tests	Treatment
Coon-hound paralysis	Probable immune reaction to virus in raccoon saliva or environment	Fairly high in some areas, dogs	Ascending LMN paralysis. May last approximately 6 weeks. Ventral roots and peripheral nerves have segmental demyelination and some axon loss.	Acute onset, lasts approximately 6 weeks, good prognosis with good nursing	History, EMG and NCV	Supportive
Postvaccinal rabies	CNS tissues in vaccine	Rare—these vaccines no longer are used	Ascending paralysis. Demyelination from immune reaction to myelin in brain-origin vaccines.	Acute onset, progressive, poor prognosis	None	None

Table 17–21. UNCLASSIFIED INFLAMMATORY DISEASES OF THE CNS IN THE DOG AND THE CAT

Disease	Cause	Incidence	Clinical Signs and Pathology	Course and Prognosis	Diagnostic Tests	Treatment
Inflammatory reticulosis	Unknown	Probably common	Differentiation of inflammatory and neoplastic reticulosis is controversial. Produces mass lesions as well as perivascular infiltrates. May produce focal, multifocal or, more rarely, disseminated signs. Cerebrum and rostral brain stem commonly are affected.	Acute to chronic, prognosis poor	CSF (↑ protein, ↑ mononuclear cells), anaplastic reticulum cells are diagnostic	Steroids may be beneficial but not curative
Granulomatous meningo-encephalomyelitis	Unknown	Probably common	Differentiation from inflammatory reticulosis not resolved. Tends to be disseminated, rather than focal or multifocal. More acute. Brain stem commonly is affected. Meningeal signs often are present.	Acute with rapid progression, prognosis poor	CSF (↑ protein, ↑ mononuclear cells)	Steroids may be beneficial but not curative
Feline polioencephalomyelitis	Unknown	Unknown	Pelvic limb ataxia and paresis progressive to brain signs. Spinal cord neurons and white matter are predominantly affected. Brain lesions scattered.	Chronic, prognosis poor	EEG, CSF	None
Polioencephalomalacia	Unknown—some may be viral, metabolic, toxic, or nutritional	Uncommon, dogs and other species	Variable cerebral signs. Necrosis of cerebral cortex.	Variable, usually chronic progressive	Histopathology	None
Neuritis of the cauda equina	Unknown—possibly viral (herpes) or sarcocysts	Sporadic in horses	LMN signs of cauda equina. Cranial nerves may be affected.	Chronic progressive, prognosis poor	History, CSF (lumbar tap, ↑ protein, ↑ neutrophils), necropsy	None

Table 17–22. DISTRIBUTION OF LESIONS AND CLINICAL SIGNS IN INFLAMMATORY DISEASES

Disease	Diffuse	Focal or Multifocal
Viral	Most	Feline infectious peritonitis, postvaccinal rabies, herpesvirus (horses)
Bacterial	Meningitis, meningoencephalomyelitis, tetanus, botulism, thromboembolic meningoencephalitis	Abscess, diskospondylitis, listeriosis
Mycotic	Most	
Protozoal	Most	Toxoplasmosis, protozoal myeloencephalitis of horses
Rickettsial	Most	
Parasitic		Most
Immune-mediated	Late	Early
Unclassified	Granulomatous meningoencephalomyelitis, polioencephalomalacia of dogs	Inflammatory reticulosis, feline polioencephalomyelitis

Table 17–23. COMMON TOXICANTS

Use	Toxicant	Primary Effect
Pesticides	Chlorinated hydrocarbons	CNS stimulation
	Organophosphates	Binding of acetylcholinesterase
	Metaldehyde	CNS stimulation
	Arsenic	Gastrointestinal irritation
Rodenticides	Strychnine	Blocking of inhibitory interneurons
	Thallium	Gastrointestinal irritation, CNS stimulation, peripheral neuropathy, skin lesion
	Alphanaphthyl thiourea (ANTU)	Gastrointestinal irritation, pulmonary edema, depression, coma
	Sodium fluoroacetate (1080)	CNS stimulation
	Warfarin	Anticoagulation
	Zinc phosphide	Gastrointestinal irritation, depression
	Phosphorus	Gastrointestinal irritation, CNS stimulation, depression, coma
Herbicides and fungicides	Numerous	Gastrointestinal irritation, CNS depression: some are stimulants
Heavy metals	Lead (see *Arsenic* and *Thallium* above)	Gastrointestinal irritation, CNS stimulation, or depression
Drugs	Narcotics	CNS depression
	Amphetamines	CNS stimulation
	Barbiturates	CNS depression
	Tranquilizers	CNS depression
	Aspirin	Gastrointestinal irritation, coma
	Marijuana	Abnormal behavior, depression
	Anthelmintics	CNS stimulation
Garbage	Staphylococcal toxin	Gastrointestinal irritation, CNS stimulation
	Botulinus toxin	LMN paralysis
Poisonous plants	Various	Various
Antifreeze	Ethylene glycol	Gastrointestinal irritation, CNS depression, renal failure
Soap	Hexachlorophene	CNS depression or stimulation, tremors
Animal origin	Snake bite	Necrotizing wound, shock, CNS depression
	Toad (*Bufo* species)	Digitoxin-like action, CNS stimulation
	Lizards	Gastrointestinal irritation, CNS stimulation or depression
	Tick paralysis (*Dermacentor* species)	LMN paralysis

(for example, intoxication from strychnine and organophosphates). Other agents, such as lead and drugs, may require laboratory confirmation (Tables 17–24 through 17–27).

Toxicants Causing Seizures

The most common sign of poisoning in small animals is seizures (see Table 17–24). The animal may present with continuous or closely spaced convulsions (e.g., from organophosphates or strychnine) or with a history of intermittent seizures (e.g., from lead). Animals in status epilepticus must be treated immediately, or they will die (see Chapter 15).

The tetany produced by strychnine is easily differentiated from the seizures produced by the other agents in this group. In spite of the severe muscle spasms, the animal is conscious. Tetany caused by strychnine may be confused with hypocalcemic tetany that is seen in nursing bitches or with tetanus. Intravenous calcium provides immediate relief in cases of hypocalcemia. Tetanus is much slower in onset than is strychnine poisoning. Seizures from other agents produce clonus (alternate flexion and extension).

Organophosphates may be distinguished from chlorinated hydrocarbons by their profound effect on the autonomic nervous system, including profuse salivation, constricted pupils, and diarrhea. Chlorinated hydrocarbons frequently produce fine muscle fasciculations, even between seizures.

CNS signs of lead intoxication are seen most often in cases of chronic exposure. The seizures are intermittent. The differential diagnosis of recurrent seizure disorders has been discussed in Chapter 15. A laboratory analysis of the blood for evidence of lead is diagnostic.

The other intoxicants causing seizures are seen infrequently.

Toxicant Causing Depression or Coma

Depression or coma may be seen with almost any poison in the terminal stages. Drugs, such as narcotics, barbiturates, and tranquilizers, are the most frequent cause of depression or coma as the primary problem (see Table 17–25). The diagnosis may be easy if the source is known (such as in cases of accidental overdosing with an anticonvulsant or of an animal that ate a bottle of the owner's tranquilizers). Reports of animals that have ingested "street" drugs are increasing, and the owner is usually reluctant to admit the source of the intoxication in these cases. A laboratory

analysis of blood or urine may be necessary in order to confirm the diagnosis.

Toxicants Causing Tremors, Ataxia, and Paresis

Chronic organophosphate poisoning from the use of flea collars and topical or systemic insecticides frequently causes signs that are suggestive of cerebellar disease or muscle weakness (see Table 17–26). The finding of weakness is not consistent with pure cerebellar disease, so when both are present, poisoning must be considered. Chronic lead poisoning also may cause tremors and ataxia (see Chapter 11).

Hexachlorophene toxicity has been seen in puppies with signs of tremors and ataxia. Severe depression may follow. The usual source has been repeated washing of the bitch's mammary glands with a soap containing hexachlorophene. Bathing young dogs or cats of any age in hexachlorophene soap also has produced the syndrome.

Metaldehyde poisoning, which produces tremors and ataxia progressing to depression and coma, is seen frequently in areas in which the substance is used for snail bait.

Toxicants Causing LMN Signs

Botulism and tick paralysis cause a generalized LMN paralysis by blockade of the neuromuscular junction (see Table 17–27). These conditions have been discussed in Chapter 10.

Some drugs (such as the nitrofurans) and some chronic toxicities (such as lead and arsenic poisoning) may produce peripheral neuropathies. Other signs usually predominate, however.

TREATMENT

Removal of the toxic substance is the most important part of the treatment for many toxicities. Agents that have entered the animal's system through the skin, such as insecticides, should be removed by thorough washing and rinsing. Ingested agents may be removed by inducing emesis, performing gastric lavage, or administering laxatives or enemas. Activated charcoal is an effective adsorbing agent.

Status epilepticus is a life-threatening emergency and must be treated accordingly (see Chapter 15).

Specific treatments for the various toxicities are outlined in Tables 17–24 through 17–27. The reader should consult the references for details.[2,22,24–27]

Text continued on page 351

Table 17–24. COMMON TOXICANTS CAUSING SEIZURES

Toxicants	Diagnosis	Management	Prognosis
Chlorinated hydrocarbons	Exposure. Muscle fasciculations common. Laboratory confirmation difficult.	Removal of toxicant—washing, gastric lavage. Sedation or anesthesia with barbiturates.	Poor with seizures
Organophosphates and carbamates	Exposure. Salivation, diarrhea, constricted pupils, muscle weakness. Blood cholinesterase level decreased. Tissue analysis poor.	Removal of toxicant. Atropine. Pralidoxime chloride (2-PAM) (not for carbamates).	Good if treated early
Strychnine	Exposure. Tetany without loss of consciousness, increased by stimulation or noise. Laboratory analysis of stomach contents, urine, tissues.	Removal of toxicant—gastric lavage or emesis. Sedation—barbiturates. Respiratory support if needed.	Good if treated early
Sodium fluoroacetate (1080)	Exposure. Seizures are clonic as compared with those in cases of strychnine. Laboratory confirmation difficult.	Removal of toxicant. Sedation—barbiturates.	Poor with seizures
Thallium	Exposure, gastrointestinal signs, seizures only in severe poisonings. Laboratory analysis of urine, tissues.	Removal of toxicant. Dithenylthiocarbazone (Dithion) early. Ferric ferrocyanide (Prussian Blue) late.	Poor with seizures, fair with other signs, good with treatment
Lead	Exposure (may be difficult to document). Chronic intoxication may cause intermittent seizures, behavioral change, tremors, gastrointestinal signs. Blood lead level >0.4 part per million. Basophilic stippling and anemia may be present.	Removal of toxicant. Calcium EDTA.	Good with treatment
Staphylococcal toxin	Exposure to garbage. Severe gastrointestinal signs. Isolation of toxins and testing in laboratory animals.	Removal of toxicant. Sedation.	Poor with seizures, animals usually die rapidly
Toad (*Bufo* species); reported only in southern Florida	Exposure. Severe buccal irritation.	Wash mouth. Sedation—anesthesia.	Fair if treated within 15 to 30 minutes, otherwise poor
Amphetamines	Exposure, medicinals or "street" drugs. Hyperactivity, dilated pupils. Analysis of urine for amphetamine.	Removal of toxicant. Sedation or anesthesia—barbiturates.	Good if treated early
Zinc phosphide	Exposure, rodenticide. Behavioral changes, hysteria followed by convulsions. Gastrointestinal irritation. Laboratory analysis of stomach contents and tissues.	Removal of toxicant. Oral and intravenous sodium bicarbonate. Sedation—barbiturates.	Poor

Table 17–25. COMMON TOXICANTS CAUSING CNS DEPRESSION OR COMA

Toxicants	Diagnosis	Management	Prognosis
Drugs— narcotics, barbiturates, tranquilizers, marijuana	Degree of depression depends on dose. Source of pharmaceuticals or "street" drugs. Laboratory analysis of blood or urine.	Removal of toxicant, narcotic antagonists, diuresis, support respiration	Good with treatment
Alphanaphthyl thiourea (ANTU)	Exposure. Pulmonary edema. Depression and coma terminal. Laboratory analysis of stomach contents and tissues.	Removal of toxicant, treatment of pulmonary edema	Poor
Ethylene glycol	Exposure. Gastrointestinal tract irritation, renal failure. Oxalate crystals in urine.	Intravenous ethanol (20%), sodium bicarbonate to correct acidosis	Poor if coma, fair to good otherwise
Many poisons produce coma terminally			

Table 17–26. COMMON TOXICANTS CAUSING TREMORS, ATAXIA, OR PARESIS

Toxicants	Diagnosis	Management	Prognosis
Hexachlorophene	Exposure. Usually young, nursing animal. Large dose causes gastrointestinal irritation, severe depression. Chronic exposure causes cerebellar signs and CNS edema.	Removal of toxicant, supportive care. Treatment for cerebral edema might be beneficial.	Fair, may be residual deficits
Metaldehyde	Exposure, snail bait. Progresses from tremors and ataxia to coma. Laboratory analysis of stomach contents.	Removal of toxicant. Sedation or anesthesia. Support respiration.	Fair
Lead	Chronic lead poisoning may produce cerebellar signs, dementia, and so forth. See Table 17–24.	See Table 17–24.	Good
Organophosphates	Chronic low doses (flea collar, dips) may produce tremors and muscle weakness. See Table 17–24.	See Table 17–24.	Good
Chlorinated hydrocarbons	Low-dose exposure may produce weakness and muscle fasciculations. See Table 17–24.	See Table 17–24.	Fair to good
Tranquilizers	Ataxia common with tranquilizers. See Table 17–25.	None needed.	Good
Marijuana	Behavioral changes and ataxia common.	Removal of toxicant.	Good
Ergot alkaloids	Cattle and other herbivores grazing on Dallis grass or Ryegrass. Ataxia, uncoordinated gait.	Removal from pasture.	Good
Nitro-bearing plants, e.g., *Astragalus* species locoweed	Cattle, sheep, and horses. Ataxia, weakness or hyperexcitability, death.	Removal from pasture.	Fair in ruminants, may be permanent CNS damage
Yellow star thistle	Horses have an acute onset of rigidity of muscles of mastication. Ataxia, circling, and pacing may occur. Lesions are necrosis of the globus pallidus and the substantia nigra.	No treatment known.	Poor

Table 17–27. COMMON TOXICANTS CAUSING LMN SIGNS

Toxicant	Diagnosis	Management	Prognosis
Botulinus toxin	Exposure to contaminated food, carrion, and so forth. Ascending LMN paralysis. See Chapter 10.	See Chapter 10	Good
Tick paralysis (*Dermacentor* species)	Presence of ticks. Ascending LMN paralysis. See Chapter 10.	Removal of ticks, see Chapter 10	Good
Drug reaction (nitrofurantoins, and so forth)	Exposure.	Removal of source	Fair
Cyanide (from Sorghum or Sudan grass)	Cauda equina syndrome with dysuria, flaccid anus and tail, prolapsed penis. May progress to paraplegia. Usually occurs in horses.	No treatment available.	Poor

CASE HISTORIES

This chapter covers systemic and multifocal diseases, so you should expect these cases to involve the same disorders. However, since this is the last chapter, we might include something else to be sure you have learned the process of making a neurologic diagnosis!

Case History 17A

Signalment

Canine, German shepherd, male, 10 months old.

History

Vaccinations were given on schedule. The dog had a "cold" 6 weeks ago, which lasted for 1 week. One week ago, the owner noticed a lack of coordination and falling to the left side. Yesterday, the dog developed a head tilt to the left side.

Physical Examination

No abnormalities.

Neurologic Examination *

A. Observation
  1. Mental status: Depressed.
  2. Posture: Head tilt to left.
  3. Gait: Ataxia. The dog stumbles on the left thoracic limb at times.
B. Palpation
C. Postural Reactions

Left	Reactions	Right
	Proprioceptive positioning	
+1	PL	+2
+1	TL	+2
NE	Wheelbarrowing	NE
+1	Hopping, PL	+2
+1	Hopping, TL	+2
+1	Extensor postural thrust	+2
0 to +1	Hemistand-hemiwalk	+2
NE	Tonic neck	NE
	Placing, tactile	
+1	PL	+2
+1	TL	+2
	Placing, visual	
+1	PL	+2
+1	TL	+2

*Key: 0 = absent, +1 = decreased, +2 = normal, +3 = exaggerated, +4 = very exaggerated or clonus, PL = pelvic limb, TL = thoracic limb, NE = not evaluated.
†Nystagmus changes to vertical when the head is elevated.

D. Spinal Reflexes

Left	Reflex / Spinal Segment	Right
+3	Quadriceps L4−L6	+2
+2	Extensor carpi radialis C7−T1	+2
+2	Triceps C7−T1	+2
+2	Flexion, PL L5−S1	+2
+2	Flexion, TL C6−T1	+2
0	Crossed extensor	0
+2	Perineal S1−S2	+2

E. Cranial Nerves

Left	Nerve + Function	Right
+2	C.N. II vision menace	+2
+2	C.N. II + C.N. III pupil size	+2
+2	Stim. left eye	+2
+2	Stim. right eye	+2
NE	C.N. II fundus	NE
+2	C.N. III, C.N. IV, C.N. VI Strabismus	+2
Horizontal†	Nystagmus	Fast phase right
+2	C.N. V sensation	+2
+2	C.N. V mastication	+2
+2	C.N. VII facial muscles	+2
+2	Palpebral	+2
+2	C.N. IX, C.N. X swallowing	+2
+2	C.N. XII tongue	+2

F. Sensation: Location
  Hyperesthesia The dog resents palpation of the neck
  Superficial pain   +2
  Deep pain   +2

Complete sections G and H before reviewing Case Summary.
G. Assessment (Anatomic diagnosis and estimation of prognosis)

H. Plan (Diagnostic)
  Rule-outs   Procedure
  1.
  2.
  3.
  4.

Case History 17B

Signalment

Yorkshire terrier litter: two female puppies, one male puppy, 4 weeks old.

History

Second litter of a 3-year-old bitch. The sire is different from that of the first litter. The bitch was the only dog in the household. One week ago, the puppies were observed shaking. The condition progressed to coarse muscular twitching. The puppies are still nursing. The bitch is in good health and has had all immunizations. No vaccinations were given during pregnancy.

Physical Examination

Normal.

Neurologic Examination *

A. Observation
  1. Mental status: Alert.
  2. Posture: Generalized tremor, worse when the puppies are active, usually stops when they are at rest.
  3. Gait: Dysmetria.
B. Palpation
  Normal.
C. Postural Reactions

Left	Reactions	Right
	Proprioceptive positioning	
Dysmetric	PL	Dysmetric
	TL	
	Wheelbarrowing	
	Hopping, PL	
	Hopping, TL	
	Extensor postural thrust	
	Hemistand-hemiwalk	
	Tonic neck	
	Placing, tactile PL	
	TL	
	Placing, visual PL	
	TL	

Key: 0 = absent, +1 = decreased, +2 = normal, +3 = exaggerated, +4 = very exaggerated or clonus, PL = pelvic limb, TL = thoracic limb.

D. Spinal Reflexes

Left	Reflex Spinal Segment	Right
+2	Quadriceps L4—L6	+2
	Extensor carpi radialis C7—T1	
	Triceps C7—T1	
	Flexion, PL L5—S1	
	Flexion, TL C6—T1	
	Crossed extensor	
	Perineal S1—S2	

E. Cranial Nerves

Left	Nerve + Function	Right
+2	C.N. II vision menace	+2
	C.N. II + C.N. III pupil size	
	Stim. left eye	
	Stim. right eye	
	C.N. II fundus	
	C.N. III, C.N. IV, C.N. VI Strabismus	
	Nystagmus	
	C.N. V sensation	
	C.N. V mastication	
	C.N. VII facial muscles	
	Palpebral	
	C.N. IX, C.N. X swallowing	
	C.N. XII tongue	

F. Sensation: Location

Hyperesthesia	No
Superficial pain	+2
Deep pain	+2

Complete sections G and H before reviewing Case Summary.

G. Assessment (Anatomic diagnosis and estimation of prognosis)

H. Plan (Diagnostic)

Rule-outs	Procedure
1.	
2.	
3.	
4.	

Case History 17C

Signalment

Canine, Doberman pinscher, male, 3 years old.

History

Intermittent lameness for several weeks.

Physical Examination

Neurologic Examination *

A. Observation
1. Mental status: Alert.
2. Posture: Normal.
3. Gait: The dog walks gingerly, as if he does not want to bear weight. Slight sway of pelvis.

B. Palpation

C. Postural Reactions

Left	Reactions	Right
+2	Proprioceptive positioning PL	+2
	TL	
	Wheelbarrowing	
	Hopping, PL	
	Hopping, TL	
	Extensor postural thrust	
	Hemistand-hemiwalk	
	Tonic neck	
	Placing, tactile PL	
	TL	
	Placing, visual PL	
	TL	

D. Spinal Reflexes

Left	Reflex Spinal Segment	Right
+2	Quadriceps L4–L6	+2
	Extensor carpi radialis C7–T1	
	Triceps C7–T1	
	Flexion, PL L5–S1	
	Flexion, TL C6–T1	
	Crossed extensor	
	Perineal S1–S2	

E. Cranial Nerves

Left	Nerve + Function	Right
+2	C.N. II vision menace	+2
	C.N. II + C.N. III pupil size	
	Stim. left eye	
	Stim. right eye	
	C.N. II fundus	
	C.N. III, C.N. IV, C.N. VI Strabismus	
	Nystagmus	
	C.N. V sensation	
	C.N. V mastication	
	C.N. VII facial muscles	
	Palpebral	
	C.N. IX, C.N. X swallowing	
	C.N. XII tongue	

F. Sensation: Location
Hyperesthesia _____
Superficial pain _____
Deep pain _____
Complete sections G and H before reviewing Case Summary.
G. Assessment (Anatomic diagnosis and estimation of prognosis)

H. Plan (Diagnostic)
Rule-outs   Procedure
1.
2.
3.
4.

*Key: 0 = absent, +1 = decreased, +2 = normal, +3 = exaggerated, +4 = very exaggerated or clonus, PL = pelvic limb, TL = thoracic limb.

Case History 17D

Signalment

English pointer, male, 6 years old.

History

The dog has been depressed and ataxic for 1 week. His appetite is poor. Vaccinations are current.

Physical Examination

The dog is depressed and thin.

Neurologic Examination *

A. Observation
1. Mental status: Alert.
2. Posture: Normal.
3. Gait: Slight truncal ataxia.

B. Palpation
Normal.

C. Postural Reactions

Left	Reactions	Right
+2	Proprioceptive positioning PL	+2
+2	TL	+2
+2	Wheelbarrowing	+2
+1	Hopping, PL	+1
+1	Hopping, TL	+1
+2	Extensor postural thrust	+2
+2	Hemistand-hemiwalk	+2
NE	Tonic neck	NE
+2	Placing, tactile PL	+2
+2	TL	+2
+2	Placing, visual PL	+2
+2	TL	+2

D. Spinal Reflexes

Left	Reflex Spinal Segment	Right
+2	Quadriceps L4–L6	+2
	Extensor carpi radialis C7–T1	
	Triceps C7–T1	
	Flexion, PL L5–S1	
	Flexion, TL C6–T1	
	Crossed extensor	
	Perineal S1–S2	

E. Cranial Nerves

Left	Nerve + Function	Right
+2	C.N. II vision menace	+2
	C.N. II + C.N. III pupil size	
	Stim. left eye	
	Stim. right eye	
	C.N. II fundus	
	C.N. III, C.N. IV, C.N. VI Strabismus	
	Nystagmus	
	C.N. V sensation	
	C.N. V mastication	
	C.N. VII facial muscles	
	Palpebral	
	C.N. IX, C.N. X swallowing	
	C.N. XII tongue	

F. Sensation: Location

Hyperesthesia	Resists turning of neck
Superficial pain	+2
Deep pain	+2

Complete sections G and H before reviewing Case Summary.

G. Assessment (Anatomic diagnosis and estimation of prognosis)

H. Plan (Diagnostic)

Rule-outs   Procedure
1.
2.
3.
4.

*Key: 0 = absent, +1 = decreased, +2 = normal, +3 = exaggerated, +4 = very exaggerated or clonus, PL = pelvic limb, TL = thoracic limb, NE = not evaluated.

Case History 17E

Signalment

Canine, Cairn terrier, male, 4 months old.

History

The dog is one of a litter of four; the others are normal. At 9 weeks he had a wide-based gait that gradually progressed to a swaying of the pelvis and a stumbling on the pelvic limbs. An examination by another veterinarian was otherwise negative. Now there is pelvic limb paresis.

Physical Examination

Normal.

Neurologic Examination *

A. Observation
   1. Mental status: Alert.
   2. Posture: The dog cannot stand. Tremor of head, trunk, and limbs when the dog is active.
   3. Gait: The dog pulls around with the thoracic limbs. Some voluntary movements of the pelvic limbs, primarily hip flexion, are present.
B. Palpation

C. Postural Reactions

Left	Reactions	Right
	Proprioceptive positioning PL	
0	PL	0
+1	TL	+1
+1	Wheelbarrowing	+1
0	Hopping, PL	0
+1	Hopping, TL	+1
0	Extensor postural thrust	0
NE	Hemistand-hemiwalk	NE
NE	Tonic neck	NE
0	Placing, tactile PL	0
+1	TL	+1
0	Placing, visual PL	0
+1	TL	+2

*Key: 0 = absent, +1 = decreased, +2 = normal, +3 = exaggerated, +4 = very exaggerated or clonus, PL = pelvic limb, TL = thoracic limb, NE = not evaluated.

D. Spinal Reflexes

Left	Reflex Spinal Segment	Right
+3	Quadriceps L4−L6	+2
+2	Extensor carpi radialis C7−T1	+2
NE	Triceps C7−T1	NE
+2	Flexion, PL L5−S1	+2
+2	Flexion, TL C6−T1	+2
0	Crossed extensor	0
+2	Perineal S1−S2	+2

E. Cranial Nerves

Left	Nerve + Function	Right
+2	C.N. II vision menace	+2
	C.N. II + C.N. III pupil size	
	Stim. left eye	
	Stim. right eye	
	C.N. II fundus	
	C.N. III, C.N. IV, C.N. VI Strabismus	
	Nystagmus	
	C.N. V sensation	
	C.N. V mastication	
	C.N. VII facial muscles	
	Palpebral	
	C.N. IX, C.N. X swallowing	
	C.N. XII tongue	

F. Sensation: Location
   Hyperesthesia _____ No _____
   Superficial pain _____ +2 _____
   Deep pain _____ +2 _____

Complete sections G and H before reviewing Case Summary.

G. Assessment (Anatomic diagnosis and estimation of prognosis)

H. Plan (Diagnostic)
   Rule-outs   Procedure
   1.
   2.
   3.
   4.

ASSESSMENT 17A

The dog has ataxia and hemiparesis from central vestibular disease on the left side (see Chapter 11 for a review of localization). The only finding not explained by a single lesion is the suggestion of hyperesthesia along the spinal column. The disease has a moderately acute onset and is progressive. In a young dog, the most common cause of an acute progressive disease is inflammation. The hyperesthesia suggests meningitis. The history of a respiratory problem several weeks ago should not be ignored. An alternative cause might be neoplasia, but this condition is much less likely. The primary question is the kind of infection: viral, bacterial, fungal, or protozoal. Canine distemper has to be considered in spite of the apparent focal neurologic deficit. Focal brain stem disease and meningitis also could be bacterial (abscess plus subarachnoid involvement).

Localization: Left brain stem, vestibular nuclei, meninges.

Rule-outs: Inflammation: viral (distemper), bacterial, or other.

How are you going to differentiate these types of infection?

If you start with simple, noninvasive methods, fundic and otoscopic examinations might reveal chorioretinitis from distemper or a middle ear infection that has progressed medially. The results of both examinations are normal, however. Laboratory data might be of value but are frequently normal when either of our choices are present, as they are in this case. An EEG might be useful if there is also cerebral disease, but it would not really differentiate viral from bacterial inflammations. The best test is an examination of the CSF. In this case, a cisternal sample produced the following results:

Protein: 65 mg/dl,
RBCs: 2 per cu cm,
WBCs: 12 per cu cm,
Differential: all lymphocytes.

These findings are indicative of a viral infection. A bacterial infection usually would cause more protein and more cells to be present, and the cells would be predominantly neutrophils. A fluorescent antibody examination of blood, conjunctival scrapings, or cells in the CSF might be used to confirm the diagnosis of distemper.

This dog was placed on chloramphenicol. The day following hospitalization, head tremors were observed, indicating involvement of the cerebellum. The third day, the dog started to have generalized seizures. The owners requested euthanasia. Necropsy confirmed the diagnosis of distemper encephalomyelitis.

ASSESSMENT 17B

The signs are compatible with cerebellar disease. Cerebellar hypoplasia or in utero damage to the cerebellum must be considered; however, toxic products also can produce cerebellar signs. The progressive nature of the syndrome would suggest something other than a congenital defect, which is usually static with some improvement as compensation occurs. Other progressive diseases, such as storage diseases, are degenerative. None have been reported in the Yorkshire terrier.

Localization: Cerebellum.
Rule-outs:
1. toxic disorders,
2. degenerative diseases, and
3. cerebellar hypoplasia.

Further questioning of the owners revealed that they did not believe there were any toxic products available, because they had small children and were very careful. They were specifically asked to describe their management routine of the bitch and the puppies. They said that they were extremely careful, and, in fact, washed the bitch's mamary glands every day because she went outside and got dirty. It turned out that they were using a hexachlorophene soap to wash the bitch. They were instructed to wash her with a mild soap, rinse thoroughly, and discontinue cleaning the mammary glands. The pups gradually improved until they were normal, approximately 4 weeks later.

Diagnosis: Hexachlorophene toxicity.

ASSESSMENT 17C

A normal neurologic examination in the case of a gait abnormality should make you ask, "How about musculoskeletal disease?" Although the history and the breed are suggestive of cervical spondylopathy or cervical disk disease, the neurologic examination is not. A vital portion of the examination—sensation—was left out. Palpation of the head and the spine was normal, but the dog experienced much pain on palpation of the long bones of the limbs. A radiographic examination confirmed the diagnosis of panosteitis.

It is very important to differentiate musculoskeletal problems from neurologic diseases. Dogs with musculoskeletal problems and no neurologic disease will have a normal neurologic examination. Severe hip dysplasia will not cause a proprioceptive deficit. Conversely, if a deficit is found on the neurologic examination, it almost never can be explained by musculoskeletal disease.

ASSESSMENT 17D

The neurologic findings are not localizing. Depression and slowing of the hopping reactions could be indicative of generalized disease not affecting the CNS or a mild CNS disease. Resistance to manipulation of the neck and the strong panniculus reaction may be indicative of pain. Deep palpation along the spinal column elicits strong guarding reactions of the paraspinal muscles. Absolute evidence of pain cannot be demonstrated, but the breed must be considered. Hunting dogs are often very stoic. Systemic disease must be considered, with meningitis included as a strong possibility. Laboratory data are needed in order to rule out the former and CSF analysis in order to rule out the latter.

Rule-outs:
1. systemic disease or
2. meningitis, possibly with mild encephalomyelitis.

Laboratory examination: The results of a blood chemistry profile and a urinalysis are normal.

WBCs: 31,000   per cu mm
    Neutrophils   24,500
    Bands   240
    Lymphocytes   6,260
CSF: Protein   235 mg/dl
    RBCs: 5 per cu mm
    WBCs: 2,435 per cu mm
      Neutrophils   94 per cent
      Mononuclear cells   6 per cent

Blood and CSF cultures were submitted.

The findings are indicative of a bacterial meningitis, probably with a septicemia. Intravenous ampicillin therapy was started, pending the results of the cultures. The dog improved in 48 hours. Blood cultures were negative, but CSF cultures revealed the presence of *Staphylococcus aureus*, which was sensitive to ampicillin. Intravenous therapy was continued for 4 days and was followed by the oral administration of ampicillin for 3 weeks. The dog recovered completely. The source of the infection was not found.

ASSESSMENT 17E

The head tremor suggests cerebellar disease. The paresis is caused by either brain stem or spinal cord dysfunction. There are no other signs of brain stem disease. The progression from pelvic limb paresis to tetraparesis can be seen with cervical spinal cord lesions or with progressive generalized myelopathy. The progression from spinal cord signs to cerebellar signs should suggest multifocal or systemic disease. The disorder is chronic and progressive in a young dog. These characteristics should make you think of one of the inherited degenerative diseases. The next step is to check and see which diseases might be present in Cairn terriers. Globoid cell leukodystrophy, a demyelinating disease, has been reported in this breed. Your rule-outs might also include viral diseases, such as distemper. Lead toxicity should be considered, although paresis is unusual with this condition.

Localization: Cerebellum, spinal cord.
Rule-outs:
1. degenerative disease (globoid cell leukodystrophy),
2. inflammation (viral), or
3. toxicity (lead).

Laboratory examination: The hemanalysis, serum chemistry profile, and urinalysis are normal.

CSF: Protein: 95 mg/dl
    Cells:
      RBCs: 4 per cu mm
      WBCs: 2 per cu mm
Blood lead level: .02 part per million

The blood lead level is normal. The CSF is indicative of a degenerative process without active inflammation (increased protein, normal cells). This finding does not rule out viral diseases of the CNS, especially canine distemper, because the active inflammatory process may have been present several weeks earlier. Globoid cells may be seen in the CSF in some cases, but their absence is not significant. A biopsy of the peripheral nerve may reveal the pathologic changes that are characteristic of globoid cell leukodystrophy. The owners elected euthanasia, since all of the possible diseases had a very poor prognosis. No significant lesions were found on gross necropsy. Histopathology confirmed the diagnosis of globoid cell leukodystrophy.

REFERENCES

1. Escourolle, R., and Poirier, J.: Manual of Basic Neuropathology, 2nd ed. Philadelphia, W. B. Saunders Co., 1978.
2. Hoerlein, B. F.: Canine Neurology: Diagnosis and Treatment, 3rd ed. Philadelphia, W. B. Saunders Co., 1978.
3. Baker, H. J., Mole, J. A., Lindsey, J. R., and Creel, R. M.: Animal models of ganglioside storage disease. Fed. Proc. 35:1193–1201, 1976.
4. Baker, H. J., Reynolds, G. D., Walkley, S. U., et al.: The gangliosidoses: Comparative features and research applications. Vet. Pathol. 16:635–649, 1979.
5. Koppang, N.: Neuronal ceroid-lipofuscinosis in English setters. J. Small Anim. Pract. 10:639–644, 1970.
6. Hegreberg, G. A., and Padgett, G. A.: Inherited progressive epilepsy of the dog with comparisons to Lafora's disease of man. Fed. Proc. 35:1202–1205, 1976.
7. Fletcher, T. F., Kurtz, H. J., and Low, D. G.: Globoid cell leukodystrophy (Krabbe type) in the dog. JAVMA 149:165–172, 1966.
8. Fletcher, T. F., and Kurtz, H. J.: Animal model for human disease: Globoid cell leukodystrophy, Krabbe's disease. Am. J. Pathol. 66:375–378, 1972.
9. deLahunta, A.: Diseases of the cerebellum. Vet. Clin. North Am. 10:91–101, 1980.
10. Sherding, R. G.: Hepatic encephalopathy in the dog. Comp. Cont. Ed. 1:55–63, 1979.
11. Barrett, R. E.: Canine hepatic encephalopathy. In Kirk, R. W.: Current Veterinary Therapy VII. Philadelphia, W. B. Saunders Co., 1980.
12. Braund, K. G.: Encephalitis and meningitis. Vet. Clin. North Am. 10:31–56, 1980.
13. Hayes, H. M., Jr., Priester, W. A., and Pendergras, T. W.: Occurrence of nervous tissue tumors in cattle, horses, cats, and dogs. Int. J. Cancer 15:39–47, 1975.
14. Luginbuhl, H., Fankhauser, R., and McGrath, J. T.: Spontaneous neoplasms of the nervous system in animals. Prog. Neurol. Surg. 2:85–164, 1968.
15. Prata, R. G.: Diagnosis of spinal cord tumors in the dog. Vet. Clin. North Am. 7:165–185, 1977.
16. Palmer, A. C., Malinowski, W., and Barnett, K. C.: Clinical Signs including papilloedema associated with brain tumors in twenty-one dogs. J. Small Anim. Pract. 15:359–386, 1974.
17. Palmer, A. C.: Comparative aspects of tumours of the central nervous system in the dog. Proc. R. Soc. Med. 69:49–51, 1976.
18. Loew, F. M.: Nutrition and bovine neurologic disease. JAVMA 166:219–221, 1975.
19. Read, D. H., Jolly, R. D., and Alley, M. R.: Polioencephalomalacia of dogs with thiamine deficiency. Vet. Pathol. 14:103–112, 1977.
20. Read, D. H., and Harrington, D. D.: Experimentally induced thiamine deficiency in beagle dogs: clinical observations. Am. J. Vet. Res. 42:984–991, 1981.
21. Palmer, A. C.: Introduction to Animal Neurology, 2nd ed. Oxford, Blackwell Scientific Pub., 1976.

22. Howard, J. L.: Current Veterinary Therapy: Food Animal Practice. Philadelphia, W. B. Saunders Co., 1981.
23. Oliver, J. E., Jr., and Greene, C. E.: Diseases of the brain. *In* Ettinger, S. J.: Textbook of Veterinary Internal Medicine, 2nd ed. Philadelphia, W. B. Saunders Co., in press.
24. Kirk, R. W.: Current Veterinary Therapy VII, Philadelphia, W. B. Saunders Co., 1980.
25. Buck, W. B., Osweiler, G. D., and Van Gelder, G. A.: Clinical and Diagnostic Veterinary Toxicology. Dubuque, Iowa, Kendall Hunt Publishing Co., 1973.
26. Oehme, F. W.: Toxicologic Disorders. *In* Ettinger, S. J.: Textbook of Veterinary Internal Medicine. Philadelphia, W. B. Saunders Co., 1975.
27. Osweiler, G. D.: Incidence and diagnostic considerations of major small animal toxicoses. JAVMA 155:2011–2014, 1969.
28. Baker, H. J.: Inherited metabolic disorders of the nervous system in dogs and cats. *In* Kirk, R. W.: Current Veterinary Therapy IV. Philadelphia, W. B. Saunders Co., 1977.
29. Jolly, R. D., and Hartley, W. J.: Storage diseases of domestic animals. Aust. Vet. J. 53:1–8, 1977.
30. Jolly, R. D.: Lysosomal storage diseases. Neuropathol. Appl. Neurobiol. 4:419–427, 1978.
31. Hardy, R. M., and Stevens, J. B.: Chronic progressive hepatitis in Bedlington terriers. *In* Kirk, R. W.: Current Veterinary Therapy VI. Philadelphia, W. B. Saunders Co., 1977.

INDEX